NATURAL PRODUCTS AND THERAPEUTICS

CURCUMA LONGA AND ITS HEALTH EFFECTS

VOLUME 1

NATURAL PRODUCTS AND THERAPEUTICS

Additional books and e-books in this series can be found on Nova's website under the Series tab.

NATURAL PRODUCTS AND THERAPEUTICS

CURCUMA LONGA AND ITS HEALTH EFFECTS

VOLUME 1

NOBORU MOTOHASHI
EDITOR

nova
Medicine & Health
New York

Library of Congress Cataloging-in-Publication Data

ISBN: 978-1-53618-083-1

Published by Nova Science Publishers, Inc. † New York

Contents

PREFACE

Curcumin, a yellow edible pigment in turmeric, has been widely used as a flavor and dye in India and its surrounding countries since ancient times. In particular, among curcumonoids (diarylheptanoids), curcumin I, curcumin II, and curcumin III have been elucidated by many researchers not only in the food area but also in human health effects.

Curcumonoids are roughly classified into linear-diarylheptanoids and cyclic-diarylheptanoids. In addition, because there are more glycosides of these two diarylheptanoids, diarylheptanoids form an enormous derivative.

Both Chapter 1 and Chapter 2 in volume 1 will be discussed according to the following classification. First, plants containing diarylheptanoids were alphabetically started from the eyes, followed by family, genus, and plant name.

Chapter 1, at least 9 orders, 12 families and 27 genera are known to contain plant diarylheptanoids as follows: **Order Fagales** contain the most versatile 3 families 8 genera including family Betulaceae 5 genera (Alnus, Betula, Carpinus, Corylus and Ostrya), family Myricaceae 2 genera (Morella and Myrica), and family Casuarinaceae 1 genus (Casuarina). This is followed by **Order Zingiberales**: 1 family 6 genera (Alpinia, Amomum, Curcuma, Hedychium, Renealmia, and Zingiber) of family Zingiberaceae; **Order Sapindales**: 2 families 3 genera of family Burseraceae 2 genera (Boswellia and Garuga), and family Sapindaceae 1 genus (Acer); **Order**

Juglandales: 2 families 4 genera of Juglandaceae 3 genera (Juglans, Platycarya, and Pterocarya) and Rhoipteleaceae 1 genus (Rhoiptelea); **Order Fabales**: 1 family Leguminosae 1 genus (Centrolobium); **Order Dioscoreales**: 1 family Dioscoreaceae 2 genera (Dioscorea and Tacca); **Order Ericale**: 1 family Actinidiaceae 1 genus (Clematoclethra); **Order Gentiales**: 1 family Rubiaceae 1 genus (Pyrostria); and **Order Santalales**: 1 family Santalaceae 1 genus (Viscum), respectively.

In Chapter 2, at least 2 orders, 3 families and 3 genera are known to contain seaweed diarylheptanoids as follows: **Order Alismatales**: 2 families 2 genera of family Cymodoceaceae 1 genus (Cymodoceaceae) and family Zosteraceae 1 genus (Zostera); and **Order Poecilosclerida**. 1 family Tedaniidae 1 genus (Tedania), respectively.

Chapter 3, biological activity of diarylheptanoids were typically described as follows: Leishmanicidal and antiprotozoal activities, antitumor activities, anti-inflammatory effects, and inhibitory on nitric oxide production.

Chapter 4, some selective extractions of curcumin was discussed.

Noboru Motohashi, PhD
March 27, 2020

In: *Curcuma longa* and Its Health Effects ISBN: 978-1-53618-083-1
Editor: Noboru Motohashi

Chapter 1

PLANTS CONTAINING CURCUMINOIDS (DIARYLHEPTANOIDS)

Noboru Motohashi[1,*], Anuradha Vanam[2†], Jyothirmayi Vadapalli[3,‡] and Rao Gollapudi[4,§]

[1]Meiji Pharmaceutical University, Tokyo, Japan
[2]Sri Venkateswara University, Tirupathi, AP, India
[3]Acharya Nagarjuna University, Nagarjunanagar, AP, India
[4]University of Kansas, Lawrence, Kansas, USA

ABSTRACT

Naturally occurring plant-derived diarylheptanoids are diarylheptanids contained in 9 orders 13 families from order Fabales, 1 family; order Fagales, 3 families; order Dioscoreales, 1 family; order Ericale, 1 family; order Gentiales, 1 family; order Juglandales, 2 families; order; Santalales, 1 family; Sapindales, 2 families; and order Zingiberales 1 family.

---

* Corresponding Author's Email: noborumotohashi@jcom.home.ne.jp.
† Corresponding Author's Email: agollapdr@gmail.com.
‡ Corresponding Author's Email: jyothi.galactica@gmail.com.
§ Corresponding Author's Email: gollapudirao@ku.edu.

Chapter 1 focused on clarifying the structure-activity relationship of plant-derived diarylheptanoids. For this purpose, the structural formulas were listed as much as possible, and the structures listed in the literature and the biological activities were listed as much as possible to make it easier to understand the correlation between the structures and activities.

Keywords: diarylheptanoids, curcuminoids, plant-derived diarylheptanoids, biological activity of plant-derived diarylheptanoids

Chemical Constituents in Plants Containing Curcuminoids (Diarylheptanoids)

(-)-centrolobine (**1**)
(-)-de-*O*-methylcentrolobine (**2**)
(-)-centrolobol (**3**)
(+)-centrolobine (**4**)
(+)-de-*O*-methylcentrolobine (**5**)
(+)-centrolobol (**6**)
centrolobol (3*S*. **7**) (-11°)
centrolobol (3*S*,7*R*. **8**) (-96°)
(-)-hannokinol (**9**) (-19°)
centrolobol (3*S*,7*R*. **10**) (-98°)
(+)-centrolobine (3*R*. **11**) (+11°)
centrolobol (3*R*,7*S*. **12**) (+95°)
centrolobol (3*R*,7*S*. **13**) (+97°)
yashabushiketol (**14**)
didydroyashabushiketol (**15**)
6'-*O*-vanilloylisotachioside (**16**)
dehydrohirsutanonol (hirsutanone. hirsutenone. **17**)
5-hydroxy-3-platyphyllone (**18**)
platyphylloside (**19**)
(5*S*)-5-hydroxy-1,7-*bis*-(4-hydroxyphenyl)-3-heptanone-5-*O*-β-D-apiofuranosyl-(1→6)-β-D-glucopyranoside (**20**)

(5*S*)-5-hydroxy-7-(3,4-dihydroxyphenyl)-1-(4-hydroxyphenyl)-3-heptanone-5-*O*-β-D-xylopyranoside (**21**)
(5*R*)-5-methoxy-1,7-*bis*-(3,4-dihydroxyphenyl)-3-heptanone (**22**)
oregonin (**23**)
(3*R*)-1,7-*bis*-(4-hydroxyphenyl)-3-heptanol-3-*O*-β-D-apiofuranosyl-(1→6)-β-D-glucopyranoside (**24**)
(3*R*)-1,7-*bis*-(3,4-dihydroxyphenyl)-3-heptanol-3-*O*-β-D-glucoopyranoside (**25**)
(3*R*)-1,7-*bis*-(3,4-dihydroxyphenyl)-3-heptanol-3-*O*-β-D-glucopyranosyl-(1→3)-β-D-xylopyranoside (**26**)
(3*R*)-1,7-*bis*-(3,4-dihydroxyphenyl)-3-heptanol-3-*O*-β-D-xylopyranoside (**27**)
ω-nitro-L-argininemethyl ester (L-NAME. **28**)
oregonin (1,7-*bis*-(3,4-dihydroxyphenyl)-heptane-3-on-5-*O*-β-D-xylopyranoside. **29**)
a mixture of 1,7-*bis*-(3,4-dihydroxyphenyl)-3-hydroxyheptane-5-*O*-β-D-xylopyranoside (**30**) epimer alcohols
rubranoside A (**31**)
rubranoside B (**32**)
hirsutanonol (**33**)
hirsutenone (**34**)
hirsutanonol-5-*O*-β-D-glucopyranoside (**35**)
platyphyllonol-5-*O*-β-D-xylopyranoside (**36**)
aceroside VII (**37**)
alnuside A (**38**)
alnuside B (**39**)
1,7-*bis*-(3,4-dihydoxyphenyl)-5-hydroxy-heptane-3-*O*-β-D-xylopyranoside (**40**)
(5*S*)-1-(4-hydroxyphenyl)-7-(3,4-dihydroxyphenyl)-5-*O*-β-D-glucopyranosyl-heptan-3-one (**41**)
(5*S*)-1,7-*bis*-(3,4-dihydroxyphenyl)-5-*O*-β-D-[6-(3,4-dimethoxycinnamoylglucopyranosyl)]-heptan-3-one (**42**)
mitomycin C (MMC. **43**)
amifhostin WR-2721 (**44**)

5(*S*)-1,7-di(4-hydroxyphenyl)-5-*O*-β-D-[6-(*E*-*p*-coumaroylglucopyranosyl)]heptane-3-one (**45**)
5(*S*)-1,7-di(4-hydroxyphenyl)-5-*O*-β-D-[6-(*E*-3,4-dimethoxycinnamoylglucopyranosyl)]heptane-3-one (**46**)
5(*S*)-1-(4-hydroxyphenyl)-7-(3,4-dihydroxyphenyl)-5-*O*-β-D-[6-(*E*-3,4-dimethoxycinnamoylglucopyranosyl)]heptane-3-one (**47**)
5(*S*)-1-(3,4-dihydroxyphenyl)-7-(4-hydroxyphenyl)-5-*O*-β-D-[6-(*Z*-3,4-dimethoxycinnamoylglucopyranosyl)]heptane-3-one (**48**)
5(*S*)-1,7-di(3,4-dihydroxyphenyl)-5-*O*-β-D-[6-(*E*-*p*-coumaroylglucopyranosyl)]heptane-3-one (**49**)
5(*S*)-1,7-di(3,4-dihydroxyphenyl)-5-*O*-β-D-[6-(*E*-3,4-dimethoxycinnamoylglucopyranosyl)] heptane-3-one (**50**)
5(*S*)-1,7-di(3,4-dihydroxyphenyl)-5-*O*-β-D-[6-(*Z*-3,4-dimethoxycinn amoylglucopyranosyl)]heptane-3-one (**51**)
5(*S*)-1,7-di(3,4-dihydroxyphenyl)-5-*O*-β-D-[6-(*E*-3,4,5-trimethoxycinnamoylglucopyranosyl)]heptane-3-one (**52**)
3(*R*)-1,7-di(3,4-dihydroxyphenyl)-3-*O*-β-D-[6-(*E*-3,4-dimethoxycinnamoylglucopyranosyl)]heptane (**53**)
3(*R*)-1,7-di(3,4-dihydroxyphenyl)-5-*O*-β-D-[6-(*Z*-3,4-dimethoxycinnamoylglucopyranosyl)] heptane (**54**)
3(*R*)-1,7-di(3,4-dihydroxyphenyl)-5-*O*-β-D-[6-(*E*-3,4,5-trimethoxycinnamoy lglucopyranosyl)]heptane (**55**)
5(*S*)-methylhirsutanonol (**56**)
3(*R*)-1,7-di(3,4-dihydroxyphenyl)-3-hydroxyheptane (**57**)
curcumin (**58**)
5(*S*)-hirsutanonol-5-*O*-β-D-glucopyranoside (**59**)
doxorubicin (**60**)
a hirsutoside 1,7-di-(3',4'-dihydroxyphenyl)heptan-3-on-5-xyloside (**61**)
2-oxatrycyclo[13.2.2.13,7]-eicosa-3,5,7(20),15,17,18-hexaen-10-16-diol (**62**)
2-oxatrycyclo [13.2.2.13,7]-eicosa-3,5,7-(20),15,17,18-hexaen-10-one (**63**)

(5*S*)-1,7-*bis*(3,4-dihydroxyphenyl)-5-hydroxyheptan-3-one (**64**)
(5*S*)-1,7-*bis*(3,4-dihydroxyphenyl)-5-(β-D-xylopyranosyloxy)heptan-3-one (**65**)
alnusonol (**66**)
(5*S*)-1,7-*bis*(4-hydroxyphenyl)-5-hydroxyheptan-3-one (**67**)
(5*S*)-l-(3,4-dihydroxyphenyl)-7-(4-hydroxyphenyl)-5-hydroxyheptan-3-one (**68**)
alnuside C (1,7-*bis*-(3,4-dihydroxyphenyl)-5-hydroxy-3-heptanone-5-*O*-[2-(2-methylbutenoyl)]-β-D-xylopyranoside. **69**)
5-*O*-methylhirusutanonol (1,7-*bis*-(3,4-dihydroxyphenyl)-5-methoxy-3-heptanone. **70**)
5-*O*-ethylhirsutanonol (**71**)
oregonin peracetate (**72**)
alnuheptanoid A [(5*S*)-7-(3,4-dihydroxyphenyl)-1-(4-hydroxyphenyl)-5-methoxyheptan-3-one] (**73**)
platyphyllenone (**74**)
(5*S*)-1,7-*bis*(4-hydroxyphenyl)-5-methoxyheptan-3-one (**75**)
1-(3,4-dihydroxyphenyl)-7-(4-hydroxyphenyl)-4-hepten-3-one (**76**)
(5*R*)-*O*-methylhirsutanonol (**77**)
alnuheptanoid B (**78**)
myricanone (**79**)
(+)-*S*-myricanol (**80**)
myricanone 5-*O*-β-D-glucopyranoside (**81**)
(+)-*S*-myricanol 5-*O*-β-D-glucopyranoside (**82**)
propyl gallate (**83**)
indomethacin (**84**)
alnustone (1,7-diphenyl-1,3-heptadiene-5-one. **85**)
(5*S*)-1,7-*bis*(3,4-dihydroxyphenyl)-5-hydroxyheptan-3-one (**86**)
(5*S*)-l-(4-hydroxyphenyl)-7-(3,4-dihydroxyphenyl)-5-(β-D-xylopyranosyloxy)heptan-3-one (**87**)
(5*S*)-1-(3,4-dihydroxyphenyl)-7-(4-hydroxyphenyl)-5-(β-D-xylopyranosyloxy)heptan-3-one (**88**)
(5*S*)-1,7-*bis*(3,4-dihydroxyphenyl)-5-(β-D-xylopyranosyloxy)heptan-3-one (**89**)

(5*S*)-1,7-*bis*(3,4-dihydroxyphenyl)-5-(β-D-glucopyranosyloxy)heptan-3-one (**90**)
2,3-digalloyl oregonin (**91**)
2,2-diphenyl-1-picrylhydrazyl (DPPH. **92**)
L-ascorbic acid (vitamin C. **93**)
allopurinol (**94**)
yashabushidiol A (*meso*-1,7-diphenylheptane-3,5-diol. **95**)
yashabushidiol B (1,7-diphenylheptane-(3*R*),(5*R*)-diol. **96**)
yashabushiketodiol A (1,7-diphenylheptane-3-keto-(1*R*),(5*S*)-diol. **97**)
yashabushiketodiol B (1,7-diphenylheptane-3-keto-(1*S*),(5*S*)-diol. **98**)
yashabushitriol (1,7-diphenylheptane-(1*R*),(3*R*),(5*S*)-triol. **99**)
3,17-dihydroxy-tricyclo[12.3.1.1^{2,6}]-nonadeca-1(18),2,4,6(19),14,16-hexaen-9,11-dione (**100**)
alnusone (**101**)
alnusonol (**102**)
acarbose (*O*-4,6-dideoxy-4-[[(1*S*,4*R*,5*S*,6*S*)-4,5,6-trihydroxy-3-(hydroxymethyl)-2-cyclohexene-1-yl]amino]-α-D-glucopyranosyl-(1→4)-*O*-α-D-glucopyranosyl-(1→4)-D-glucopyranose. **103**)
papyriferoside A ((*S*)-1,7-*bis*-(4-hydroxyphenyl)-heptan-3-one-5-*O*-α-L-arabinofuranosyl-(1→6)-β-D-glucopyranoside. **104**)
5-*O*-β-D-apiofuranosyl-(1→2)-β-D-glucopyranosyl-1,7-*bis*-(4-hydroxyphenyl)-heptan-3-one (**105**)
1,7-*bis*-(4-hydroxyphenyl)-4-hepten-3-one (**106**)
etoposide (**107**)
fluorouracil (5-Fu. **108**)
11-oxo-3,8,9,17-tetrahydroxy-[7,0]-metacyclophane (Compound I. **109**)
11-oxo-3,9,12,17-tetrahydroxy-[7,0]-metacyclophane (**110**)
11-oxo-3,7,12,13,17-pentahydroxy-[7,0]-metacyclophane (**111**)
11-oxo-3,12,17-trihydroxy-9-ene-[7,0]-metacyclophane (**112**)
11-oxo-3,8,12,17-tetrahydroxy-9-ene-[7,0]-metacyclophane (**113**)
11-oxo-3,17-dihydroxy-8,9-isopropylidene-[7,0]-metacyclophane (**114**)
platyphyllonol (**115**)

carpinontriol B (**116**)
α-tocophenol (vitamin E. **117**)
asadanin (8,11-*trans*, 11,12-*cis*. **118**)
giffonin P (**119**)
epiasadanol (8,9-*cis*. tricyclo[12.3.1.12,6]nonadeca-1(18),2,4,6(19),14,16-hexaene-3,8,9,10,12,17-hexol(8CI,9CI). **120**)
isoasadanol (all *cis-form*. **121**)
asadanol (**122**)
deoxoasadanin (**123**)
trideoxyasadanin-8-ene (**124**)
dideoxyasadanin-8-ene (**125**)
monodeoxyasadanin (**126**)
casuarinondiol (**127**)
alnusdiol (**128**)
7-hydroxymyricanol 5-*O*-β-D-glucopyranoside (**129**)
juglanin B 3-*O*-β-D-glucopyranoside (**130**)
16-hydroxyjuglanin B 17-*O*-β-D-glucopyranoside (**131**)
myricanone 5-*O*-β-D-glucopranosyl-(1→6)-β-D-glucopyranoside (**132**)
neomyricanone 5-*O*-β-D-glucopranosyl-(1→6)-β-D-glucopyranoside (**133**)
myricanone 17-*O*-α-L-arabinofuranosyl-(1→6)-β-D-glucopyranoside (**134**)
juglanin B-sulfate (**135**)
myricanol (**136**)
myricanol 5-*O*-β-D-glucopyranoside (**137**)
myricanol 11-*O*-β-D-xylopyranoside (**138**)
myricanol 5-*O*-β-D-(6'-*O*-galloyl)-glucopyranoside. **139**)
myricanone 5-*O*-β-D-(6'-*O*-galloyl)-glucopyranoside (**140**)
myricanol 5-*O*-α-L-arabinofuranosyl-(1→6)-β-D-glucopyranoside (**141**)
myricanol gentiobiosidse: myricanol 5-*O*-β-D-glucopranosyl-(1→6)-β-D-glucopyranoside (**142**)
porson (**143**)
galeon (**144**)
hydroxygaleon (**145**)

12-dehydroporson (**146**)
12-hydroxymyricanone (**147**)
myricatomentoside I (**148**)
myricatomentoside II (**149**)
(+)-galeon (**150**)
myricanol glucoside (**151**)
myricanol galloylglucoside (**152**)
myricanol 5-*O*-β-D-glucopyranosyl-(1→3)-β-D-glucopyranoside (**153**)
myricanol 11-*O*-β-D-glucopyranoside (**154**)
neomyricanone 5-*O*-β-D-glucopyranoside (**155**)
myricanol glucoside (11β-OH. **156**)
myricanene A 5-*O*-α-L-arabinofuranosyl-(1→6)-β-D-glucopyranoside (**157**)
myricanene A (**158**)
myricanene B 5-*O*-α–L-arabinofuranosyl-(1→6)-β-D-glucopyranoside (**159**)
myricanene B (**160**)
myricanane (**161**)
N^G-monomethyl-L-arginine, monoacetate salt (L-NMMA. **162**)
(+)-*S*-myricanol 5-*O*-β-D-glucopyranoside (**163**)
myricanene A 5-*O*-α-L-arabinofuranosyl(1→6)-β-D-glucopyranoside (**164**)
myricanene B 5-*O*-α-L-arabinofuranosyl(1→6)-β-D-glucopyranoside (**165**)
dioscorol A (**166**),
dioscoroside E1 (**167**)
dioscoroside E2 (**168**)
1,7-*bis*(4-hydroxyphenyl)-hepta-4*E*,6*E*-dien-3-one (**169**)
1,7-*bis*(4-hydroxyphenyl)-1,4,6-heptatrien-3-one (**170**)
3,5-dihydroxy-1,7-*bis*(4-hydroxyphenyl)heptane (**171**)

(3*R*,5*R*)-3,5-dihydroxy-1,7-*bis*(4-hydroxyphenyl)heptane 3-*O*-β-D-glucopyranoside (**172**)
(3*R*,5*R*)-3,5-dihydroxy-1,7-*bis*(4-hydroxy-3-methoxyphenyl)-heptane 3-*O*-β-D-glucopyranoside (**173**)
(1*S*,3*S*,5*R*,6*E*)-1,7-*bis*(4-hydroxyphenyl)-1,5-epoxy-3-hydroxyhept-6-ene (**174**)
(1*S*,3*S*,5*S*)-1,7-*bis*(4-hydroxyphenyl)-1,5-epoxy-3-hydroxyheptane (**175**)
(1*R*,3*R*,5*R*)-1,7-*bis*(4-hydroxyphenyl)-1,5-epoxy-3-hydroxyheptane (**176**)
(1*S*,3*R*,5*S*)-1,7-*bis*(4-hydroxyphenyl)-1,5-epoxy-3-hydroxyheptane (**177**)
(1*R*,3*S*,5*R*)-1,7-*bis*(4-hydroxyphenyl)-1,5-epoxy-3-hydroxyheptane (**178**)
(5*R*,1*E*)-1,7-*bis*(4-hydroxyphenyl)-5-hydroxyhept-1-en-3-one (**179**)
(5*R*,1*E*)-1,7-*bis*(4-hydroxyphenyl)-5-hydroxyhept-1-en-3-one (**180**)
Compound **#8** (**181**)
Compound **#9** (**182**)
Compound **#10** (**183**)
Compound **#11** (**184**)
Compound **#12** (**185**)
Compound **#13** (**186**)
Compound **#14** (**187**)
(3*R*,5*R*)-3,5-dihydroxy-1-(3,4-dihydroxyphenyl)-7-(4-hydroxyphenyl)heptane (**188**)
(3*R*,5*R*)-3,5-dihydroxy-1,7-*bis*-(3,4-dihydroxyphenyl)heptane (**189**)
(3*R*,5*R*)-3,5-dihydroxy-1-(3,4-dihydroxyphenyl)-7-(4-hydroxyphenyl)-heptane 3-*O*-β-D-glucopyranoside (**190**)
(3*R*,5*R*)-3,5-dihydroxy-1-(3,4-dihydroxyphenyl)-7-(4-hydroxyphenyl)heptane 5-*O*-β-D-glucopyranoside (**191**)
(3*R*,5*R*)-3,5-dihydroxy-1-(4-hydroxy-3-methoxyphenyl)-7-(4-hydroxyphenyl)heptanc 3-*O*-β-D-glucopyranoside (**192**)
(3*R*,5*R*)-3,5-dihydroxy-1,7-*bis*(3,4-dihydroxyphenyl)heptane 3-*O*-β-D-glucopyranoside (**193**)
(3*R*,5*R*)-3,5-dihydroxy-1-(4-hydroxy-3-methoxyphenyl)-7-(3,4-dihydroxyphenyl)heptane 3-*O*-β-D-glucopyranoside (**194**)
(3*R*,5*R*)-3,5-dihydroxy-1,7-*bis*(4-hydroxy-3-methoxyphenyl)-heptane 3-*O*-β-D-glucopyranoside (**195**)

(3*R*,5*R*)-3,5-dihydroxy-1,7-*bis*(4-hydroxyphenyl)heptane 3-*O*-β-D-glucopyranoside (**196**)
actinidione (**197**)
irinotecan (**198**)
(3*S*,5*S*)-3,5-dihydroxy-1,7-*bis*(4-methoxyphenyl)heptyl 3-*O*-β-D-glucopyranoside (**199**)
(3*S*,5*S*)-3,5-dihydroxy-1-(3-hydroxy-4-methoxyphenyl)-7-(4-methoxyphenyl)heptyl 3-*O*-β-D-glucopyranoside (**200**)
(3*S*,5*S*)-1-(3,4-dihydroxyphenyl)-3,5-dihydroxy-7-(4-methoxyphenyl)heptyl 3-O-β-D-glucopyranoside (**201**)
(3*S*,5*S*)-3,5-dihydroxy-1,7-*bis*(3,4-dihydroxyphenyl)heptyl 3-*O*-β-D-glucopyranoside (**202**)
(3*S*,5*S*)-3,5-dihydroxy-7-(3-hydroxy-4-methoxyphenyl)-1-(4-methyoxyphenyl)heptyl 3-*O*-β-D-glucopyranoside (**203**)
1-(3,4-dihydroxyphenyl)-3,5-dihydroxy-7-(3-hydroxy-4-methoxyphenyl)heptyl 3-*O*-β-D-glucopyranoside (**204**)
1-(3,4-dihydroxyphenyl)-5-formyl-3-hydroxy-7-(4-methoxyphenyl)heptyl 3-O-β-D-glucopyranoside (**205**)
1,7-*bis*(3,4-dihydroxyphenyl)-5-formyl-3-hydroxyheptyl 3-*O*-β-D-glucopyranoside (**206**)
chloroquine (**207**)
pentamidine (**208**)
amphotericin B (**209**)
docetaxel (DTX. TXT. **210**)
juglanin A (JA. **211**)
rhoiptelol (RH. **212**)
juglanin C (JC. **213**)
juglanin B (JB. **214**)
platycarynol (**215**)
pterocarine (**216**)
myricatomentogenin ((+)-3’,4”-epoxy-1-(4’-hydroxylphenyl)-7-(3”-hydroxyphenyl)heptane-3-one. **217**)

rhoiptelol A (**218**)
rhoiptelol B (**219**)
rhoiptelol C (**220**)
hirsutanone (1,7-di-(3',4'-dihydroxyphenyl)-4-hepten-3-one. **221**)
etoposide (VP-16. **222**)
curcumin I (curcumin. diferuloylmethane. 1,7-*bis*-4-hydroxy-3-methoxyphenyl-1,6-heptadiene-3,5-dione. **223**)
curcumin II (demethoxycurcumin. (1*E*,6*E*)-1-(4-hydroxy-3-methoxyphenyl)-7-(4-hydroxyphenyl)hepta-1,6-diene-3,5-dione. **224**)
curcumin III (bisdemethoxycurcumin. (1*E*,6*E*)-1,7-*bis*(4-hydroxyphenyl)hepta-1,6-diene-3,5-dione. **225**)
yakuchinone A (1-[4'-hydroxy-3'-methoxy-phenyl]-7-phenylhept-3-one. **226**)
yakuchinone B (1-[4'-hydroxy-3'-methoxyphenyl]-7-phenylhept-1-en-3-one. **227**)
1,7-*bis*(4-hydroxyphenyl)-1,4-heptadien-3-one (**228**)
cisplatin (C-DDP. **229**)
ovalifoliolatin A (**230**)
ovalifoliolatin B (**231**)
acerogenin C (**232**)
garugamblin-1 (**233**)
garugamblin-2 (**234**)
garuganin I (**235**)
garuganin III (**236**)
16-hydroxygaruganin V (**237**)
11-desmethylgarugamblin I (**238**)
2,11-didesmethylgaruganin III (**239**)
1-desmethylgaruganin III (**240**)
acerogenin A (**241**)
aceroside I (acerogenin A β-D-glucopyranoside. **242**)
aceroside B1 (**243**)
aceroside B2 (**244**)
aceroketoside (**245**)
acerogenin A (**246**)

acerogenin B (**247**)
acerogenin E (**248**)
acerogenin K (**249**)
L-arginine (**250**)
(5*R*)-*trans*-1,7-diphenyl-5-hydroxy-6-hepten-3-one (**251**)
(3*S*,5*S*)-*trans*-1,7-diphenyl-3,5-dihydroxy-1-heptene (**252**)
trans-1,7-diphenyl-5-hydroxy-1-heptene (**253**)
trans,trans-1,7-diphenyl-5-hydroxy-4,6-heptadien-3-one (**254**)
(3*S*,5*R*)-3,5-dihydroxy-1,7-diphenylheptane (**255**)
trans,trans-1,7-diphenyl-4,6-heptadien-3-one (**256**)
trans,trans-1(3'-methoxy-4'-hydroxyphenyl)-7-phenyl-5-ol-4,6-dien-3-heptanone (**257**)
trans,trans-1,7-diphenyl-5-ol-4,6-dien-3-heptanone (**258**)
1,7-diphenyl-5-ol-3-heptanone (**259**)
1,7-diphenyl-4-en-3-heptanone (**260**)
7-(4"-hydroxyphenyl)-1-phenyl-5-ol-3-heptanone (**261**)
7-(4"-hydroxy-3"-methoxyphenyl)-1-phenyl-5-ol-3-heptanone (**262**)
(5*S*)-5-hydroxy-7-(3,4-hydroxyphenyl)-1-phenyl-3-heptanone (**263**)
(5*R*)-5-hydroxy-7-(3-methoxy-4,5-dihydroxyphenyl)-1-phenyl-3-heptanone (**264**)
(5*R*)-5-hydroxy-1-(3,4-hydroxyphenyl)-7-(4-hydroxy-3-methoxyphenyl)-3-heptanone (**265**)
7-(3,4-hydroxyphenyl)-1-(4-hydroxy-3-methoxyphenyl)-4-en-3-heptanone (**266**)
alpinin B (**267**)
1,7-diphenyl-3,5-heptanedione (unit-I. **268**)
1,7-diphenyl-heptan-3-one (unit-II. **269**)
(4*E*)-1,7-diphenylhept-4-en-3-one (**270**)
(4*E*)-7-(4-hydroxyphenyl)-1-phenylhept-4-en-3-one (**271**)
5-fluorouracil (5-FU. **272**)
alpinin C (**273**)
alpinin D (**274**)

7-(4-hydroxyphenyl)-1-phenyl-3-heptanone (**275**)
5*S*-ethoxyl-7-(4-hydroxy-3-methoxyphenyl)-1-phenyl-3-heptanone (**276**)
5*R*-hydroxy-7-(4-hydroxy-3-methoxyphenyl)-1-phenyl-3-heptanone (**277**)
(4*E*,6*E*)-5-hydroxy-1-(4-hydroxy-3-methoxyphenyl)-7-phenylhepta-4,6-dien-3-one (**278**)
alpinnanin A (**279**)
muricarpone A ((5*R*)-5-methoxy-1,7-*bis*(3,4-dihydroxyphenyl)-3-heptanone. **280**)
muricarpone B (1,7-*bis*(3,4-dihydroxyphenyl)-3-heptanone. **281**)
1,7-di-(3',4'-dihydroxyphenyl)-4-hepten-3-one (**282**)
1-(3',4'-dihydroxyphenyl)-7-(4"-hydroxyphenyl)-4-hepten-3-one (**283**)
muricarpin (1-(4'-hydroxyphenyl)-7-(3",4"-dihydroxyphenyl)-heptan-3-one. **284**)
1,7-*bis*(3,4-dihydroxyphenyl)heptan-3-yl acetate (**285**)
1-(4'-hydroxyphenyl)-7-(3",4"-dihydroxyphenyl)heptan-3-yl acetate (**286**)
1-(3',4'-hydroxyphenyl)-7-(4"-hydroxyphenyl)-heptan-3-one (**287**)
(5*R*)-5-hydroxy-1,7-*bis*(4-hydroxyphenyl)-3-heptanone (**288**)
rel-(3*R*,5*S*)-3,5-dihydroxy-1-(3,4-dihydroxyphenyl)-7-(4-hydroxyphenyl)-heptane (**289**)
rel-(3*R*,5*S*)-3,5-dihydroxy-1-(4-hydroxy-3-methoxyphenyl)-7-(4-hydroxyphenyl)-heptane (**290**)
rel-(3*R*,5*S*)-3,5-dihydroxy-1-(3-methoxy-4,5-dihydroxyphenyl)-7-(4-hydroxyphenyl)-heptane (**291**)
(5*S*)-5-hydroxy-1-(4-hydroxyphenyl)-7-phenyl-3-heptanone (**292**)
(5*S*)-5-hydroxy-1-(4-hydroxyphenyl)-7-(3,4-dihydroxyphenyl)-3-heptanone (**293**)
(5*S*)-5-hydroxy-1-(4-hydroxy-3-methoxyphenyl)-7-(4-hydroxyphenyl)-3-heptanone (**294**)
(3*R*,5*R*)-3-acetoxy-5-hydroxy-1,7-*bis*(4-hydroxyphenyl)-heptane (**295**)
(3*R*,5*R*)-3-acetoxy-5-hydroxy-1,7-*bis*(3,4-dihydroxyphenyl)-heptane (**296**)
(3*R*,5*R*)-3,5-diacetoxy-1-(3,4-dihydroxyphenyl)-7-(4-hydroxyphenyl)-heptane (**297**)
(3*S*,5*S*)-3-acetoxy-5-hydroxy-1-(3,4-dihydroxyphenyl)-7-(4-hydroxyphenyl)-heptane (**298**)

(3*R*,5*S*)-3-acetoxy-5-hydroxy-1-(3,4-dihydroxyphenyl)-7-(4-hydroxyphenyl)-heptane (**299**)
(3*R*,5*R*)-3,5-dihydroxy-1,7-*bis*(4-hydroxyphenyl)-heptane (**300**)
(3*R*,5*R*)-3,5-dihydroxy-1-(3,4-dihydroxyphenyl)-7-(4-hydroxyphenyl)-heptane (**301**)
(3*R*,5*R*)-3,5-dihydroxy-1-(4-hydroxy-3-methoxyphenyl)-7-(3,4-dihydroxyphenyl)-heptane (**302**)
(3*R*,5*R*)-3,5-diacetoxy-1,7-*bis*(3,4-dihydroxyhenyl)-heptane (**303**)
(3*R*,5*S*)-3,5-dihydroxy-1,7-*bis*(4-hydroxyhenyl)-heptane (**304**)
(5*S*)-5-hydroxy-1,7-*bis*(4-hydroxyhenyl)-heptane-3-one (**305**)
(5*S*)-5-hydroxy-1-(4-hydroxy-3-methoxy-henyl)-7-(3,4-dihydroxyphenyl)-heptane-3-one (**306**)
indomethacin (**307**)
hydrocortisone (**308**)
hedycoropyran A (**309**)
hedycoropyran B (**310**)
hedycoropyran C (**311**)
hedycorofuran A (**312**)
hedycorofuran B (**313**)
hedycorofuran C (**314**)
hedycorofuran D (**315**)
renealtin A (**316**)
renealtin B (**317**)
(1*R*,2*S*,5*S*)-2-hydroxy-1,7(*p*-hydroxyphenyl)-centrolobine (**318**)
1,7-*bis*(4-hydroxyphenyl)-(1*E*)-1-hepten-3-one (**319**)
5*R*-1,7-*bis*(4-hydroxyphenyl)-1*E*-hepten-5-ol (**320**)
3,5-dioxo-1,7-*bis*(3-methoxy-4-hydroxy)-phenyl-heptane (1,7-*bis*(4-hydroxy-3-methoxyphenyl)heptanes-3,5-dione. **321**)
gingerenone A ((*E*)-1,7-*bis*(4-hydroxy-3-methoxyphenyl)hept-4-en-3-one. **322**)
3,5-diacetoxy-1-(3-methoxy-4,5-dihydroxy-phenyl)-7-(4-hydroxy-3-methoxyphenyl)heptane (1-(3,4-dihydroxy-5-methoxyphenyl)-7-(4-hydroxy-3-methoxyphenyl)heptane-3,5-diyl diacetate. **323**)

1,7-*bis(*4-hydroxy-3- methoxyphenyl)heptane-3,5-diol (**324**)

7-(3,4-dihydroxy-5-methoxyphenyl)-5-hydroxy-1-(4-hydroxy-3-methoxyphenyl)heptan-3-one (**325**)

1,5-epoxy-3-hydroxy-1-(3,4-hydroxy-5-methoxyphenyl)-7-(4-hydroxy-3-methoxyphenyl)heptane. (5-((2*S*,4*S*,6*S*)-4-hydroxy-6-(3-hydroxy-4-methoxyphenethyl)tetrahydro-2*H*-pyran-2-yl)-3-methoxybenzene-1,2-diol (**326**)

1,5-epoxy-3-hydroxy-1-(3,4-hydroxy-5-methoxyphenyl)-7-(4-hydroxy-3-methoxyphenyl)heptane (5-((2*S*,4*R*,6*S*)-4-hydroxy-6-(3-hydroxy-4-methoxyphenethyl)tetrahydro-2*H*-pyran-2-yl)-3-methoxybenzene-1,2-diol (**327**)

5-[4-hydroxy-6-(4-hydroxyphenethyl)tetrahydro-2*H*-pyran-2-yl]-3-methoxybenzene-1,2-diol (5-((2*S*,4*R*,6*S*)-4-hydroxy-6-(4-hydroxyphenethyl)tetrahydro-2*H*-pyran-2-yl)-3-methoxybenzene-1,2-diol (**328**)

quercetin (**329**)

(4*E*,6*E*)-7-(3,4-dihydroxy-5-methoxyphenyl)-1-(4-hydroxy-3-methoxyphenyl)-hepta-4,6-dien-3-one (**330**)

tetrahydrocurcumin (**331**)

5-hydroxy-1,7-*bis*(4-hydroxy-3-methoxyphenyl)heptan-3-one (**332**)

7-(3,4-dihydroxyphenyl)-5-hydroxy-1-(4-hydroxy-3-methoxyphenyl)heptan-3-one (**333**)

(*E*)-1,7-*bis*(4-hydroxy-3-methoxyphenyl)hept-1-ene-3,5-dione (**334**)

(*E*)-7-(4-hydroxy-3-methoxyphenyl)-1-(4-hydroxyphenyl)-hept-1-ene-3,5-dione (**335**)

shogasulfonic acid A (**336**)

1,5-epoxy-3-hydroxy-1-(3,4-dihydroxy-5-methoxyphenyl)-7-(4-hydroxy-3-methoxyphenyl)heptane (**337**)

(3*S*,5*S*)-3,5-diacetoxy-1,7-*bis*(3,4-dihydroxyphenyl)heptane (**338**)

galanganol C (**339**)

7-(3,4-dihydroxy-5-methoxyphenyl)-5-hydroxy-1-(4-hydroxy-3-methoxyphenyl)-3-heptanone (**340**)
1-(3,4-dihydroxy-5-methoxyphenyl)-5-hydroxy-7-(4-hydroxy-3-methoxyphenyl)-3-heptanone (**341**)

ABBREVIATIONS IN PLANTS CONTAINING CURCUMINOIDS (DIARYLHEPTANOIDS)

BV2 microglial cells	C57BL/6, brain, microglial cells
CBMN	cytokinesis-block micronucleus
CBPI	cytokinesis-block proliferation index
DNP-BSA	dinitrophenylated bovine serum albumin
DPPH	2,2-diphenyl-1-picrylhydrazyl
EC_{50}	50% effective concentration
GI_{50}	50% growth inhibitions
HGF	human gingival fibroblasts
IgE	immunoglobulin E
% IN	% inhibition
iNOS	inducible nitric oxide synthase
LPO	lipid peroxidation
LPS	lipopolysaccharide
IC_{50}	50% inhibitory concentration
MAO-A	monoamine oxidase-A
MDR	multidrug resistance
MEC	minimum effective concentration
MN	micronucleus
NBT	nitroblue tetrazolium test
NO	nitric oxide
NOS	nitric oxide synthase
NSCLC	human non-small-cell lung cancer
PET	paw edema thickness
P-gp	P-glycoprotein
QSAR	quantitative structure-activity relationships

SAR	structure- activity relationship
SI	selective index
SOSA	superoxide anion radical scavenging activities
TPC	total phenol content
VL (kala-azar)	visceral leishmaniasis
XO	xanthine oxidase

1. Introduction

Since ancient times, curcumin has been widely used for food pigments and spices in many parts of the world including India and neighboring countries. Recently, it has been identified that curcumin and diarylheptanoids (curcuminoids) in turmeric are also present in other genus genera and species. Therefore, Chapter 1 describes about diarylheptanoids (curcuminoids) derived from plants, and the correlation between diarylheptanoids and their antitumor and anti-inflammatory properties, including some isolation methods for selective extraction of diarylheptanoids.

2. Plants Containing Curcuminoids (Diarylheptanoids)

2.1. Order Fabales

2.1.1. Leguminosae

2.1.1.1. Centrolobium

2.1.1.1.1. *Centrolobium robusturn* Mart. and *Centrolobium tomentosum* Benth.

In 1970, Craveiro *et al.* confirmed three types of diarylheptanoids: (-)-centrolobine (**1**), (-)-de-*O*-methylcentrolobine (**2**) and (-)-centrolobol (**3**) (Figure 1) from the heartwood of *Centrolobium robusturn* Mart.

In 1970, Craveiro *et al.* also confirmed three types of diarylheptanoids: (+)-centrolobine (**4**), (+)-de-*O*-methylcentrolobine (**5**) and (+)-centrolobol (**6**) (Figure 1) from the heartwood of *Centrolobium tomentosum* Benth [1].

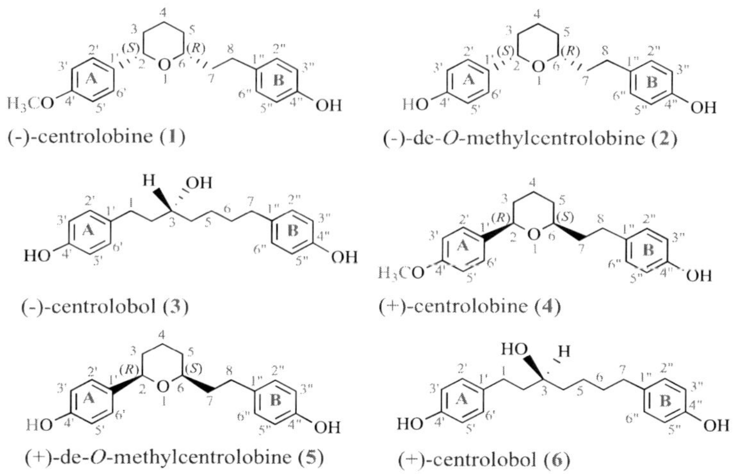

Figure 1. (-)-Centrolobine (**1**), (-)-de-*O*-methylcentrolobine (**2**), (-)-centrolobol (**3**), (+)-centrolobine (**4**), (+)-de-*O*-methylcentrolobine (**5**), and (+)-centrolobol (**6**) from the heartwood of *Centrolobium robusturn* Mart. or *Centrolobium tomentosum* Benth..

2.1.1.1.2. *Centrolobium paraense* var. *paraense* Tull, *Centrolobium sclerophyllum* Lima sp. nova, *Centrolobium tomentosum* Guillem. ex Benth. and *Centrolobium robustum* (Veil.) Benth. ex Mart.

In 1989, Alegrio *et al.* confirmed levorotatory diarylheptanoids from three *Centrolobium paraense* var. *paraense* Tull, *Centrolobium sclerophyllum* Lima sp. nova and *Centrolobium tomentosum* Guillem. ex Benth., and dextrorotatory diarylheptanoids from one *Centrolobium robustum* (Veil.) Benth. ex Mart., as follows:

Centrolobium paraense var. *paraense* Tull contained all levorotatory diarylheptanoids such as centrolobol (3*S*. **7**) (-11°), and centrolobol (3*S*,7*R*. **8**) (-96°), followed by centrolobol (3*S*. **7**) (-11°), (-)-hannokinol (**9**) (-19°) and centrolobol (3*S*,7*R*. **8**) (-96°) for *Centrolobium sclerophyllum* Lima sp. nova, centrolobol (3*S*. **7**) (-11°), centrolobol (3*S*,7*R*. **8**) (-96°) and centrolobol (3*S*,7*R*. **10**) (-98°) (Figure 2) for *Centrolobium tomentosum* Guillem. ex Benth.

Centrolobium robustum (Veil.) Benth. ex Mart. also contained all dextrorotatory diarylheptanoids from (+)-centrolobine (3*R*. **11**) (+11°), centrolobol (3*R*,7*S*. **12**) (+95°) and centrolobol (3*R*,7*S*. **13**) (+97°) (Figure 2) [2].

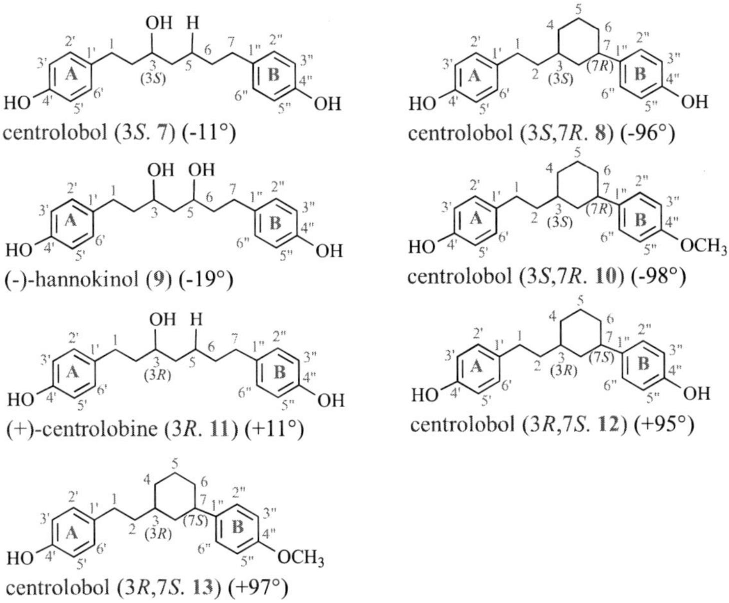

Figure 2. Centrolobol (3*S*. 7) (-11°), centrolobol (3*S*,7*R*. #8) (-96°), (-)-hannokinol (9) (-19°), centrolobol (3*S*,7*R*. #10) (-98°), (+)-centrolobine (3*R*. #11) (+11°), centrolobol (3*R*,7*S*. 12) (+95°) and centrolobol (3*R*,7*S*. 13) (+97°) from three *Centrolobium paraense* var. *paraense* Tull, *Centrolobium sclerophyllum* Lima sp. nova and *Centrolobium tomentosum* Guillem. ex Benth., and one *Centrolobium robustum* (Veil.) Benth. ex Mart..

2.2. Order Fagales

2.2.1. Betulaceae

*2.2.1.1. Alnus (*Alnus mill. *Common Name: Alder) [The Family Betulaceae, Genus Betula, Alder]*

Since ancient times, Alnus plants have been used in many traditional medicines such as stimulant, vomit, galactogogues (milk secretion promoting substance. milk producing substance), febrifuges (antipyretic agent), hemostatic agent, parasite control agent, pest control agent, skin tonic agent and astringents [3].

The genus *Alnus mill.* is one of six genera of the family Betulaceae that has nitrogen fixation ability through symbiotic relationship with actinomycetes of the soil filamentous fungus called Frankia, and it is the only genus with nitrogen fixation capacity among the birchidae. Therefore, the actinomycetes that make up the genus Frankia are distinguished from other actinomycetes because they have the ability to induce N2 fixed root nodules in certain non-legumes.

Alder species are widely distributed in temperate regions of the northern hemisphere. The exception is *Alnus glutinosa* (L.), which is an Alder species scattered throughout the South American Andes and in small areas of North Africa [4, 5].

2.2.1.1.1. *Alnus firma*

2.2.1.1.1.1. *Alnus firma*/1969

In 1969, Asakawa Y *et al.* identified yashabushiketol (**14**) (Figure 3) from benzene extract of the buds of *Alunus firma* Sieb. et Zucc. (Betulaceae) [6].

2.2.1.1.1.2. *Alnus Firma*/1970

In 1970, Asakawa Y identified novel didydroyashabushiketol (**15**) (Figure 3) along with known yashabushiketol (**14**) from benzene extract of the young shoots of *Alunus firma* Sieb. et Zucc. (Betulaceae) [7].

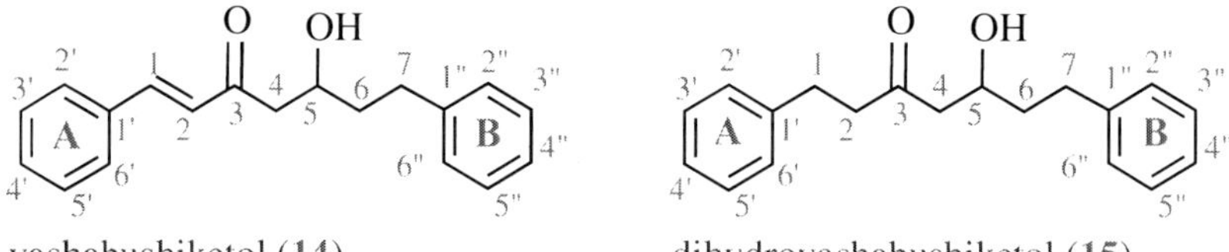

yashabushiketol (**14**) dihydroyashabushiketol (**15**)

Figure 3. Yashabushiketol (**14**) and dihydroyashabushiketol (**15**) from benzene extracts of *Alunus firma* Sieb. et Zucc.(Betulaceae).

2.2.1.1.1.3. *Alnus firma*/2010

In 2010, Lee MA *et al.* studied the chemical constituents of *Alnus firma* and their inhibitory activity on lipopolysaccharide (LPS)-induced nitric oxide (NO) production in BV2 microglia (BV2 microglial cells where as C57BL/6, brain, microglial cells served as an alternative model system for primary microglia cultures or for animal experiments for the examination of brain inflammation.

First, 6'-*O*-vanilloylisotachioside (**6**) [8] and 11 known diarylheptanoids (**17 - 27**) were isolated from the methanolic extract of *Alnus firma* barks (Betulaceae).

11 known diarylheptanoids have the following name: dehydrohirsutanonol (hirsutanone. hirsutenone. **17**) [9], 5-hydroxy-3-platyphyllone (**18**) [10], platyphylloside ((5*S*)-1,7-*bis*(4-hydroxyphenyl)-5-[(2*R*,3*R*,4*S*,5*S*,6*R*)-3,4,5-trihydroxy-6-(hydroxymethyl)oxan-2-yl]oxyheptan-3-one. **19**) [11], (5*S*)-5-hydroxy-1,7-*bis*-(4-hydroxyphenyl)-3-heptanone-5-*O*-β-D-apiofuranosyl-(1→6)-β-D-glucopyranoside (**20**) [12], (5*S*)-5-hydroxy-7-(3,4-dihydroxyphenyl)-1-(4-hydroxyphenyl)-3-heptanone-5-*O*-β-D-xylopyranoside (**21**) [9], (5*R*)-5-methoxy-1,7-*bis*-(3,4-dihydroxyphenyl)-3-heptanone (**22**) [13], oregonin (**23**) [9] (Figure 4), (3*R*)-1,7-*bis*-(4-hydroxyphenyl)-3-heptanol-3-*O*-β-D-apiofuranosyl-(1→6) -β-D-glucopyranoside (**24**) [12], (3*R*)-1,7-*bis*-(3,4-dihydroxyphenyl)-3-heptanol-3-*O*-β-D-glucoopyranoside (**25**) [14], (3*R*)-1,7-*bis*-(3,4-dihydroxyphenyl)-3-heptanol-3-*O*-β-D-glucopyranosyl-(1→3)-β-D-xylopyranoside (**26**) [15], and (3*R*)-1,7-*bis*-(3,4-dihydroxyphenyl)-3-heptanol-3-*O*-β-D-xylopyranoside (**27**) [15] (Figure 4(continued 1)), respectively.

Second, on radical scavenging effects of LPS-induced NO production for 11 known diarylheptanoids (**17-27**) by using positive control ω-nitro-L-argininemethyl ester (L-NAME. **28**) (Figure 4(continued 1)), 7 known diarylheptanoids (**17-23**) significantly inhibited the NO production by LPS in BV2 microglial cells (mouse, C57BL/6, brain, microglial cells) at concentrations ranging from 10 μM to 100 μM. Among 11 known diarylheptanoids (**17-27**), dehydrohirsutanonol (**17**) showed cytotoxicity at 50 μM and 100 μM except 10 μM. These results suggest that the presence of C-3 carbonyl group in diarylheptanoids plays an important role in inhibitory activity of LPS-induced NO production. To determine a more relevant structure-activity relationship, more diarylheptanoids should be evaluated for their inhibitory activities on NO production.

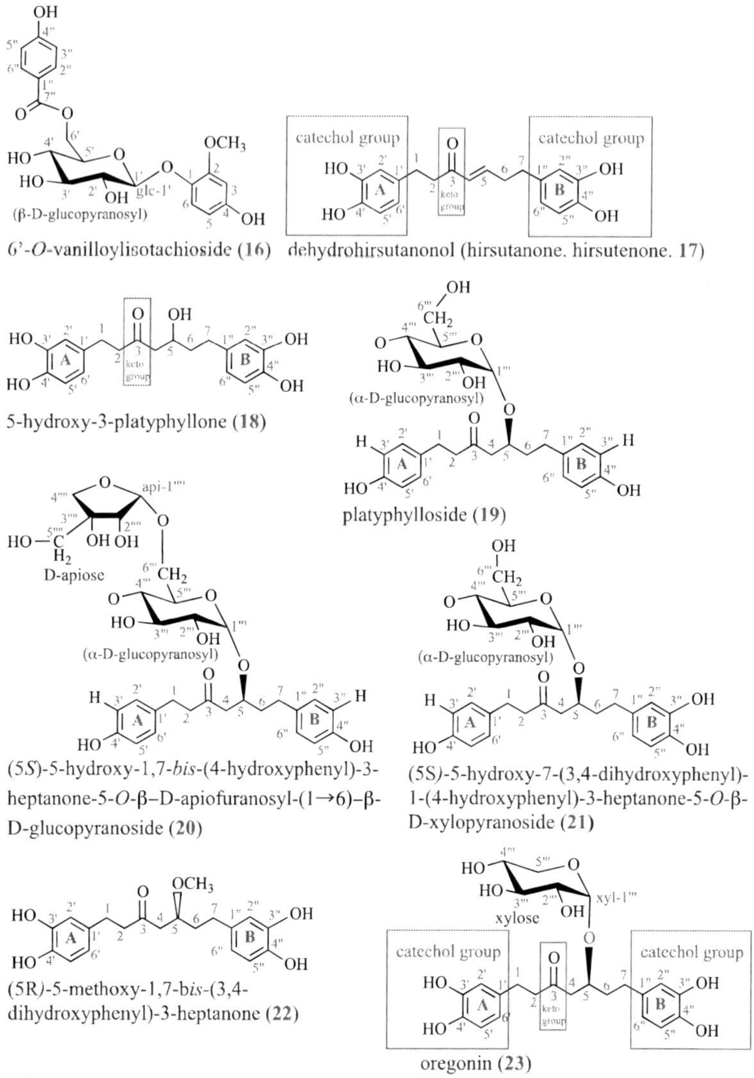

Figure 4. 6'-*O*-Vanilloylisotachioside (16) and eleven diarylheptanoids from barks of *Alnus firma* barks (Betulaceae): dehydrohirsutanonol (hirsutanone. hirsutenone. 17), 5-hydroxy-3-platyphyllone (18 platyphylloside (19), (5*S*)-5-hydroxy-1,7-*bis*-(4-hydroxyphenyl)-3-heptanone-5-*O*-β–D-apiofuranosyl-(1→6)–β-D-glucopyranoside (20), (5S)-5-hydroxy-7-(3,4-dihydroxyphenyl)-1-(4-hydroxyphenyl)-3-heptanone-5-*O*-β-D-xylopyranoside (21), (5R)-5-methoxy-1,7-bi*s*-(3,4-dihydroxyphenyl)-3-heptanone (22), and oregonin (23).

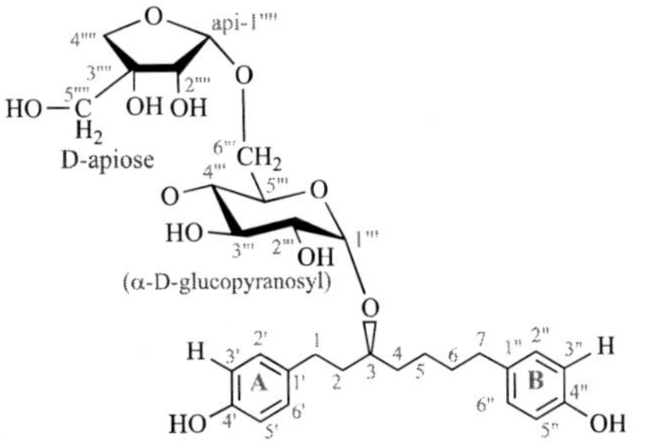

(3*R*)-1,7-*bis*-(4-hydroxyphenyl)-3-heptanol-3-*O*-β-D-apiofuranosyl-(1→6)-β-D-glucopyranoside (**24**)

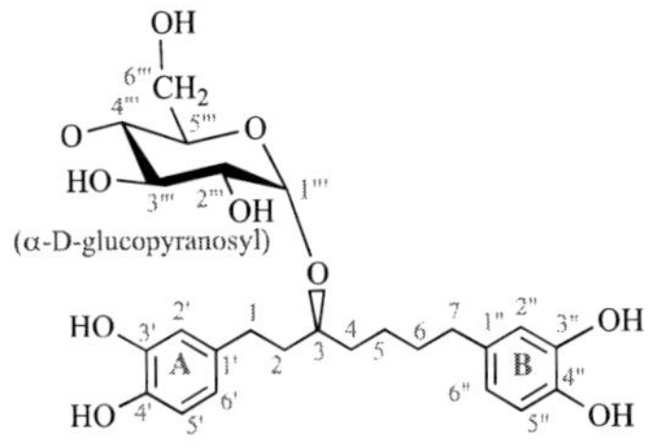

(3*R*)-1,7-*bis*-(3,4-dihydroxyphenyl)-3-heptanol-3-*O*-β-D-glucoopyranoside (**25**)

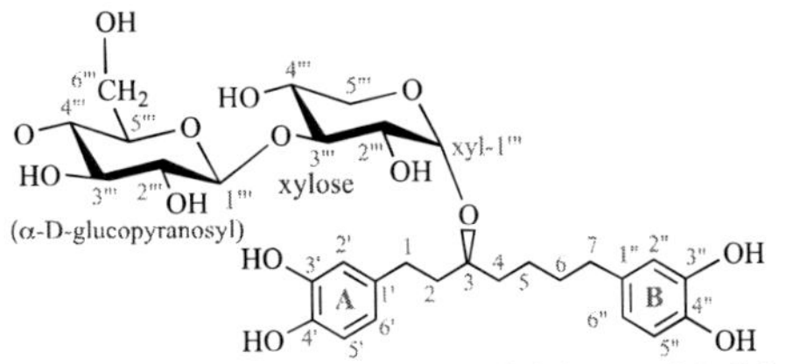

(3*R*)-1,7-*bis*-(3,4-dihydroxyphenyl)-3-heptanol-3-*O*-β-D-glucopyranosyl-(1→3)-β-D-xylopyranoside (**26**)

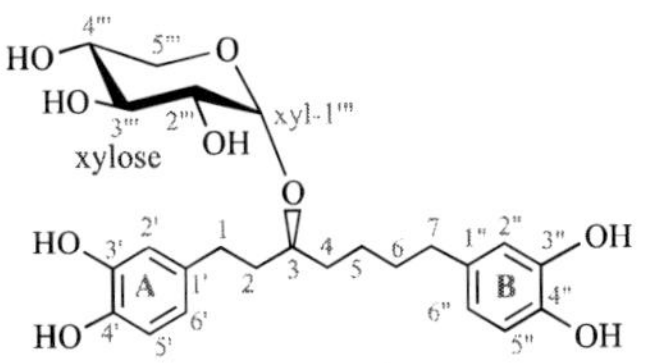

(3*R*)-1,7-*bis*-(3,4-dihydroxyphenyl)-3-heptanol-3-*O*-β-D-xylopyranoside (**27**)

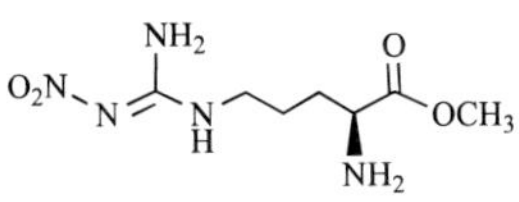

ω-nitro-L-argininemethyl ester (**L-NAME**, **28**)

Figure 4(continued 1). Eleven diarylheptanoids from barks of *Alnus firma* barks (Betulaceae): (3*R*)-1,7-*bis*-(4-hydroxyphenyl)-3-heptanol-3-*O*-β-D-apiofuranosyl-(1→6)-β-D-glucopyranoside (**24**), (3*R*)-1,7-*bis*-(3,4-dihydroxyphenyl)-3-heptanol-3-*O*-β-D-glucoopyranoside (**25**), (3*R*)-1,7-*bis*-(3,4-dihydroxyphenyl)-3-heptanol-3-*O*-β-D-glucopyranosyl-(1→3)-β-D-xylopyranoside (**26**), and (3*R*)-1,7-*bis*- (3,4-dihydroxyphenyl)-3-heptanol-3-*O*-β-D-xylopyranoside (**27**). Positive control: ω-nitro-L-argininemethyl ester (**L-NAME**, **28**).

However, in this experiment, since the structure-activity relationship was only for 11 known diarylheptanoids (**17-27**), in order to obtain even more reliable structure-activity relationships, it may be necessary to confirm the radical scavenging effects of LPS-induced NO production on more diverse diarylheptanoids [16].

2.2.1.1.2. *Alnus glutinosa*

2.2.1.1.2.1. *Alnus glutinosa*/2011

In 2011, Roze L *et al.* identified two known diarylheptanoids: oregonin (1,7-*bis*-(3,4-dihydroxyphenyl)-heptane-3-on-5-*O*-β-Dxylopyranoside. **29**) and a mixture of 1,7-*bis*-(3,4- dihydroxyphenyl)-3-hydroxyheptane-5-*O*-β-D-xylopyranoside (**30**) epimer alcohols (Figure 5) from the bark of two Alder species of grey alder (*Alnus incana*) and black alder (*Alnus glutinosa*) [17].

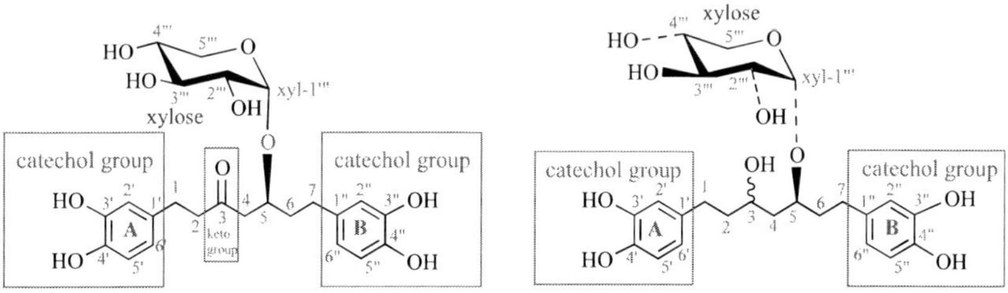

oregonin (**29**)

a mixture of 1,7-*bis*-(3,4- dihydroxyphenyl)-3-hydroxyheptane-5-*O*-β-D-xylopyranoside (**30**) epimer alcohols

Figure 5. Two diarylheptanoids - oregonin (**29**), and a mixture of 1,7-*bis*-(3,4-dihydroxyphenyl)-3-hydroxyheptane-5-*O*-β-D-xylopyranoside (**30**) epimer alcohols from the bark of two *Alder* species of grey alder (*Alnus incana*) and black alder (*Alnus glutinosa*).

2.2.1.1.2.2. *Alnus glutinosa*/2013

In 2013, a group of Institute of Chemistry, Technology and Metallurgy, University of Belgrade, Belgrade, Serbia, first, examined fourteen diarylheptanoids: oregonin (**23**), platyphylloside (**19**), rubranoside A (**31**), rubranoside B (**32**), hirsutanonol (**33**), hirsutenone (**34**), hirsutanonol-5-*O*-β-D-glucopyranoside (**35**), platyphyllonol-5-*O*-β-D-xylopyranoside (**36**) (Figure 6), aceroside VII (**37**), alnuside A (**38**), alnuside B (**39**), 1,7-*bis*-(3,4-dihydoxyphenyl)-5-hydroxy-heptane-3-*O*-β-D-xylopyranoside (**40**), (5*S*)-1-(4-hydroxyphenyl)-7-(3,4-dihydroxyphenyl)-5-*O*-β-D-glucopyranosyl-heptan-3-one (**41**), and (5*S*)-1,7-*bis*-(3,4-dihydroxyphenyl)-5-*O*-β-D-[6-(3,4-dimethoxycinnamoylglucopyranosyl)]-heptan-3-one (**42**) (Figure 6(continued 1) from the bark of *Alnus glutinosa*.

Among these 14 diarylheptanoids, 12 other diarylheptanoids except diarylheptanoids: oregonin (**23**) and hirsutanonol (**33**) were first identified in *Alnus glutinosa*. Meanwhile, two diarylheptanoids of (5*S*)-1-(4-hydroxyphenyl)-7-(3,4-dihydroxyphenyl)-5-*O*-β-D-glucopyranosyl-heptan-3-one (**41**) and (5*S*)-1,7-*bis*-(3,4-dihydroxyphenyl)-5-*O*-β-D-[6-(3,4-dimethoxycinnamoylglucopyranosyl)]-heptan-3-one (**42**) were catacorized as novel compounds.

Second, these fourteen diarylheptanoids were examined for their *in vitro* for the protection against chromosomal aberrations in human peripheral lymphocytes using the cytokinesis-block micronucleus (CBMN) assay. Whole blood lymphocytes were treated with two concentrations of diarylheptanoid (1.0 and 2.0 μg/mL). Diarylheptanoid-untreated cells served as a blank control (blank). One cell culture containing only the known chromosome aberration inducer mitomycin C (MMC. **43**) (Figure 7) whereas 0.1 μg /mL in phosphate buffer was used as a negative control. The known DNA protectant amifhostin WR-2721 (**44**) (Figure 7) (0.1 μg /mL) was used as a radioprotectant for positive control. The human lymphocyte micronucleus assay (MN) was performed according to the cytokinesis-block method [18].

First, the inhibitory effect of cell proliferation on diarylheptanoids was determined by the cytokinesis-block proliferation index (CBPI).

Second, the micronucleus (MN) frequency (occurrence rate of cells having micronucleus (MN)) (%) in cell cultures of human lymphocytes treated with fourteen diarylheptanoids, mitomycin C (MMC. **43**), and amifhostin WR-2721 (**44**) were as follows:

Control: 100%; amifhostin WR-2721 (**44**): 82.8% at concentration of 1.0 μg/mL); mitomycin C (MMC. **43**): 130% (0.1 μg/mL); oregonin (**23**): 47.2% (1.0 μg/mL) and 57.2% (2.0 μg/mL); platyphylloside (**19**): 57.2% (1.0 μg/mL) and 66.4% (2.0 μg/mL); rubranoside A (**31**): 75.2% (1.0 μg/mL) and 83.6% (2.0 μg/mL); rubranoside B (**32**): 67.6% (1.0 μg/mL) and 74.4% (2.0 μg/mL); hirsutanonol (**33**): 36.4% (1.0 μg/mL) and 42.0% (2.0 μg/mL); hirsutenone (**34**): 60.4% (1.0 μg/mL) and 66.0% (2.0

μg/mL); hirsutanonol-5-*O*-β-D-glucopyranoside (**35**): 76.8% (1.0 μg/mL) and 88.4% (2.0 μg/mL); platyphyllonol-5-*O*-β-D-xylopyranoside (**36**): 94.0% (1.0 μg/mL) and 104.0% (2.0 μg/mL); aceroside VII (**37**): 86.4% (1.0 μg/mL) and 89.2% (2.0 μg/mL); alnuside A (**38**): 67.2% (1.0 μg/mL) and 69.2% (2.0 μg/mL); alnuside B (**39**): 72.4% (1.0 μg/mL) and 76.0% (2.0 μg/mL); 1,7-*bis*-(3,4-dihydoxyphenyl)-5-hydroxy-heptane-3-*O*-β-D-xylopyranoside (**40**): 76.8% (1.0 μg/mL) and 81.6% (2.0 μg/mL); (5*S*)-1-(4-hydroxyphenyl)-7-(3,4-dihydroxyphenyl)-5-*O*-β-D-glucopyranosyl-heptan-3-one (**41**): 55.6% (1.0 μg/mL) and 71.6% (2.0 μg/mL); and (5*S*)-1,7-*bis*-(3,4-dihydroxyphenyl)-5-*O*-β-D-[6-(3,4-dimethoxycinnamoyl-glucopyranosyl)]-heptan-3-one (**42**): 44.0% (1.0 μg/mL) and 52.0% (2.0 μg/mL).

According to the human lymphocyte micronucleus (MN) test, diarylheptanoids having remarkable protective activity among 14 kinds of diarylheptanoids *invariably* have a 3-keto group and two 3,4-dihydroxyphenyl (catechol) sites in the diarylheptanoids. Interestingly, flavonoids and other secondary metabolites with strong antioxidants also have catechol moieties and keto groups in their structure [19]. In light of the structural features presented for this structure-bioactivity relationship, the protective effect in this human lymphocyte micronucleus (MN) test is strongly correlated with antioxidant activity [20, 21], it is clear that the reason why 3 kinds of diarylheptanoids such as oregonin (**29**), hirsutanonol (**33**), and (5*S*)-1,7-*bis*-(3,4-dihydroxyphenyl)-5-*O*-β-D-[6-(3,4-dimethoxy-cinnamoylglucopyranosyl)]-heptan-3-one (**42**) in 14 diaryl heptanoids showed the best activity. However, hirsutenone (**34**) also has these structural elements, but its keto group is conjugated, which may be due to its slightly lower activity. Six diarylheptanoids (**31, 32, 38, 39, 40, 41**) lacking one of the mentioned groups (*i.e.*, having a keto group and one catechol group or only two catechol groups) showed weaker activity than three diarylheptanoids (**23**, **33**, **42**). Platyphyllonol-5-*O*-β-D-xylopyranoside (**36**) with only a keto group, and aceroside VII (**37**) not containing any of these groups showed the lowest activity [22].

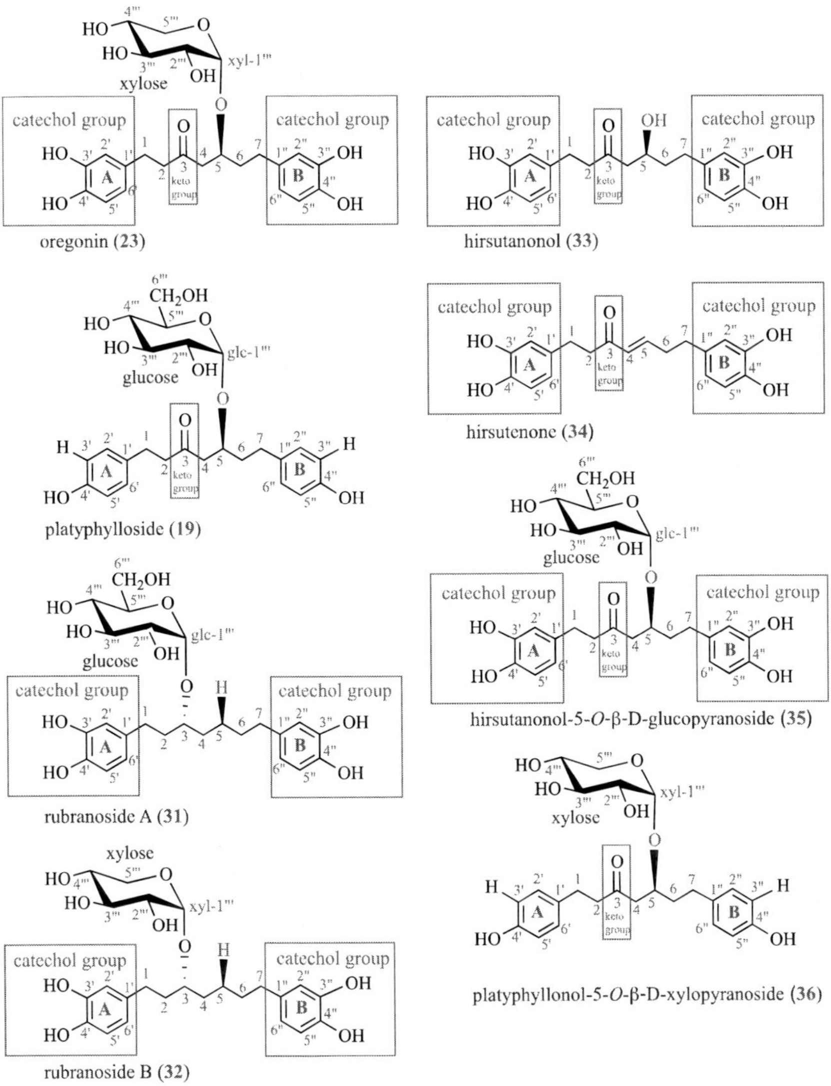

Figure 6. Fourteen diarylheptanoids - oregonin (**23**), platyphylloside (**19**), rubranoside A (**31**), rubranoside B (**32**, hirsutanonol (**33**), hirsutenone (**34**), hirsutanonol-5-*O*-β-D-glucopyranoside (**35**), and platyphyllonol-5-*O*-β-D-xylopyranoside (**36**) - from the bark of *Alnus glutinosa*.

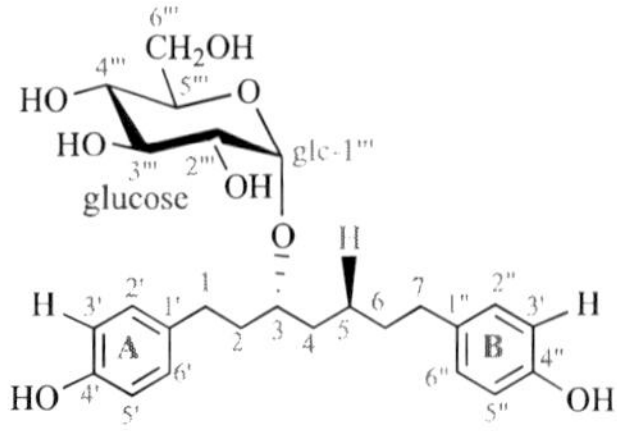

aceroside VII (**37**)

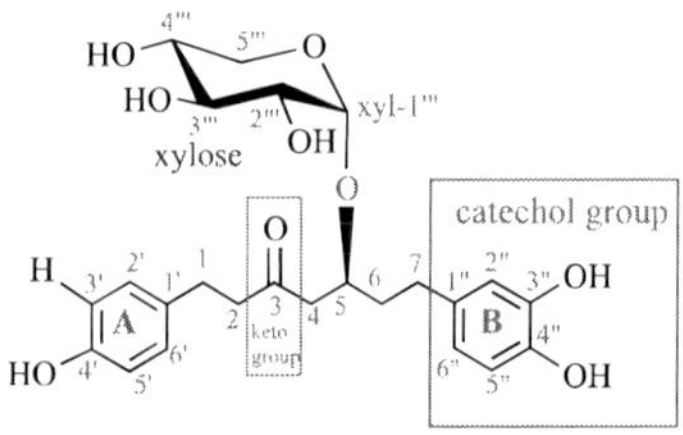

alnuside A (**38**)

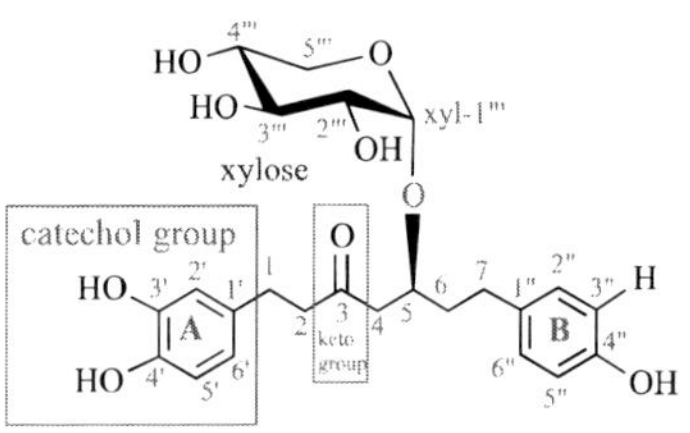

alnuside B (**39**)

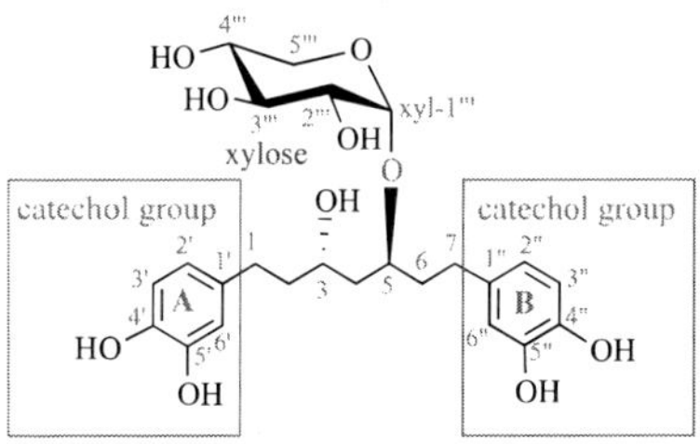

1,7-b*is*-(3,4-dihydoxyphenyl)-5-hydroxy-heptane-3-*O*-β–D-xylopyranoside (**40**)

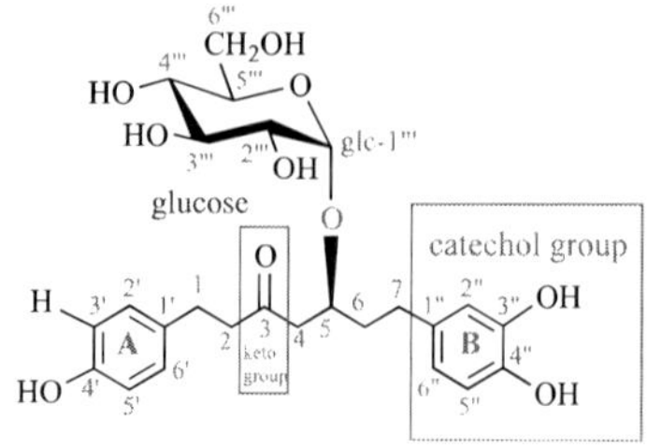

(5*S*)-1-(4-hydroxyphenyl)-7-(3,4-dihydroxyphenyl)-5-*O*-β-D-glucopyranosyl-heptan-3-one (**41**)

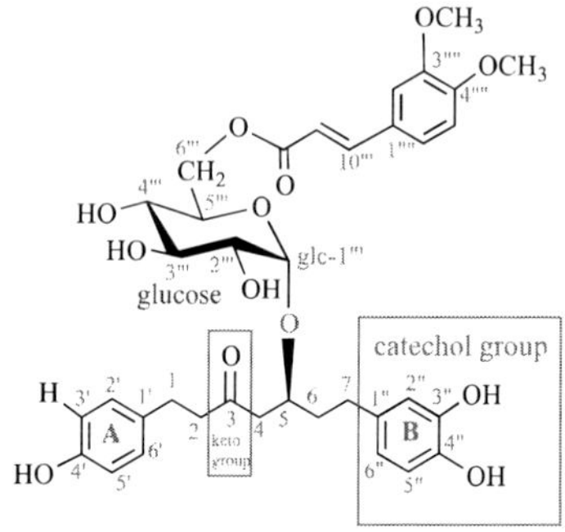

(5*S*)-1,7-*bis*-(3,4-dihydroxyphenyl)-5-*O*-β-D-[6-(3,4-dimethoxycinnamoylglucopyranosyl)]-heptan-3-one (**42**)

Figure 6(continued 1). Fourteen diarylheptanoids - aceroside VII (**37**), alnuside A (**38**), alnuside B (**39**), 1,7-*bis*-(3,4-dihydoxyphenyl)-5-hydroxy-heptane-3-*O*-β-D-xylopyranoside (**40**), (5*S*)-1-(4-hydroxyphenyl)-7-(3,4-dihydroxyphenyl)-5-*O*-β-D-glucopyranosyl-heptan-3-one (**41**), and (5*S*)-1,7-*bis*-(3,4-dihydroxyphenyl)-5-*O*-β-D-[6-(3,4-dimethoxycinnamoylglucopyranosyl)]-heptan-3-one (**42**) - from the bark of *Alnus glutinosa*.

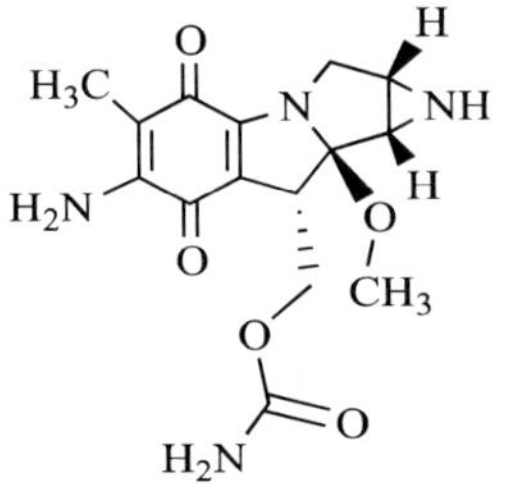

mitomycin C (MMC. 43)

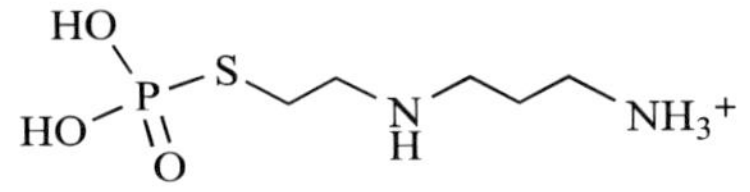

amifhostin WR-2721 (44)

Figure 7. Mitomycin C (MMC. 43) and amifhostin WR-2721 (44).

2.2.1.1.2.3. *Alnus glutinosa*/2014

In 2014, Novaković *et al.* confirmed a total of 20 diarylheptanoids with 10 novel diarylheptanoids (**45-49 51-55**) (Figure 8) (Figure 8(continued 1)) together with 10 known diarylheptanoids (**19, 36, 38, 39, 33, 56, 23, 34, 57, 50**) (Figure 9) from the chloroform/methanol (1:1) extract of the bark of *Alnus glutinosa* (black alder).

Each of the 20 diarylheptanoids has the following names:

Ten novel diarylheptanoids (**45-49, 51-55**) are 5(*S*)-1,7-di(4-hydroxyphenyl)-5-*O*-β-D-[6-(*E*-*p*-coumaroylglucopyranosyl)]heptane-3-one (**45**), 5(*S*)-1,7-di(4-hydroxyphenyl)-5-*O*-β-D-[6-(*E*-3,4-dimethoxy-cinnamoylglucopyranosyl)]heptane-3-one (**46**), 5(*S*)-1-(4-hydroxyphenyl)-7-(3,4-dihydroxyphenyl)-5-*O*-β-D-[6-(*E*-3,4-dimethoxycinnamoylgluco-pyranosyl)]heptane-3-one (**47**), 5(*S*)-1-(3,4-dihydroxyphenyl)-7-(4-hydroxyphenyl)-5-*O*-β-D-[6-(*Z*-3,4-dimethoxycinnamoylglucopyrano-syl)]heptane-3-one (**48**), 5(*S*)-1,7-di(3,4-dihydroxyphenyl)-5-*O*-β-D-[6-(*E*-p-coumaroylglucopyranosyl)]heptane-3-one (**49**), 5(*S*)-1,7-di(3,4-dihydro-xyphenyl)-5-*O*-β-D-[6-(*Z*-3,4-dimethoxycinn amoylglucopyrano-syl)]hep-tane-3-one. (**51**), 5(*S*)-1,7-di(3,4-dihydroxyphenyl)-5-*O*-β-D-[6-(*E*-3,4,5-trimethoxycinnamoylglucopyranosyl)]heptane-3-one (**52**), 3(*R*)-1,7-di(3,4-dihydroxyphenyl)-3-*O*-β-D-[6-(*E*-3,4-dimethoxycinnamoylglucopy-rano-syl)]heptane (**53**), 3(*R*)-1,7-di(3,4-dihydroxyphenyl)-5-*O*-β-D-[6-(*Z*-3,4-dimethoxycinnamoylglucopyranosyl)] heptane (**54**) and 3(*R*)-1,7-di(3,4-dihydroxyphenyl)-5-*O*-β-D-[6-(*E*-3,4,5-trimethoxycinnamoylglucopyrano-syl)]heptane (**55**).

Ten known diarylheptanoids (**19, 36, 38, 39, 33, 56, 23, 34, 57, 50**) are platyphylloside (**19**) [12], platyphyllonol-5-*O*-β-D-xylopyranoside (**36**) [23], alnuside A (**38**), alnuside B (**39**), 5(*S*)-methylhirsutanonol (**56**), oregonin (**23**) [9], hirsutanonol (**33**) [24], hirsutenone (**34**) [25], 3(R)-1,7-di(3,4-dihydroxyphenyl)-3-hydroxyheptane (**57**), and 5(*S*)-1,7-di(3,4-dihydroxyphenyl)-5-*O*-β-D-[6-(*E*-3,4-dimethoxycinnamoylglucopyranosyl)] heptane-3-one (**50**) [22].

On the structure- activity relationship (SAR) between their structures and cytotoxic effects of diarylheptanoids, human non-small-cell lung cancer (NSCLC) cell line (NCI-H460), its corresponding multidrug resistance (MDR) variant (NCI-H460/R), and normal human keratinocytes (HaCaT) were examined by the sulforhodamine B assay after 72 hr treatments with a positive control curcumin (**58**) (Figure 10). The results of cytotoxic effects are expressed as concentrations of diarylheptanoids that inhibited cell growth by 50% (50% inhibitory concentration (IC_{50})).

In addition to the above 20 types of diarylheptanoids, the cytotoxicity of the following 4 known diarylheptanoids (**59, 9, 31, 32**) (Figure 10) was examined: 55(*S*)-hirsutanonol-5-*O*-β-D-glucopyranoside (**59**) [25], aceroside VII (**9**) [26], rubranoside A (**31**) [27], and 1,7-di(3,4-dihydroxyphenyl)-5-hydroxy-heptane-3-*O*-β-D-xylopyranoside (**32**) [9] are diarylheptanoids previously isolated from black alder [22].

First, regarding cytotoxic effect (IC_{50} (μM)) on human NSCLC cell line (NCI-H460) among the 24 isolated diarylheptanoids, platyphyllonol-5-*O*-β-D-xylopyranoside (**36**) (IC_{50}: 14.9±1.1 μM), alnuside B (**39**) (IC_{50}: 17.8±1.9 μM), and hirsutenone (**34**) (IC_{50}: 19.2±0.3 μM) was more cytotoxic when compared to tha t(cytotoxic toxicity) of the positive control curcumin (**58**) (IC_{50}: 38.4±2.9 μM).

Second, on two cancer cell lines (NCI-H460 と NCI-H460/R), two new diarylheptanoids 5(*S*)-1,7-di(4-hydroxyphenyl)-5-*O*-β-D-[6-(*E*-*p*-coumaroylglucopyranosyl)]heptane-3-one (**45**) (IC_{50}: 19.9±1.1 μM/NCI-H460; IC50: 25.0±2.7 μM/NCI-H460/R) and 5(*S*)-1,7-di(3,4-dihydroxyphenyl)-5-*O*-β-D-[6-(*E*-*p*-coumaroylglucopyranosyl)]heptane-3-one (**49**) (IC_{50}: 27.8±1.8 μM/NCI-H460; IC_{50}: 45.0±0.4 μM/NCI-H460/R) showed higher cytotoxicity when compared to those (IC_{50}) of positive control curcumin (**58**) (IC_{50}: 38.4±2.9 μM/NCI-H460; IC_{50}: 56.7±2.1 μM/NCI-H460/R)).

Here, the selective index (SI) was defined as the ratio of IC_{50} values between normal human keratinocytes (HaCaT) and human NSCLC cell line (NCI-H460). As a result, SI of 5(*S*)-1,7-di(4-hydroxyphenyl)-5-*O*-β-D-[6-(*E*-*p*-coumaroylglucopyranosyl)]heptane-3-one (**45**) (IC_{50}: 19.9±1.1 μM/NCI-H460; IC_{50}: 31.3±1.4 μM/HaCaT) was 1.6, and SI of 5(*S*)-1,7-di(3,4-dihydroxyphenyl)-5-*O*-β-D-[6-(*E*-*p*-coumaroylglucopyranosyl)] heptane-3-one (**49**) (IC_{50}: 19.9±1.1 μM/NCI-H460; IC_{50}: 76.3±3.1 μM/HaCaT) was 2.7, respectively. Therefore, these two 5(*S*)-1,7-di(4-hydroxyphenyl)-5-*O*-β-D-[6-(*E*-*p*-coumaroylgluco-pyranosyl)]heptane-3-one (**45**) と 5(*S*)-1,7-di(3,4-dihydroxyphenyl)-5-*O*-β-D-[6-(*E*-*p*-coumaroyl-glucopyranosyl)]heptane-3-one (**49**) showed good selectivity.

The positive control curcumin (**58**) (IC_{50}: 38.4±2.9 μM/NCI-H460; IC_{50}: 7.1±0.8 μM/HaCaT) was not selective. However, curcumin (**58**) (IC_{50}: 7.1±0.8 μM/HaCaT) showed higher cytotoxicity to normal human keratinocytes (HaCaT).

Among 24 diarylheptanoids, aceroside VII (**9**) (IC_{50}: 100.0±3.1 μM/NCI-H460; IC_{50}: 144.1±3.4 μM/NCI-H460R; IC_{50}: - (no effect) μM/HaCaT) showed the lowest cytotoxic potential. Aceroside VII (**9**) is already known to be an ineffective diarylheptanoid in anti-cancer assays [28].

Second, from the above biological activity results, the following relationship was found:

First, the presence of a carbonyl group at the C-3 position of the diarylheptanoid enhanced the cytotoxic activity of the diarylheptanoid. This correlation is consistent with the results of [29].

Second, the presence of hydroxyl groups at the C-3 'and C-3 "positions of diarylheptanoids inhibited the diarylheptanoidal cytotoxic activity. Moreover, the degree of cytotoxic activity of this diarylheptanoid was lower when compared to that (cytotoxic activity) of the absence of carbonyl groups. The cytotoxic activity of three diarylheptanoids platyphylloside (**19**), 5(*S*)-hirsutanonol-5-*O*-β-D-glucopyranoside (**59**) and rubranoside A (**31**) decreased in the following order: **19**> **59**> **31**. This fact is consistent with the following findings: Platyphylloside (**19**) has no OH group on C-3' and C-3" ($p < 0.01$) when compared to 5(*S*)-hirsutanonol-5-*O*-β-D-glucopyranoside (**59**). On the other hand, rubranoside A (**31**) does not have a carbonyl group at C-3 when compared to 5(*S*)-hirsutanonol-5-*O*-β-D-glucopyranoside (**59**) ($p < 0.001$). The same explanation is given for three diarylheptanoids 5(*S*)-1,7-di(4-hydroxyphenyl)-5-*O*-β-D-[6-(*E*-3,4-dimethoxycinnamoylglucopyranosyl)]heptane-3-one (**46**), 5(*S*)-1,7-di(3,4-dihydroxyphenyl)-5-*O*-β-D-[6-(*E*-3,4-dimethoxycinnamoylglucopyranosyl)]heptane-3-one (**50**), and dimethoxycinnamoylglucopyranosyl)]heptane (**53**) are also effective in decreasing cytotoxic activity: **46** > **50** > **53** ($p < 0.001$).

Four diarylheptanoids aceroside VII (**9**), 3(*R*)-1,7-di(3,4-dihydroxyphenyl)-3-hydroxyheptane (**57**), rubranoside A (**31**), and dimethoxycinnamoylglucopyranosyl)]heptane (**53**) does not have a carbonyl group. Therefore, these four kinds of diarylheptanoids aceroside VII (**9**), 3(*R*)-1,7-di(3,4-dihydroxyphenyl)-3-hydroxyheptane (**57**), rubranoside A (**31**), and dimethoxycinnamoylglucopyranosyl)]heptane (**53**) showed lower cytotoxic activity than platyphylloside (**19**), hirsutanonol (**33**), 5(*S*)-hirsutanonol-5-*O*-β-D-glucopyranoside (**59**), and 5(*S*)-1,7-di(3,4-dihydroxyphenyl)-5-*O*-β-D-[6-(*E*-3,4-dimethoxycinnamoylglucopyranosyl)] heptane-3-one (**50**). This fact gives strong support for *the first conclusion* ($p < 0.001$).

Three diarylheptanoids platyphylloside (**19**), platyphyllonol-5-*O*-β-D-xylopyranoside (**36**) and dimethoxycinnamoylglucopyranosyl)]heptane-3-one (**46**) with a carbonyl group at C-3 inhibited cell growth more potently than three related diarylheptanoids 5(*S*)-hirsutanonol-5-*O*-β-D-glucopyranoside (**59**) ($p < 0.01$), oregonin (**23**) ($p < 0.001$), and 5(*S*)-1,7-di(3,4-dihydroxyphenyl)-5-*O*-β-D-[6-(*E*-3,4-dimethoxycinnamoylglucopyranosyl)] heptane-3-one (**50**) ($p < 0.001$) with one carbonyl group and hydroxyl group in C-3', and C-3." This result supports *the second conclusion*.

In the presence of only one OH group on C-3 'or C-3 "of a diarylheptanoid, the diarylheptanoid adversely affected cytotoxic activity. From diarylheptanoid pairs platyphyllonol-5-*O*-β-D-xylopyranoside (**36**)/alnuside A (**38**) (p <0.01), and dimethoxycinnamoyl-glucopyranosyl)]heptane-3-one (**46**)/dimethoxycinnamoylglucopyranosyl)] heptane-3-one (**47**) (p <0.001), it confirms that 3”-OH significantly reduces cytotoxic activity. Among 24 diarylheptanoids, aceroside VII (**9**) and 3(*R*)-1,7-di(3,4-dihydroxyphenyl)-3-hydroxyheptane (**57**) have the lowest cytotoxic activity. This drop is consistent with previous findings.

Third, the presence of a carbonyl group at C-3 along with a C-5 substituent in the diarylheptanoid enhanced the cytotoxicity of the diarylheptanoid. Specifically, depending on the C-5 substituent in the diarylheptanoid, their cytotoxicity of hirsutanonol (**33**), 5(*S*)-methylhirsutanonol (**56**), 5(*S*)-hirsutanonol-5-*O*-β-D-glucopyranoside (**59**), and oregonin (**23**) decreased in the following order: OCH_3 > O-xylol (Oxyl) > O-glucose (Oglc) > OH. In addition, regarding the cytotoxic activity, the presence of the monosaccharides xylose and glucose within the diarylheptanoids also had a similar effect. Changes in cytotoxic activity due to these substituents within diarylheptanoids are supported by statistical analysis. In general, diarylheptanoid glycosides showed higher cytotoxic activity than the corresponding aglycone: 5(*S*)-hirsutanonol-5-*O*-β-D-glucopyranoside (**59**) > hirsutanonol (**33**) ($p < 0.001$); oregonin (**23**) > hirsutanonol (**33**) ($p < 0.001$); rubranoside A (**31**) > 3(*R*)-1,7-di(3,4-dihydroxyphenyl)-3-hydroxyheptane (**57**) ($p < 0.01$). Addition of cinnamoyl groups to diarylheptanoid glycosides also increased cytotoxic activity as follows: 5(*S*)-1,7-di(3,4-dihydroxyphenyl)-5-*O*-β-D-[6-(*E*-*p*-coumaroylglucopyranosyl)]heptane-3-one (**49**) > 5(*S*)-hirsutanonol-5-*O*-β-D-glucopyranoside (**59**); 3(*R*)-1,7-di(3,4-dihydroxyphenyl)-5-*O*-β-D-[6-(*Z*-3,4-dimethoxycinnamoylglucopyranosyl)] heptane (**54**), 3(*R*)-1,7-di(3,4-dihydroxyphenyl)-5-*O*-β-D-[6-(*E*-3,4,5-trimethoxycinnamoylglucopyranosyl)]heptane (**55**)> rubranoside A (**31**). Finally, among the new diarylhcptanoids, the two diarylheptanoids: 5(*S*)-1,7-di(4-hydroxyphenyl)-5-*O*-β-D-[6-(*E*-*p*-coumaroylglucopyranosyl)]heptane-3-one (**45**), and 5(*S*)-

1,7-di(3,4-dihydroxyphenyl)-5-*O*-β-D-[6-(*E*-*p*-coumaroylglucopyranosyl)] heptane-3-one (**49**) with both a carbonyl group and a *p*-coumaroyl group at C-3 showed the highest cytotoxicity.

Fourth, three diarylheptanoids (platyphylloside (**19**) (IC_{50}: 8.7±2.3 μM/HaCaT; SI: 0.3), platyphyllonol-5-*O*-β-D-xylopyranoside (**36**) (IC_{50}: 10.0±1.1 μM/HaCaT; SI: 0.7), and curcumin (**58**) (IC_{50}: 7.1±0.8 μM/HaCaT; SI: 0.2)) with high cytotoxic activity did not show selectivity for two types of cancer cells (NCI-H460, NCI-H460/R).

However, these three types of diarylheptanoids showed high cytotoxic activity against normal human HaCaT keratinocytes. On the other hand, six diarylheptanoids (alnuside B (**39**) (SI: 2.3), 5(*S*)-methylhirsutanonol (**56**) (SI: 4.8), hirsutenone (**34**) (SI: 2.3), 5(*S*)-1,7-di(4-hydroxyphenyl)-5-*O*-β-D-[6-(*E*-*p*-coumaroylglucopyranosyl)]heptane-3-one (**45**) (SI: 1.6), 5(*S*)-1,7-di(3,4-dihydroxyphenyl)-5-*O*-β-D-[6-(*E*-*p*-coumaroylglucopyranosyl)] heptane-3-one (**49**) (SI: 2.7), and 3(*R*)-1,7-di(3,4-dihydroxyphenyl)-5-*O*-β-D-[6-(*E*-3,4,5-trimethoxycinnamoy lglucopyranosyl)]heptane (**55**) (SI: 1.7)) with the high selective toxicity against two types of cancer cells (NCI-H460, NCI-H460/R) showed low cytotoxicity to HaCaT cells. And the SI values of these six diarylheptanoids showed clear selectivity.

Fifth, seven diarylheptanoids (alnuside A (**38**), 5(*S*)-methylhirsutanonol (**56**), aceroside VII (**9**), 3(*R*)-1,7-di(3,4-dihydroxyphenyl)-3-hydroxyheptane (**57**), 5(*S*)-1,7-di(4-hydroxyphenyl)-5-*O*-β-D-[6-(*E*-3,4-dimethoxycinnamoylglucopyranosyl)]heptane-3-one (**46**), 5(*S*)-1,7-di(3,4-dihydroxyphenyl)-5-*O*-β-D-[6-(*E*-*p*-coumaroylgluco-pyranosyl)]heptane-3-one (**49**), and 3(*R*)-1,7-di(3,4-dihydroxyphenyl)-5-*O*-β-D-[6-(*E*-3,4,5-trimethoxycinnamoy lglucopyranosyl)]heptane (**55**)) and the positive control curcumin (**58**) showed lower cytotoxicity against multidrug resistance (MDR) cancer cell NCI-H460/R. The cytotoxicity for other diarylheptanoides except these seven diarylheptanoids and curcumin (**58**) was independent of the presence of the MDR phenotype. Here, curcumin (**58**) is known to regulate multidrug resistance (MDR) by inhibiting P-glycoprotein (P-gp) activity [30, 31]. Thus, it was investigated whether diarylheptanoids also interact with P-glycoprotein (P-gp) overexpressed in NCI-H460/R cell membrane [31]. As a result, only two types of diarylheptanoids (alnuside A (**38**) and 5(*S*)-methylhirsutanonol (**56**)) inhibited P-glycoprotein (P-gp) function. In the P-glycoprotein (P-gp) substrates, the ability of these two diarylheptanoids to increase the accumulation of doxorubicin (**60**) (an antineoplastic agent) (Figure 10) in the NCI-H460/R cell membrane was equivalent to the curcumin (**58**) accumulation ability.

Sixth, apoptotic cell death of NCI-H460 cells by curcumin (**58**), and two diarylheptanoids (platyphylloside (**19**) and 5(*S*)-1,7-di(4-hydroxyphenyl)-5-*O*-β-D-[6-(*E*-*p*-coumaroylglucopyranosyl)]heptane-3-one (**45**)) was examined by annexin V (AV) propidium iodide (PI) staining. As a result, 5(*S*)-1,7-di(4-hydroxyphenyl)-5-*O*-β-D-[6-(*E*-*p*-coumaroyl-glucopyranosyl)]heptane-3-one (**45**) showed the highest apoptotic activity among 10 novel diarylheptanoids. Whereas platyphylloside (**19**) is a diarylheptanoid that does not have a *p*-coumaroyl group corresponding to 5(*S*)-1,7-di(4-hydroxyphenyl)-5-*O*-β-D-[6-(*E*-*p*-coumaroylglucopyranosyl)]heptane-3-one (**45**).

These results show that: After 72 hours of treatment of diarylheptanoids with NCI-H460 cells, 50 μM curcumin (**58**) induced apoptosis in almost all NCI-H460 cells. After 72 hr treatment of 50 μM platyphylloside (**19**) with NCI-H460 cells, platyphylloside (**19**) induced necrosis on 50% NCI-H460 cells.

On the other hand, after 72 hr treatment with 50 μM 5(*S*)-1,7-di(4-hydroxyphenyl)-5-*O*-β-D-[6-(*E*-*p*-coumaroylglucopyranosyl)]heptane-3-one (**45**) and NCI-H460 cells, 5(*S*)-1,7-di(4-hydroxyphenyl)-5-*O*-β-D-[6-(*E*-*p*-coumaroylglucopyranosyl)]heptane-3-one (**45**) induced apoptosis and necrosis on 50% NCI-H460 cells, respectively.

From the above results, the general structural feature of the novel diarylheptanoids was the C-6''' cinnamoyl moiety of glucose. The two new diarylheptanoids 5(*S*)-1,7-di(4-hydroxyphenyl)-5-*O*-β-D-[6-(*E*-*p*-coumaroylglucopyranosyl)]heptane-3-one (**45**) and 5(*S*)-1,7-di(3,4-dihydroxyphenyl)-5-*O*-β-D-[6-(*E*-*p*-coumaroylglucopyranosyl)]heptane-3-one (**49**) showed higher cytotoxicity (IC_{50} < 30 μM) and selectivity for non-small-cell lung cancer (NSCLC) when compared to other diarylheptanoids. The three diarylheptanoids (alnuside B (**39**), 5(*S*)-methylhirsutanonol (**56**), and hirsutenone (**34**)) also showed significant cytotoxicity and selectivity.

(10 novel diarylheptanoids: **45-49, 51**)

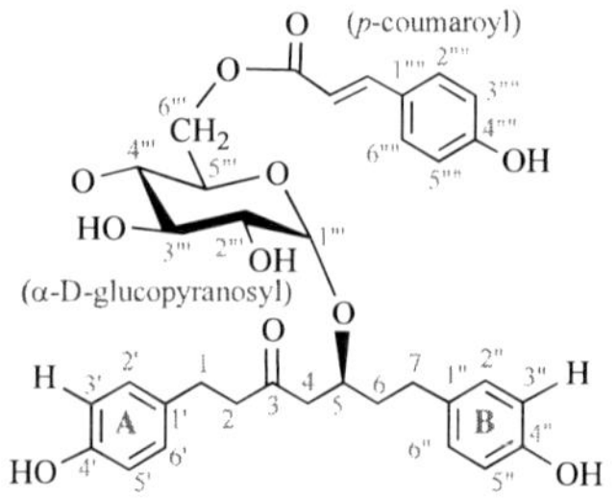

5(*S*)-1,7-di(4-hydroxyphenyl)-5-*O*-β-D-[6-(*E*-*p*-coumaroylglucopyranosyl)]heptane-3-one (**45**)

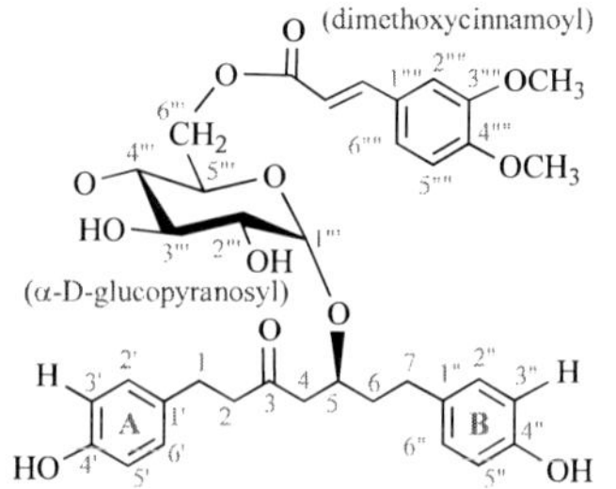

5(*S*)-1,7-di(4-hydroxyphenyl)-5-*O*-β-D-[6-(*E*-3,4-dimethoxycinnamoylglucopyranosyl)]heptane-3-one (**46**)

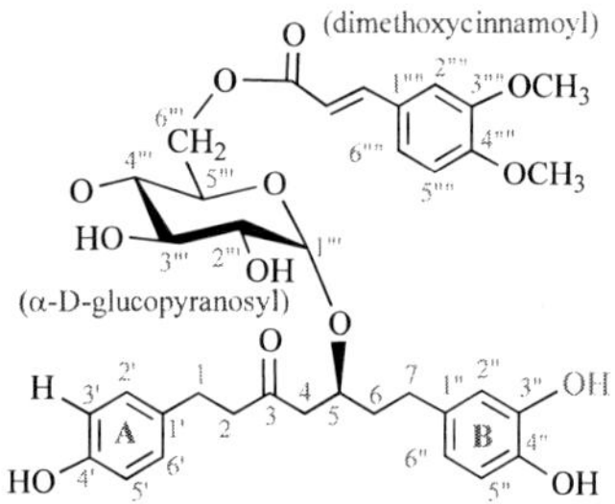

5(*S*)-1-(4-hydroxyphenyl)-7-(3,4-dihydroxyphenyl)-5-*O*-β-D-[6-(*E*-3,4-dimethoxycinnamoylglucopyranosyl)]heptane-3-one (**47**)

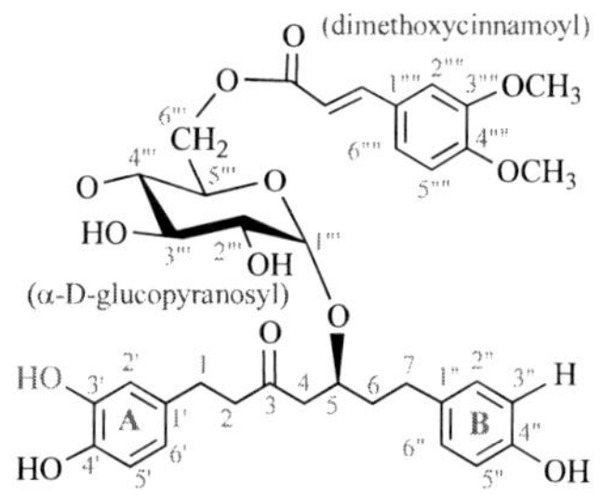

5(*S*)-1-(3,4-dihydroxyphenyl)-7-(4-hydroxyphenyl)-5-*O*-β-D-[6-(*Z*-3,4-dimethoxycinnamoylglucopyranosyl)]heptane-3-one (**48**)

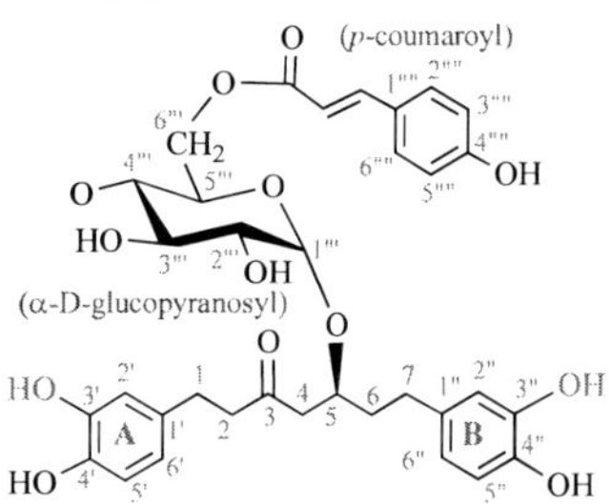

5(*S*)-1,7-di(3,4-dihydroxyphenyl)-5-*O*-β–D-[6-(*E*-p-coumaroylglucopyranosyl)]heptane-3-one (**49**)

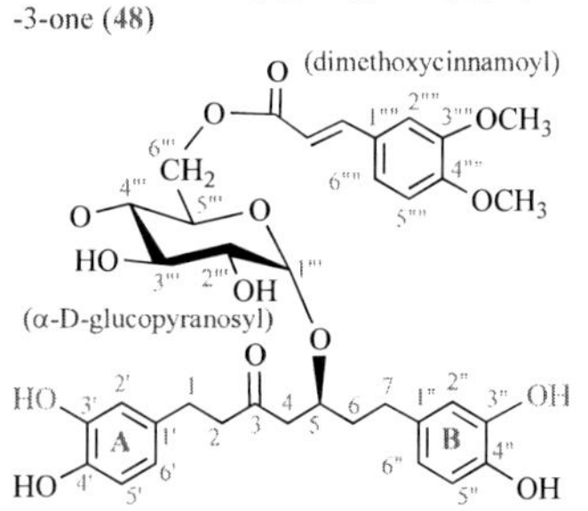

5(*S*)-1,7-di(3,4-dihydroxyphenyl)-5-*O*-β-D-[6-(*Z*-3,4-dimethoxycinnamoylglucopyranosyl)]heptane-3-one (**51**)

Figure 8. 10 Novel diarylheptanoids (**45-49, 51**) from the chloroform/methanol (1:1) extract of the bark of *Alnus glutinosa* (black alder).

(10 novel diarylheptanoids: **52-55**)

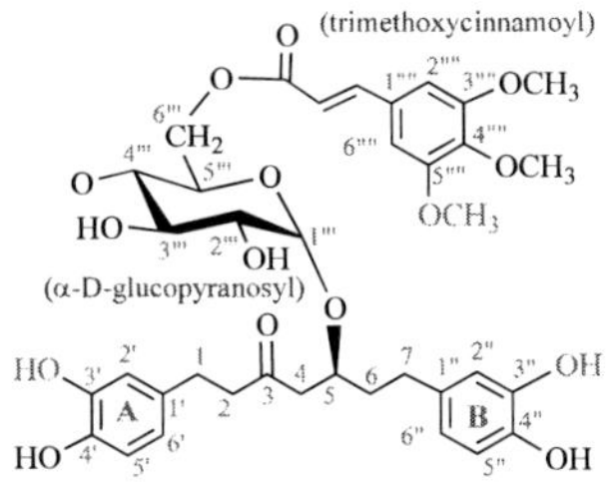

5(*S*)-1,7-di(3,4-dihydroxyphenyl)-5-*O*-β-D-[6-(*E*-3,4,5-trimethoxycinnamoylglucopyranosyl)]heptane-3-one (**52**)

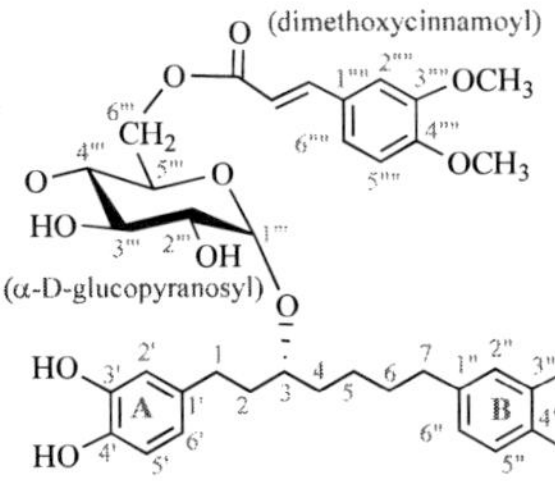

3(*R*)-1,7-di(3,4-dihydroxyphenyl)-3-*O*-β-D-[6-(*E*-3,4-dimethoxycinnamoylglucopyranosyl)]heptane (**53**)

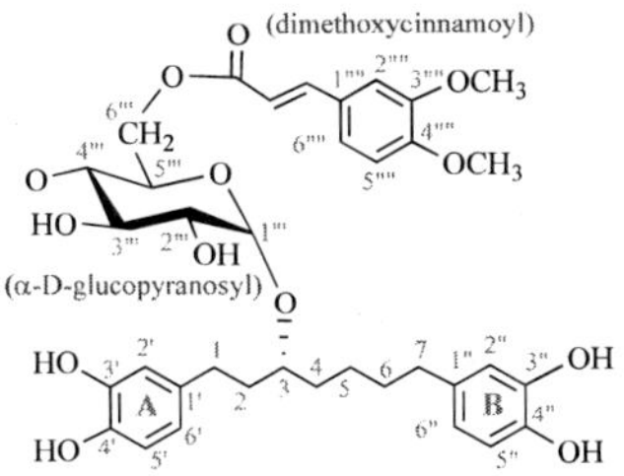

3(*R*)-1,7-di(3,4-dihydroxyphenyl)-5-*O*-β-D-[6-(*Z*-3,4-dimethoxycinnamoylglucopyranosyl)] heptane (**54**)

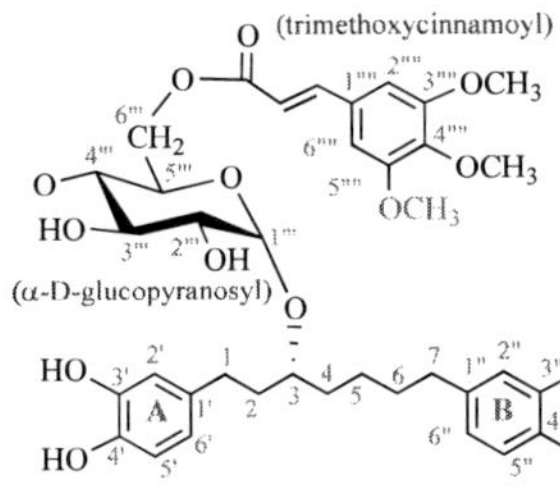

3(*R*)-1,7-di(3,4-dihydroxyphenyl)-5-*O*-β-D-[6-(*E*-3,4,5-trimethoxycinnamoy lglucopyranosyl)]heptane (**55**)

Figure 8(continued 1). 10 Novel diarylheptanoids (**52-55**) from the chloroform/methanol (1:1) extract of the bark of *Alnus glutinosa* (black alder).

5(*S*)-1,7-Di(4-hydroxyphenyl)-5-*O*-β-D-[6-(*E*-*p*-coumaroylglucopyranosyl)]heptane-3-one (**45**) efficiently induced both apoptosis and necrosis on non-small-cell lung cancer (NSCLC). The C-3 carbonyl group of diarylheptanoids had a significant positive effect on cytotoxicity. Furthermore, the coexistence of both methoxy/glucosyl/xylosyl/*p*-coumaroylglucosyl group at C-5, and the carbonyl group at C-3 of diarylheptanoid had a high positive relationship with the effectiveness of diarylheptanoids. Two kinds of diarylheptanoys (alnuside A (**38**) and 5(*S*)-methylhirsutanonol (**56**)) modulated P-gp (multidrug resistance protein 1, P-glycoprotein) activity and enhanced doxorubicin (**60**) accumulation in the cell membrane. So, two kinds of diarylheptanoys (**38** and **56**) suggest that it may overcome multidrug resistance (MDR). In addition, considering the importance of curcumin (**58**) in the development of new anticancer drugs, the two novel diarylheptanoids (5(*S*)-1,7-di(4-hydroxyphenyl)-5-*O*-

β-D-[6-(*E*-*p*-coumaroylglucopyranosyl)]heptane-3-one (**45**) and 5(*S*)-1,7-di(3,4-dihydroxyphenyl)-5-*O*-β-D-[6-(*E*-*p*-coumaroylglucopyranosyl)] heptane-3-one (**49**)) with higher cytotoxic activity and selectivity suggests to be a natural anticancer agent [32] after further chemical modification [33].

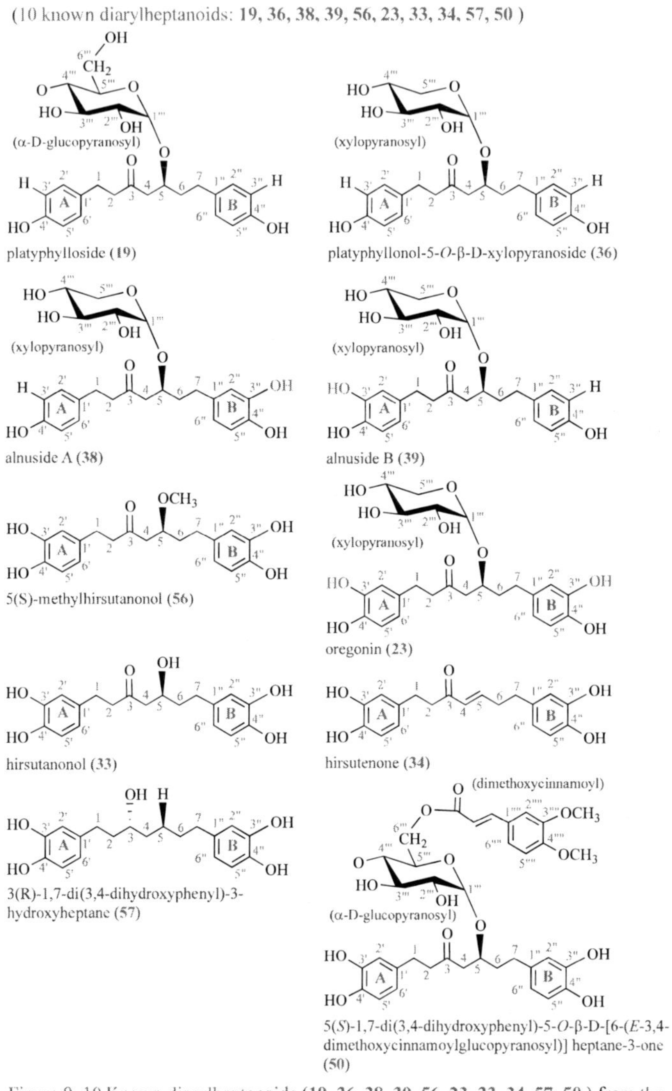

Figure 9. 10 Known diarylheptanoids (**19, 36, 38, 39, 56, 23, 33, 34, 57, 50**) from the chloroform/methanol (1:1) extract of the bark of *Alnus glutinosa* (black alder).

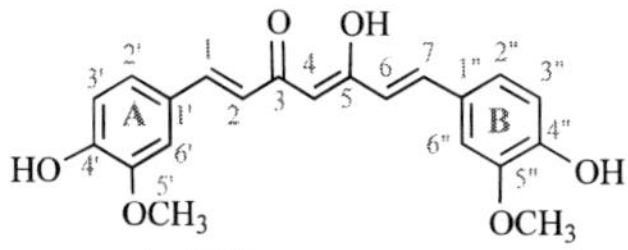

curcumin (**58**)

(four previously known diarylheptanoids: **59, 9, 31, 32**)

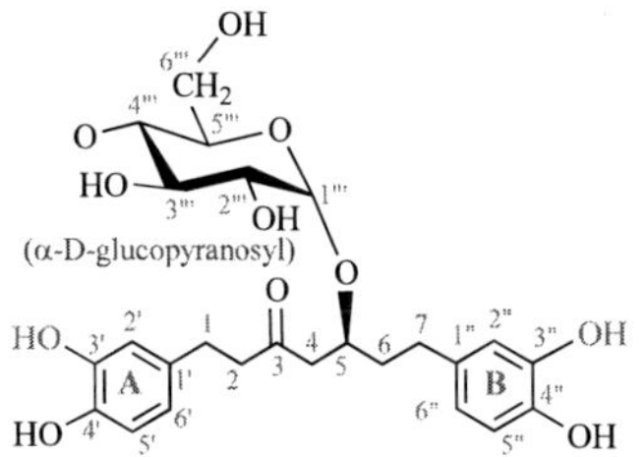

5(*S*)-hirsutanonol-5-*O*-β-D-glucopyranoside (**59**)

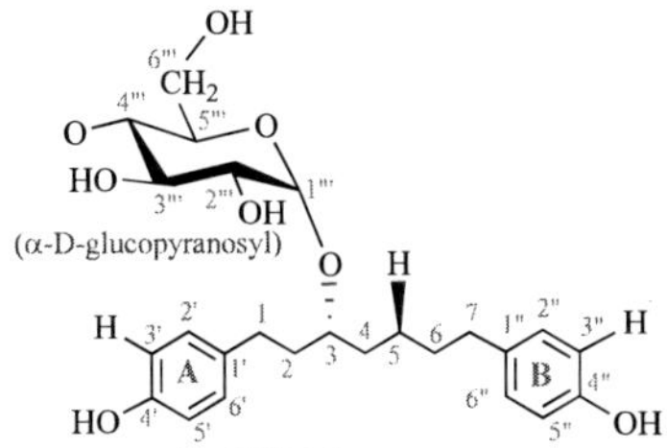

aceroside VII (**9**)

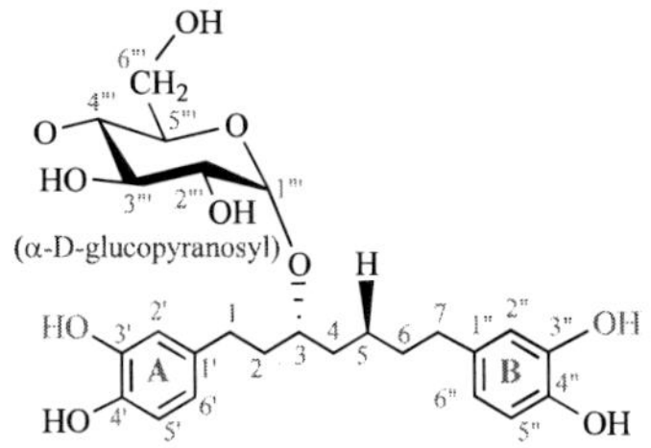

rubranoside A (**31**)

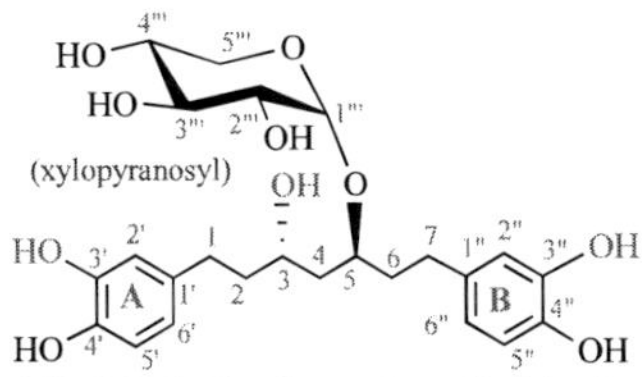

1,7-di(3,4-dihydroxyphenyl)-5-hydroxy-heptane-3-*O*-β-D-xylopyranoside (**32**)

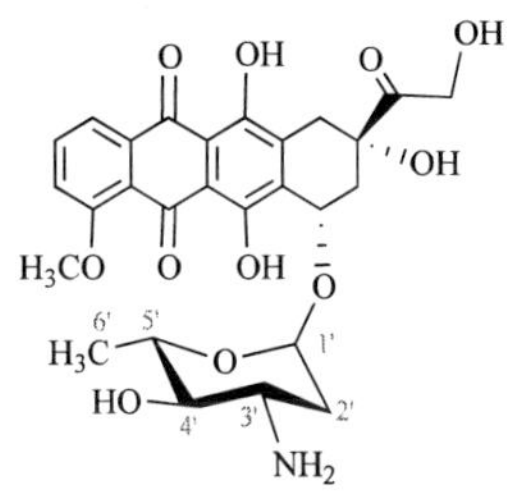

doxorubicin (**60**)

Figure 10. Curcumin (**58**) and four previously known diarylheptanoids (**59, 9, 31, 32**). An antitumor control doxorubicin (**60**).

2.2.1.1.3. *Alnus hirsuta*

2.2.1.1.3.1. *Alnus hirsuta*/1984

In 1984, Terazawa *et al.* confirmed that a dramatic reddish-orange stain on the cut surface of the xylem and inner bark of alder *Alnus hirsuta*

Turcz, and alder *Alnus japonica* Steud [Betulaceae], which begins shortly after cutting the tree, originates from interaction between catechol oxidase and platyphyllonol-5-*O*-β-D-xylopyranoside (**36**) of a new diaryl heptanoid xyloside (hirsutoside) containing two catechol nuclei by following experiments:

The results of *in vivo* experiments using reddish young sprouts of *Alnus hirsuta* Turcz and catechol oxidase inhibitors and peroxidase inhibitors showed that the enzyme responsible for the color change was catechol oxidase, not peroxidase.

Furthermore, from *in vitro* experiments using the hirsutoside and catechol oxidase in acetone powder derived from apple with or without catechol oxidase inhibitor, it was confirmed that hirsutoside is a precursor of reddish orange color change material.

However, the reason for not causing discoloration despite the birch (*Betula platyphylla* Sukatchev var. japonica Hara) contains also a diarylheptanoid such as platyphylloside (**19**) is thought to be the absence of catechol oxidase, or the presence of catechol oxidase inhibitors, or the lack of a suitable substrate supply to catechol oxidase [34, 35].

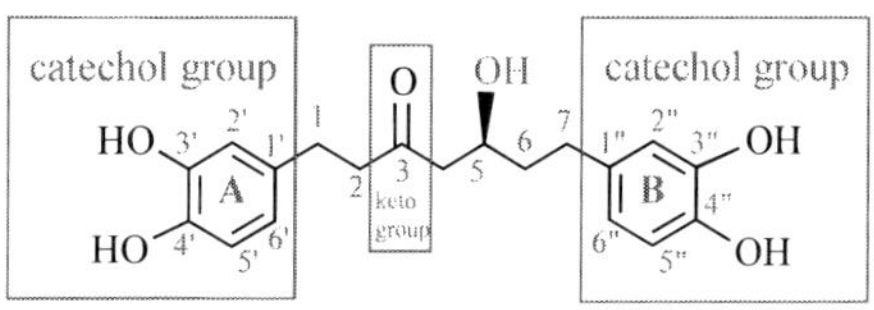

hirsutanonol (**33**)

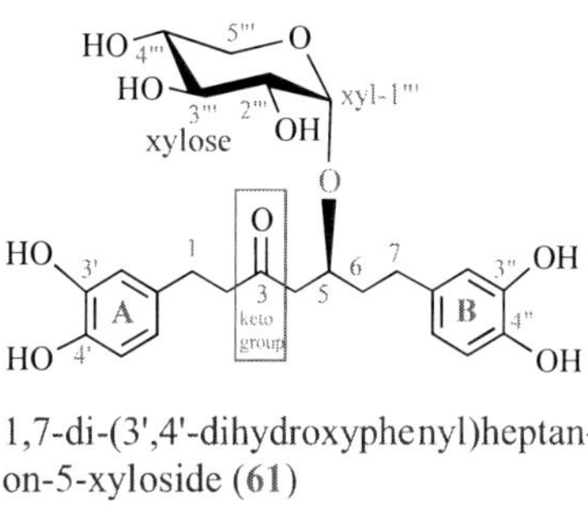

1,7-di-(3',4'-dihydroxyphenyl)heptan-3-on-5-xyloside (**61**)

Figure 11. Hirsutanonol (**33**), and a hirsutoside 1,7-di-(3 Dihydroxyphenyl)heptan-3-on-5-xyloside (**61**) from the green bark of keyamahannoki (*Alnus hirsuta*) [Betulaceae].

In 1984, Terazawa *et al.* confirmed a new diarylheptanoid 1,7-di-(3',4'-dihydroxyphenyl)heptan-3-on-5-xyloside (**61**) (Figure 11) of a glycoside hirsutoside of hirsutanonol (**33**) from the inner bark of keyamahannoki (*Alnus hirsuta* Turcz.).

On the other hand, 1,7-di-(3',4'-dihydroxyphenyl)heptan-3-on-5-xyloside (**61**) of hirsutoside was found to be the precursor for the reddish orange staining materials on the surface of the xylem and the inner bark of both woods, which formed immediately after their being cut or injured [36].

2.2.1.1.3.2. *Alnus hirsuta*/2007

In 2007, Jin *et al.* confirmed the presence of 2-oxatrycyclo [13.2.2.13,7]-eicosa-3,5,7(20),15,17,18-hexaen-10-16-diol (**62**) and 2-oxatrycyclo [13.2.2.13,7]-eicosa-3,5,7-(20),15,17,18-hexaen-10-one (**63**) (Figure 12) from the methanol extract of the stem bark of *Alnus hirsuta.*

On the effects of the hypoxia-inducible factor (HIF)-1 activation, these two diarylheptanoids (**62** and **63**) inhibited hypoxia-inducible factor (HIF)-1 activation dose-dependently with 50% inhibitory concentration (IC_{50}) values of 11.2 μM and 12.3 μM, respectively [37].

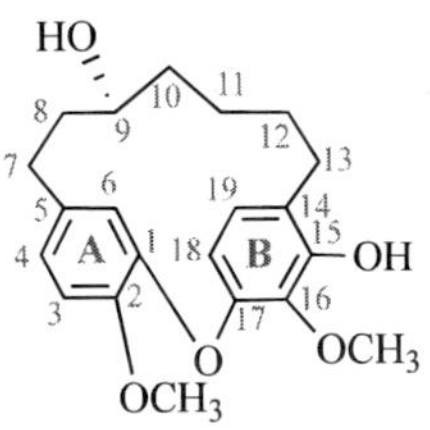

2-oxatrycyclo[13.2.2.13,7]-eicosa-3,5,7(20),15,17,18-hexaen-10-16-diol (**62**)

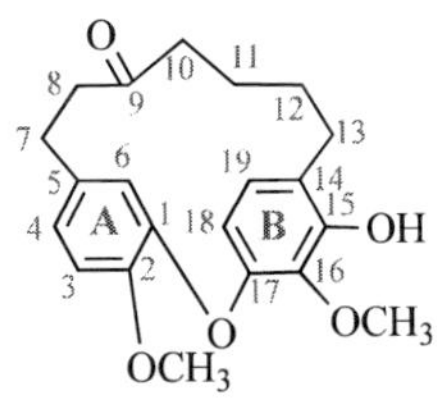

2-oxatrycyclo [13.2.2.13,7]-eicosa-3,5,7-(20),15,17,18-hexaen-10-one (**63**)

Figure 12. 2-Oxatrycyclo[13.2.2.13,7]-eicosa-3,5,7(20),15,17,18-hexaen-10-16-diol (**62**) and 2-oxatrycyclo [13.2.2.13,7]-eicosa-3,5,7-(20),15,17,18-hexaen-10-one (**63**) from the methanol extract of the stem bark of *Alnus hirsuta.*

2.2.1.1.4. *Alnus japonica*

2.2.1.1.4.1. *Alnus japonica*/1990

In 1990, Aoki *et al.* isolated and confirmed 5 diarylheptanoids of (5*S*)-1,7-*bis*(3,4-dihydroxyphenyl)-5-hydroxyheptan-3-one (**64**), (5*S*)-1,7-*bis*(3,4-dihydroxyphenyl)-5-(β-D-xylopyranosyloxy)heptan-3-one (**65**), alnusonol (**66**) [38], (5*S*)-1,7-*bis*(4-hydroxyphenyl)-5-hydroxyheptan-3-one (**67**), and (5*S*)-l-(3,4-dihydroxyphenyl)-7-(4-hydroxyphenyl)-5-hydroxyheptan-3-one (**68**) (Figure 13) from both the male and female flowers of *Alnus japonica* [39].

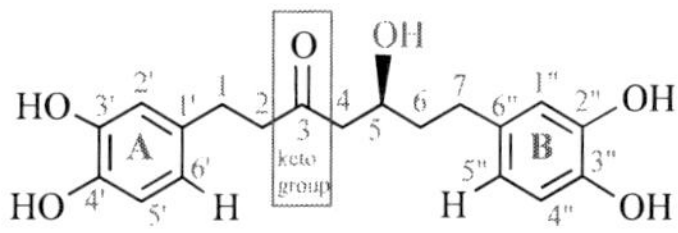

(5S*)*-1,7-*bis(*3,4-dihydroxyphenyl)-5-hydroxyheptan-3-one (**64**)

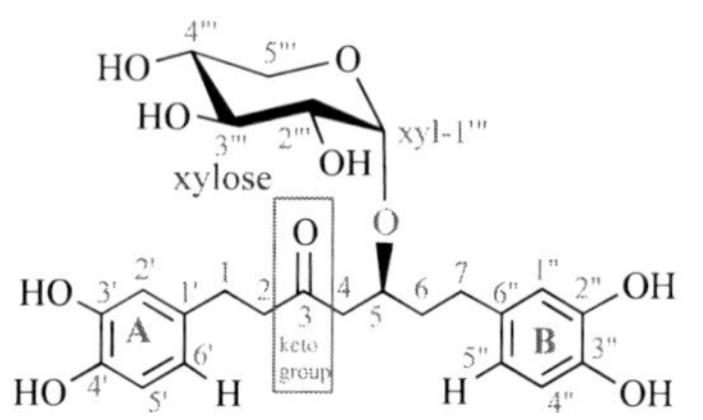

(5*S*)-1,7-*bis*(3,4-dihydroxyphenyl)-5-(β-D-xylopyranosyloxy)heptan-3-one (**65**)

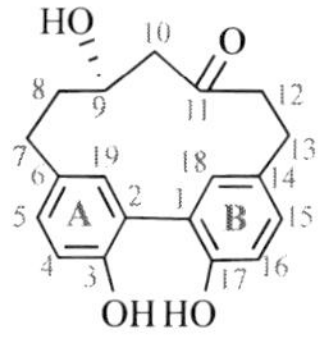

alnusonol (**66**)

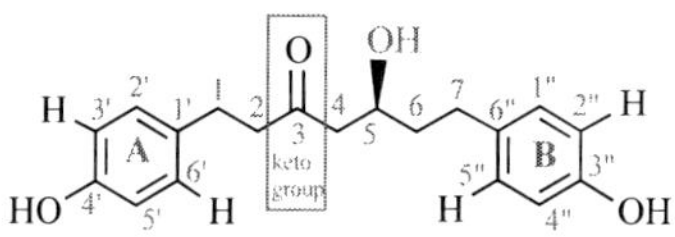

(5*S*)-1,7-*bis*(4-hydroxyphenyl)-5-hydroxyheptan-3-one (**67**)

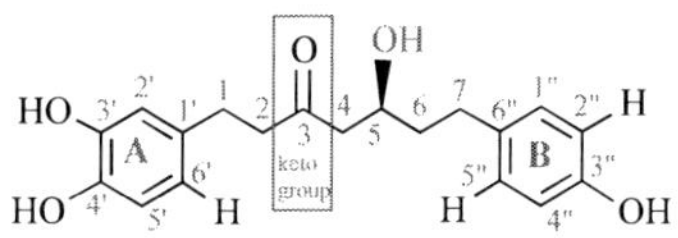

(5*S*)-l-(3,4-dihydroxyphenyl)-7-(4-hydroxyphenyl)-5-hydroxyheptan-3-one (**68**)

Figure 13. Five diarylheptanoids: (5*S*)-1,7-*bis*(3,4-dihydroxyphenyl)-5-hydroxyheptan-3-one (**64**), (5*S*)-1,7-*bis*(3,4-dihydroxyphenyl)-5-(β-D-xylopyranosyloxy)heptan-3-one (**65**), alnusonol (**66**), (5*S*)-1,7-*bis*(4-hydroxyphenyl)-5-hydroxyheptan-3-one (**67**), and (5*S*)-l-(3,4-dihydroxyphenyl)-7-(4-hydroxyphenyl)-5-hydroxyheptan-3-one (**68**) from both the male and female flowers of *Alnus japonica*.

2.2.1.1.4.2. *Alnus japonica*/2005

In 2005, Kuroyanagi M *et al.* confirmed four new diarylheptanoids - alnuside A (7-(3,4-dihydroxyphenyl)-5-hydroxy-1-(4-hydroxyphenyl)-3-heptanone-5-*O*-β-D-xylopyranoside (**38**), alnuside B (1-(3,4-dihydroxyphenyl)-5-hydroxy-7-(4-hydroxyphenyl)-3-heptanone-5-*O*-β-D-xylopyranoside. **39**), alnuside C (1,7-*bis*-(3,4-dihydroxyphenyl)-5-hydroxy-3-heptanone-5-*O*-[2-(2-methylbutenoyl)]-β-D-xylopyranoside (**69**) and 5-*O*-methylhirusutanonol (1,7-*bis*-(3,4-dihydroxyphenyl)-5-methoxy-3-heptanone. **70**) (Figure 14) - along with 7 known diarylheptanoids - oregonin (**23**), hirsutanonol-5-*O*-β-D-glucopyranoside (**35**), hirsutanonol (**33**), platyphyllonol-5-*O*-β-D-xylopyranoside (**36**), dedehydrohirsutanonol (hirsutanone. hirsutenone. **17**) [9], 5-*O*-ethylhirsutanonol (**71**) [9], and oregonin peracetate (**72**) [9] (Figure 15) - from methanol extract of the leaves of *Alnus japonica*.

The antioxidant activity of curcuminoids and their derivatives was investigated using the superoxide radical scavenging test [40] and the DPPH radical scavenging test [41].

5-*O*-Methylhirusutanonol (1,7-*bis*-(3,4-dihydroxyphenyl)-5-methoxy-3-heptanone. **70**), oregonin (**23**), hirsutanonol-5-*O*-β-D-glucopyranoside (**35**), hirsutanonol (**33**), platyphyllonol-5-*O*-β-D-xylopyranoside (**36**), dedehydrohirsutanonol (**17**), and 5-*O*-ethylhirsutanonol (**71**) with two 3,4-dihydroxyphenyl (catechol) moieties showed *strong* antioxidant activity.

Alnuside A (7-(3,4-dihydroxyphenyl)-5-hydroxy-1-(4-hydroxyphenyl)-3-heptanone-5-*O*-β-D-xylopyranoside. **38**) and alnuside B (1-(3,4-dihydroxyphenyl)-5-hydroxy-7-(4-hydroxyphenyl)-3-heptanone-5-*O*-β-D-xylopyranoside. **39**) having both one 3,4-dihydroxyphenyl (catechol) moiety and 4-hydroxyphenyl moiety showed *moderate* antioxidant activity. However, platyphyllonol-5-*O*-β-D-xylopyranoside (**36**) having two 4-hydroxyphenyl moieties, and oregonin peracetate (**72**) having a catechol ester structure did *not show* antioxidant activity. Hirsutanonol-5-*O*-β-D-glucopyranoside (**35**) showed weak antioxidant activity.

From these results, the catechol structure is suggested to be important for the *potent* antioxidant effect of diarylheptanoids (diphenylheptanoids) from *Alnus japonica* [9, 35].

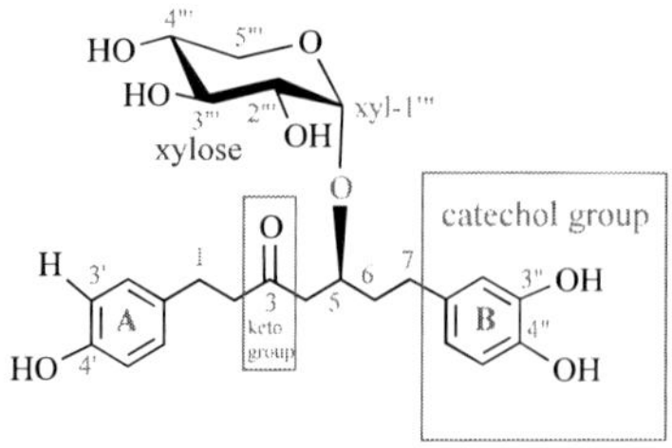

alnuside A (7-(3,4-dihydroxyphenyl)-5-hydroxy-1-(4-hydroxyphenyl)-3-heptanone-5-*O*-β-D-xylopyranoside. **38**)

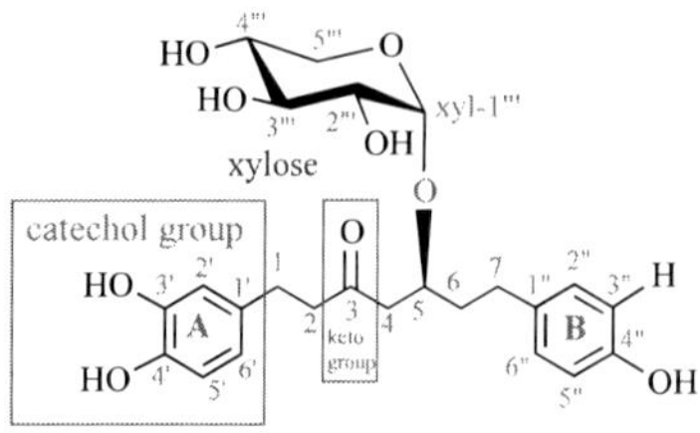

alnuside B (1-(3,4-dihydroxyphenyl)-5-hydroxy-7-(4-hydroxyphenyl)-3-heptanone-5-*O*-β-D-xylopyranoside. **39**)

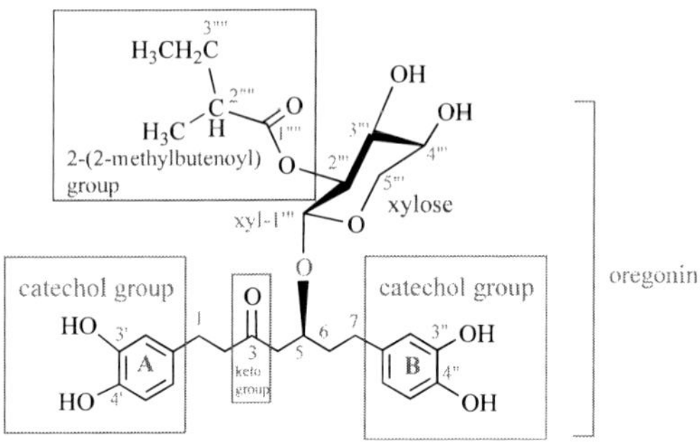

alnuside C (1,7-*bis*-(3,4-dihydroxyphenyl)-5-hydroxy-3-heptanone-5-*O*-[2-(2-methylbutenoyl)]-β-D-xylopyranoside. **69**)

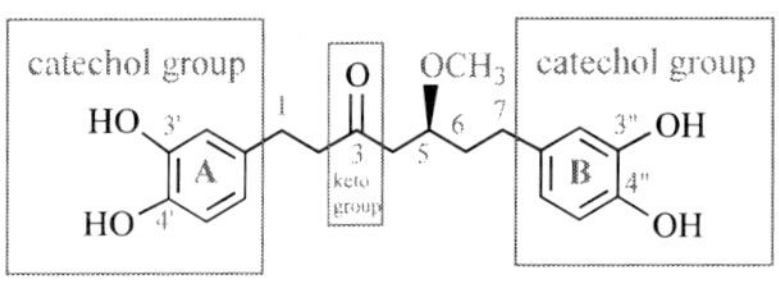

5-*O*-methylhirusutanonol (1,7-*bis*-(3,4-dihydroxyphenyl)-5-methoxy-3-heptanone. **70**)

Figure 14. Four new diarylheptanoids: alnuside A (7-(3,4-dihydroxyphenyl)-5-hydroxy-1-(4-hydroxyphenyl)-3-heptanone-5-*O*-β-D-xylopyranoside. **38**), alnuside B (1-(3,4-dihydroxyphenyl)-5-hydroxy-7-(4-hydroxyphenyl)-3-heptanone-5-*O*-β-D-xylopyranoside. **39**), alnuside C (1,7-*bis*-(3,4-dihydroxyphenyl)-5-hydroxy-3-heptanone-5-*O*-[2-(2-methylbutenoyl)]-β-D-xylopyranoside. **69**), and 5-*O*-methylhirusutanonol (1,7-*bis*-(3,4-dihydroxyphenyl)-5-methoxy-3-heptanone. **70**) from methanol extract of the leaves of *Alnus japonica*.

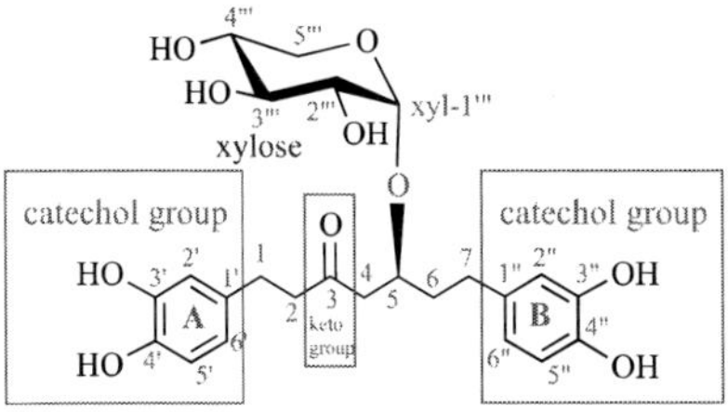

oregonin (**23**)

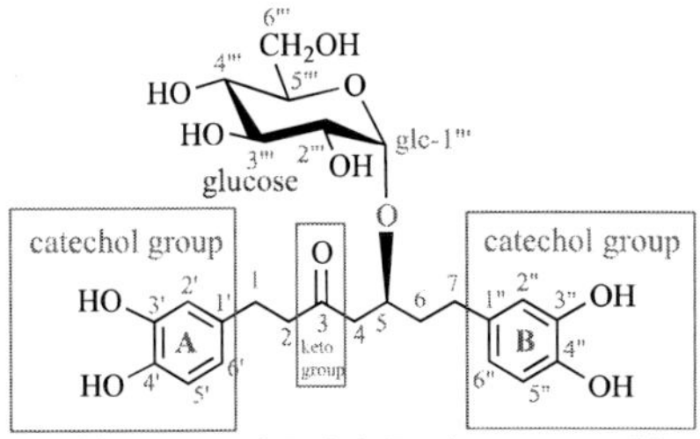

hirsutanonol-5-*O*-β-D-glucopyranoside (**35**)

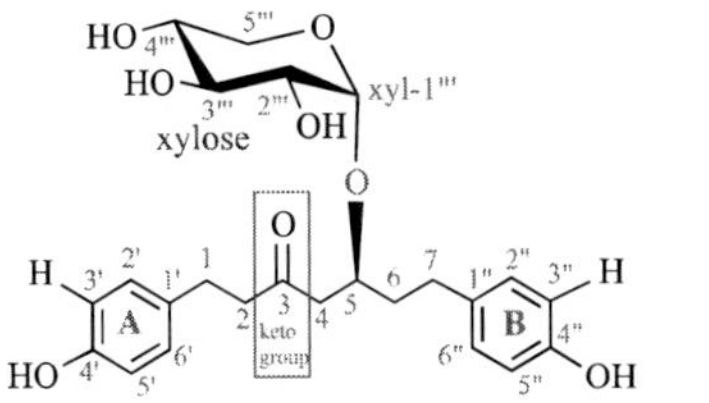

platyphyllonol-5-*O*-β-D-xylopyranoside (**36**)

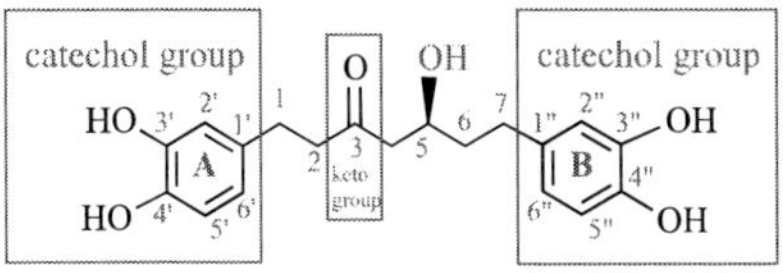

hirsutanonol (**33**)

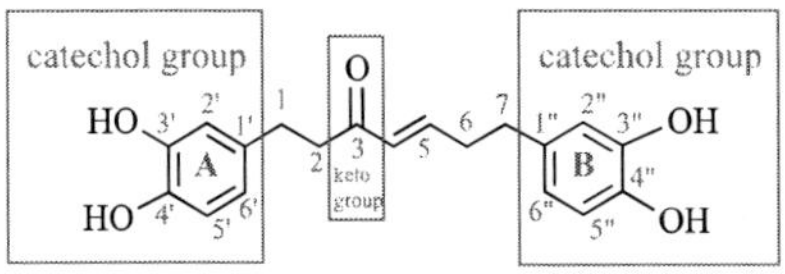

dehydrohirsutanonol (hirsutanone. hirsutenone. **17**)

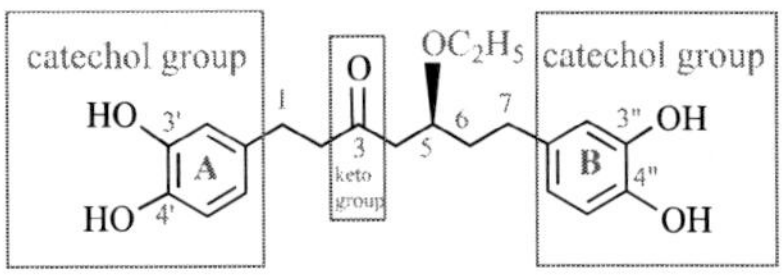

5-*O*-ethylhirsutanonol (**71**)

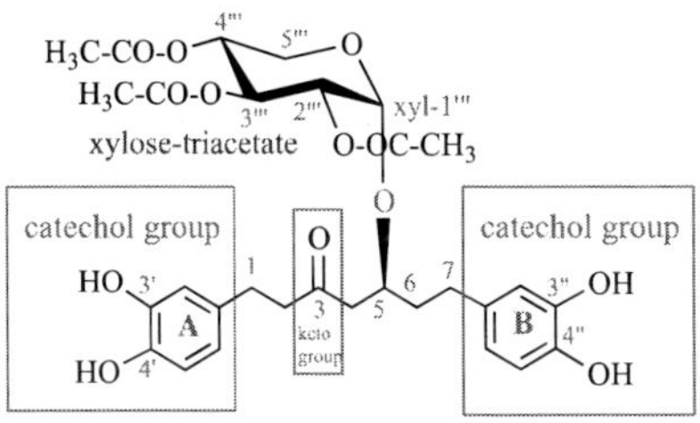

oregonin peracetate (**72**)

Figure 15. Seven known diarylheptanoids: oregonin (**23**), hirsutanonol-5-*O*-β-D-glucopyranoside (**35**), hirsutanonol (**33**), platyphyllonol-5-*O*-β-D-xylopyranoside (**36**), dedehydrohirsutanonol (**17**), 5-*O*-ethylhirsutanonol (**71**), and oregonin peracetate (**72**) from methanol extract of the leaves of *Alnus japonica*.

2.2.1.1.4.3. *Alnus japonica*/2014

In 2014, Ibrahim SR *et al.* identified a novel linear-diarylheptanoid alnuheptanoid A [(5*S*)-7-(3,4-dihydroxyphenyl)-1-(4-hydroxyphenyl)-5-methoxyheptan-3-one] (**73**), along with seven known linear-diarylheptanoids: platyphyllenone (**74**), (5*S*)-1,7-*bis*(4-hydroxyphenyl)-5-methoxyheptan-3-one (**75**), 1-(3,4-dihydroxyphenyl)-7-(4-hydroxyphenyl)-4-hepten-3-one (**76**), hirsutenone (**34**), (5*R*)-*O*-methylhirsutanonol (**77**), hirsutanonol (**33**) and oregonin (**23**) (Figure 16) from the ethanolic extract of stem bark of *Alnus japonica* Steud [42].

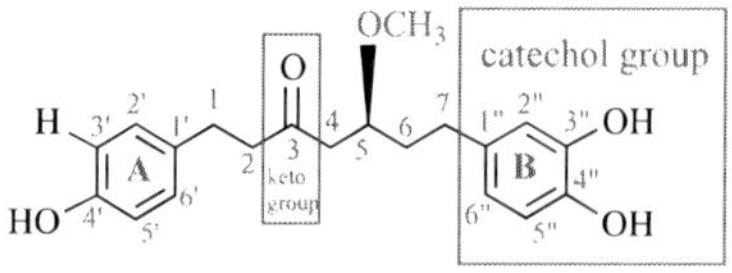

alnuheptanoid A [(5S)-7-(3,4-dihydroxyphenyl)-1-(4-hydroxyphenyl)-5-methoxyheptan-3-one] (73)

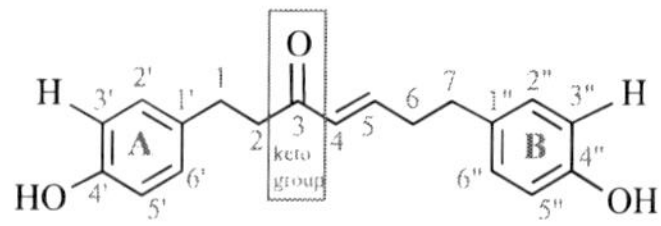

platyphyllenone (74)

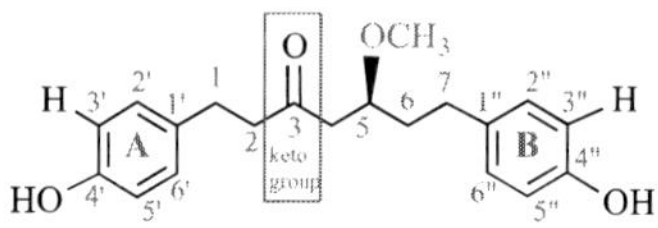

(5*S*)-1,7-*bis*(4-hydroxyphenyl)-5-methoxyheptan-3-one (75)

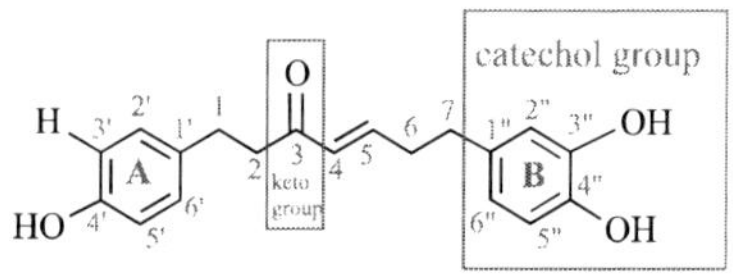

1-(3,4-dihydroxyphenyl)-7-(4-hydroxyphenyl)-4-hepten-3-one (76)

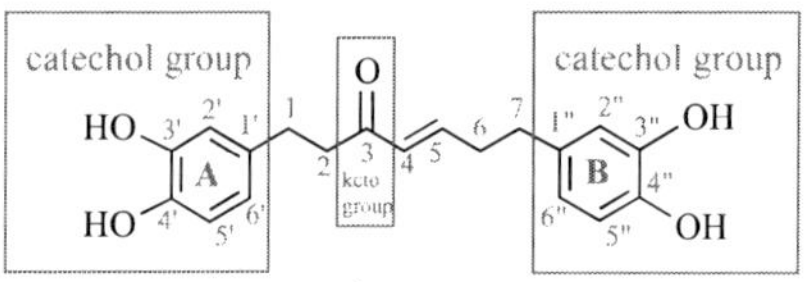

hirsutenone (34)

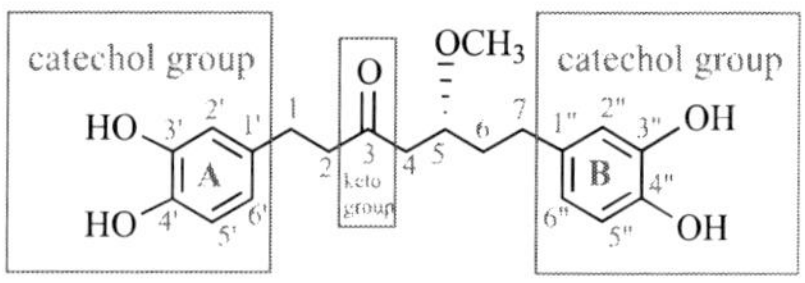

(5*R*)-*O*-methylhirsutanonol (77)

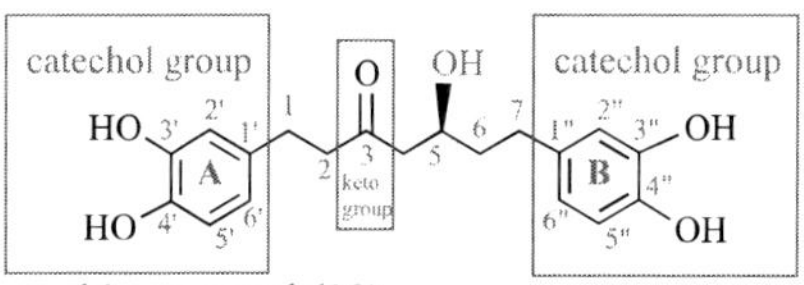

hirsutanonol (33)

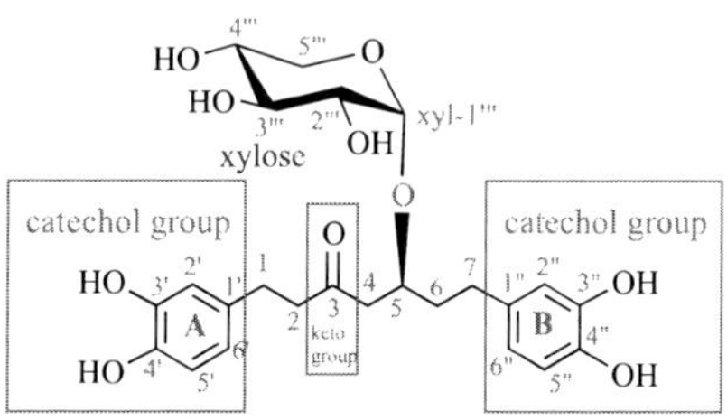

oregonin (23)

Figure 16. A novel linear-diarylheptanoid: alnuheptanoid A [(5S)-7-(3,4-dihydroxyphenyl)-1-(4-hydroxyphenyl)-5-methoxyheptan-3-one] (73), and seven known linear-diarylheptanoids: platyphyllenone (74), (5*S*)-1,7-*bis*(4-hydroxyphenyl)-5-methoxyheptan-3-one (75), 1-(3,4-dihydroxyphenyl)-7-(4-hydroxyphenyl)-4-hepten-3-one (76), hirsutenone (34), (5*R*)-*O*-methylhirsutanonol (77), hirsutanonol (33), and oregonin (23) from the ethanolic extract of stem bark of *Alnus japonica* Steud.

2.2.1.1.4.4. *Alnus japonica*/2017

In 2017, Ibrahim SRM *et al.* confimed a novel cyclic diarylheptanoid alnuheptanoid B (**78**), along with four known cyclic diarylheptanoids: myricanone (**79**), (+)-*S*-myricanol (**80**), myricanone 5-*O*-β-D-glucopyranoside (**81**), and (+)-*S*-myricanol 5-*O*-β-D-glucopyranoside (**82**) (Figure 17) from the ethyl acetate (EtOAc) fraction of the stem bark of *Alnus japonica* Steud (family: Betulaceae).

First, on DPPH radical scavenging activity (antioxidant property) using 2,2-diphenyl-1-picrylhydrazyl (DPPH) assay for each 50 □M of five cyclic diarylheptanoids (**78-82**), (+)-*S*-myricanol (**80**) showed the highest inhibition 70.14±0.55%, followed by myricanone (**79**) (63.10±0.81%), (+)-*S*-myricanol 5-*O*-β-D-glucopyranoside (**82**) (52.11±0.59%), myricanone 5-*O*-β-D-glucopyranoside (**81**) (49.09±0.76%), and alnuheptanoid B (**78**) (41.16±0.64%), respectively. A control propyl gallate (**83**) (Figure 17) displayed 97.31±0.37% inhibition.

From the above results, the antioxidant activity of five cyclic diarylheptanoids (**78-82**) was related to the number of free hydroxyl groups in each structure. In fact, myricanone (**79**), and (+)-*S*-myricanol (**80**) showed significant activity compared to the control propyl gallate (**83**) at the same concentration of 50 μM. On the other hand, blocking of the hydroxyl group by the acetyl or glucose moiety lead to a decrease in the antioxidant power like three cyclic diarylheptanoids (**78, 81, 82**) [43].

Second, on anti-inflammatory property using carrageenin-induced rat paw edema method_and adult male albino rats after 4 hr for each oral dose 10 mg/kg of five cyclic diarylheptanoids (**78-82**), anti-inflammatory properties for swollen feet of (+)-*S*-myricanol (**80**) played the highest activity: paw edema thickness (PET) 3.38±0.13 and % inhibition (% IN) 51.51, followed by myricanone (**79**) PET 3.51±0.07 and % IN 49.64, (+)-*S*-myricanol 5-*O*-β-D-glucopyranoside (**82**) PET 3.69±0.11 and % IN 47.06, myricanone 5-*O*-β-D-glucopyranoside (original **81**) PET 3.70±0.09 and % IN 46.92, and alnuheptanoid B (**78**) PET 3.74±0.11 and % IN 46.34, respectively. Control: indomethacin (**84**) (Figure 17) at 4 hr was PET 3.12±0.08 and % IN 46.34, and nontreated inflamed albino rat group was PET 6.97±0.10 and % IN 0.00, respectively.

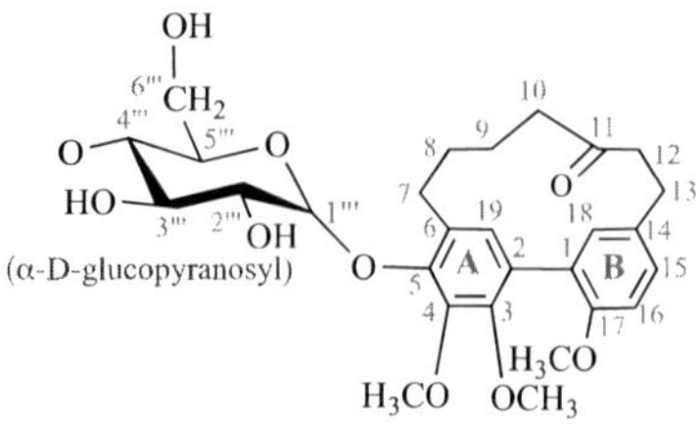

alnuheptanoid B (**78**)

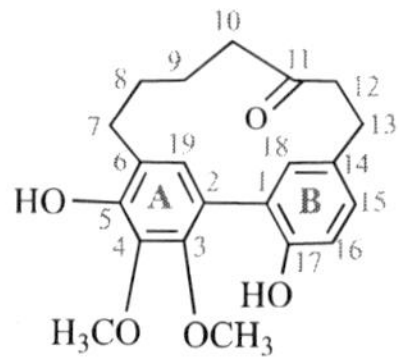

myricanone (**79**)

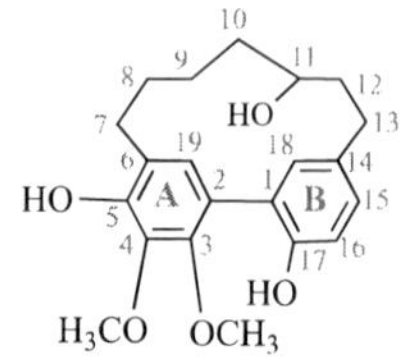

(+)-*S*-myricanol (**80**)

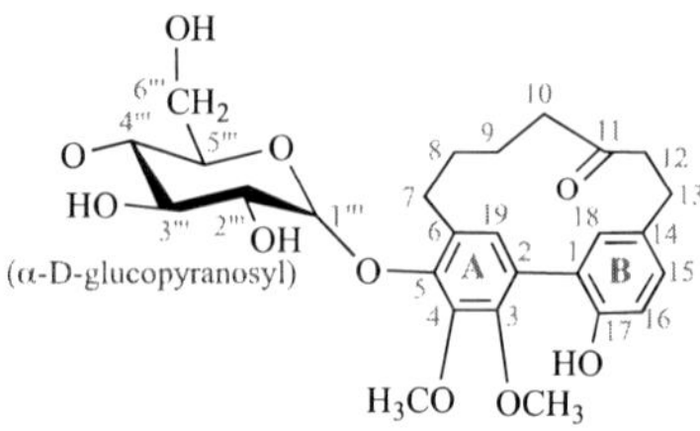

myricanone 5-*O*-β-D-glucopyranoside (**81**)

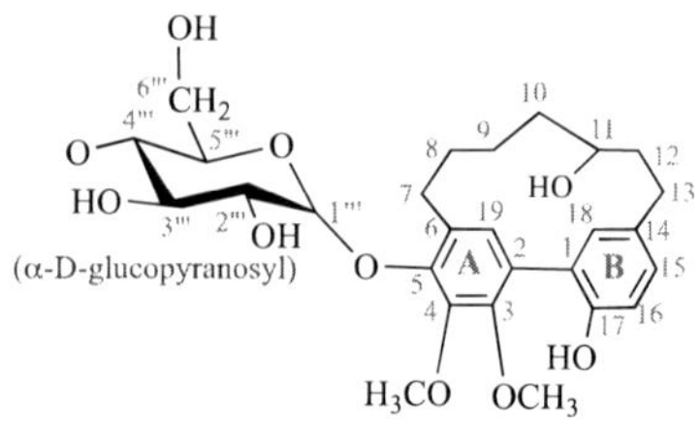

(+)-*S*-myricanol 5-*O*-β-D-glucopyranoside (**82**)

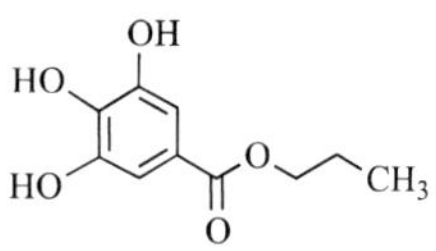

propyl gallate (**83**)

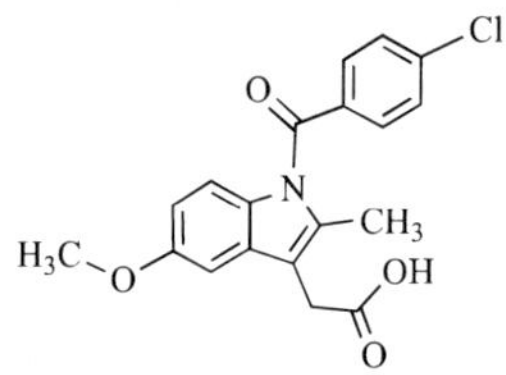

indomethacin (**84**)

Figure 17. A novel cyclic diarylheptanoid: alnuheptanoid B (**78**), and four known cyclic diarylheptanoids: myricanone (**79**), (+)-*S*-myricanol (**80**), myricanone 5-*O*-β-D-glucopyranoside (**81**), and (+)-*S*-myricanol 5-*O*-β-D-glucopyranoside (**82**) from the stem bark of *Alnus japonica* Steud (family: Betulaceae). A control propyl gallate (**83**) for DPPH radical scavenging activity. A control indomethacin (**84**) for carrageenin-induced rat paw edema method.

From the above results, (+)-*S*-myricanol (**80**) (10 mg/kg) showed the highest anti-inflammatory property comparable to indomethacin (**84**). Similarly, after 4 hr at a dose of 10 mg/kg, myricanone (**79**), alnuheptanoid B (**79**), myricanone 5-*O*-β-D-glucopyranoside (**81**), and (+)-*S*-myricanol 5-*O*-β-D-glucopyranoside (**82**) also showed strong anti-inflammatory properties. Here, phenolic compounds such as flavonol and its glycosides are known to inhibit the endoperoxide pathway by prostaglandin synthase [44]. In fact, release of prostaglandin-like substances is known to be seen in the second stage of carrageenin-induced edema [45, 46]. In addition, the anti-inflammatory properties of phenolics [47, 48] strongly suggest that the anti-inflammatory effects of five cyclic diarylheptanoids (**78-82**) may be due to inhibition of inflammatory prostanoids. Therefore, there is a clear structure-activity relationship (SAR) among five cyclic diarylheptanoids (**78-82**). In fact, phenolic hydroxyl groups have been observed to be responsible for anti-inflammatory activity, like myricanone (**79**), and (+)-*S*-myricanol (**80**) [47, 48]. Anti-inflammatory activity is obviously reduced by glucosidation of phenolic OH groups, as in three cyclic diarylheptanoids (**78, 81, 82**). Secondary alcoholic hydroxyl groups on the aliphatic chain may increase anti-inflammatory activity, like (+)-*S*-myricanol (**80**), and (+)-*S*-myricanol 5-*O*-β-D-glucopyranoside (**82**) when compared to other compounds [49].

2.2.1.1.5. *Alnus pendula*

2.2.1.1.5.1. *Alnus pendula* /1972

In 1972, Sakakibara *et al.* confirmed alnustone (1,7-diphenyl-1,3-heptadiene-5-one. **85**) (Figure 18) from the fresh catkin of *Alnus pendula* (Hime-yashabushi in Japanese) [50].

In 1972, Suga *et al.* confirmed alnustone (1,7-diphenyl-1,3-heptadiene-5-one. **85**) (Figure 18) from the flowers of *Alnus pendula* Matsum. (*A. multinervis* Call.).

Interestingly, alnustone (1,7-diphenyl-1,3-heptadiene-5-one. **85**) was found in *Alnus pendula*, but was not found in *Alnus sieboldiana*. On the other hand, yashabushiketol (**14**) (Figure 18) and dihydroyashabushiketol (**15**) (Figure 18) appeared only in *Alnus sieboldiana* [51].

2.2.1.1.5.2. *Alnus pendula* /1990

In 1990, Aoki *et al.* confirmed alnustone (1,7-diphenyl-1,3-heptadiene-5-one. **85**) (Figure 18) from both the male and female flowers of *Alnus pendula* [39].

1. alnustone (1,7-diphenyl-1,3-heptadiene-5-one. **85**) in *A. pendula*

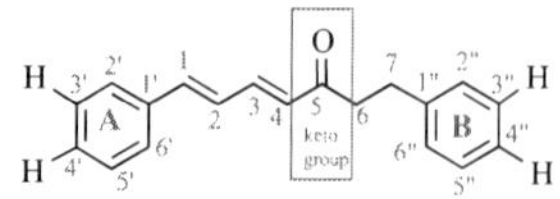

alnustone (1,7-diphenyl-1,3-heptadiene-5-one. **85**)

2. yashabushiketol (**14**) and dihydroyashabushiketol (**15**) in *only A. sieboldiana*.

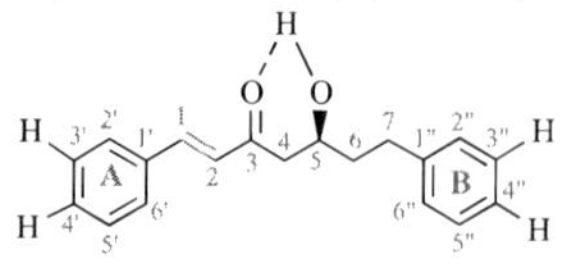

yashabushiketol (**14**)

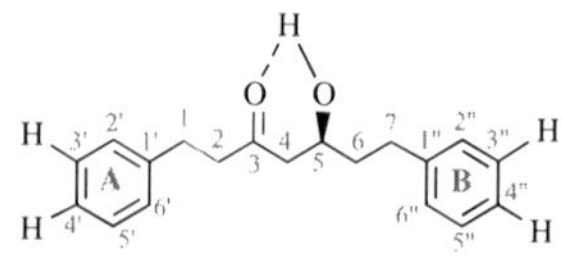

dihydroyashabushiketol (**15**)

Figure 18. Alnustone (1,7-diphenyl-1,3-heptadiene-5-one. **85**) from the fresh catkin and the flowers of *Alnus pendula*. Yashabushiketol (**14**) and dihydroyashabushiketol (**15**) found in *only Alnus sieboldiana*.

2.2.1.1.6. *Alnus rubra*

In 2000, Chen *et al.* identified platyphylloside (Compound 1. **19**) [25], 5(*S*)-hirsutanonol-5-*O*-β-D-glucopyranoside (Compound 2. **59**) [25], and platyphyllonol-5-*O*–β-D-xylopyranoside (Compound 3. **36**) (Figure 19) from the bark of *Alnus rubra* [52].

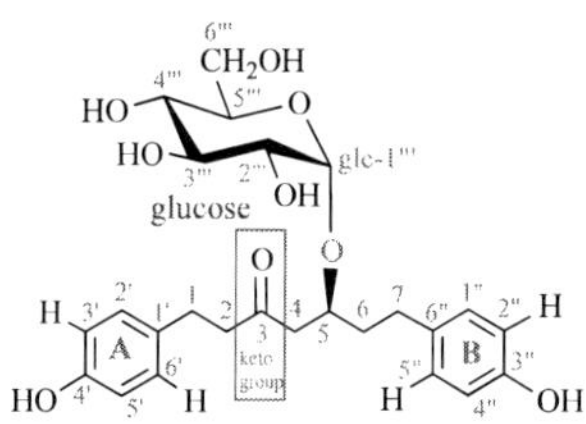

platyphylloside (Compound 1, **19**)

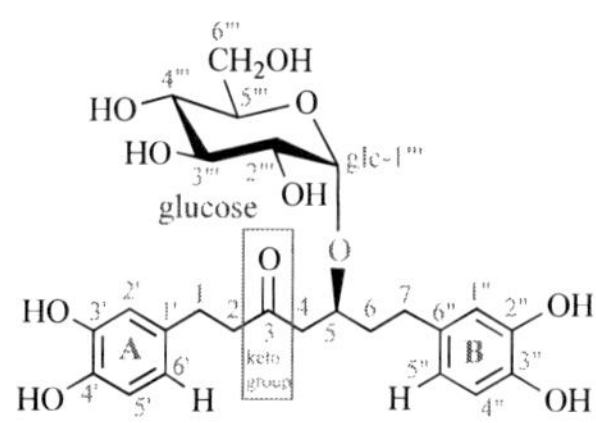

5(*S*)-hirsutanonol-5-*O*-β-D-glucopyranoside (Compound 2, **59**)

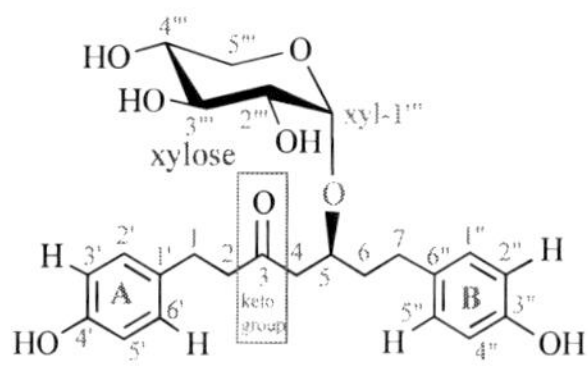

platyphyllonol-5-*O*-β-D-xylopyranoside (Compound 3, **36**)

Figure 19. platyphylloside (Compound 1, **19**), 5(*S*)-hirsutanonol-5-*O*-β-D-glucopyranoside (Compound 2, **59**), and platyphyllonol-5-*O*-β-D-xylopyranoside (Compound 3, **36**) from the bark of *Alnus rubra*.

2.2.1.1.7. *Alnus serrulatoides* (Call.)

In 1990, Aoki *et al.* isolated and confirmed 5 diarylheptanoids of (5*S*)-1,7-*bis*(3,4-dihydroxyphenyl)-5-hydroxyheptan-3-one (**86**), (5*S*)-l-(4-hydroxyphenyl)-7-(3,4-dihydroxyphenyl)-5-(β-D-xylopyranosyloxy)heptan-3-one (**87**), (5*S*)-1-(3,4-dihydroxyphenyl)-7-(4-hydroxyphenyl)-5-(β-D-xylopyranosyloxy)heptan-3-one (**88**), (5*S*)-1,7-*bis*(3,4-dihydroxyphenyl)-5-(β-D-xylopyranosyloxy)heptan-3-one (**89**) and (5*S*)-1,7-*bis*(3,4-dihydroxyphenyl)-5-(β-D-glucopyranosyloxy)heptan-3-one (**90**) (Figure 20) from both the male and female flowers of *Alms serrulatoides* [39].

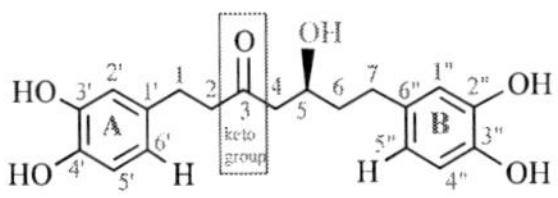

(5S)-1,7-*bis(*3,4-dihydroxyphenyl)-5-hydroxyheptan-3-one (**86**)

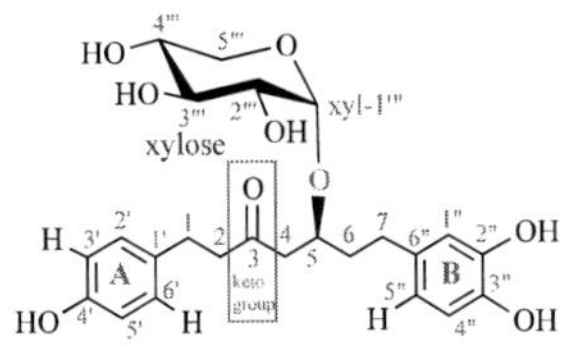

(5*S*)-l-(4-hydroxyphenyl)-7-(3,4-dihydroxyphenyl)-5-(β-D-xylopyranosyloxy)heptan-3-one (**87**)

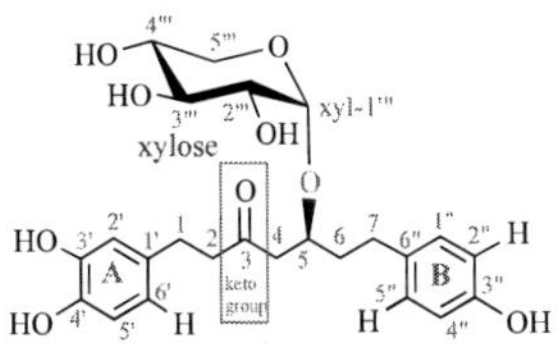

(5*S*)-1-(3,4-dihydroxyphenyl)-7-(4-hydroxyphenyl)-5-(β-D-xylopyranosyloxy)heptan-3-one (**88**)

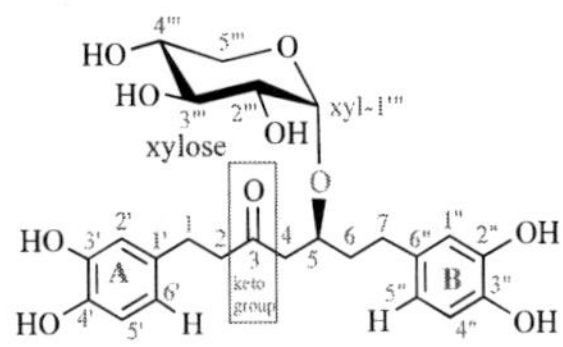

(5*S*)-1,7-*bis*(3,4-dihydroxyphenyl)-5-(β-D-xylopyranosyloxy)heptan-3-one (**89**)

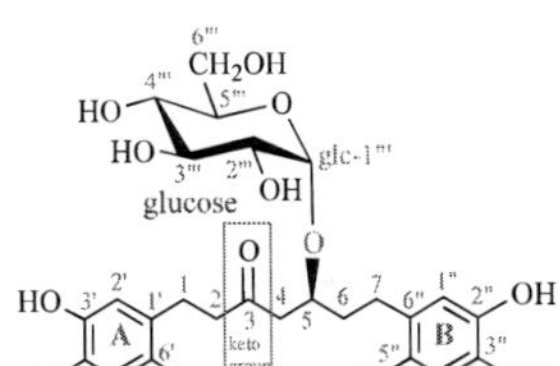

(5*S*)-1,7-*bis*(3,4-dihydroxyphenyl)-5-(β-D-glucopyranosyloxy)heptan-3-one (**90**)

Figure 20. Five diarylheptanoids of (5*S*)-1,7-*bis*(3,4-dihydroxyphenyl)-5-hydroxyheptan-3-one (**80**), (5*S*)-l-(4-hydroxyphenyl)-7-(3,4-dihydroxyphenyl)-5-(β-D-xylopyranosyloxy)heptan-3-one (**87**), (5*S*)-1-(3,4-dihydroxyphenyl)-7-(4-hydroxyphenyl)-5-(β-D-xylopyranosyloxy)heptan-3-one (**88**), (5*S*)-1,7-*bis*(3,4-dihydroxyphenyl)-5-(β-D-xylopyranosyloxy)heptan-3-one (**89**) and (5*S*)-1,7-*bis*(3,4-dihydroxyphenyl)-5-(β-D-glucopyranosyloxy)heptan-3-one (**90**) from both the male and female flowers of *Alnus serrulatoides*.

2.2.1.1.8. *Alnus sibirica* Fisch. Ex Turcz.

Alnus sibirica Fisch. ex Turcz. (AS) is geographically distributed in Korea, Japan, Northeast China and Russia, and the bark of this plant has been used as an antipyretic, expectorant, antiasthmatic and a health tea for alcoholism [53].

In 2016, a group of Laboratory of Pharmacognosy and Natural Product Derived Medicine, College of Pharmacy, Chung-Ang University, Seoul, Republic of Korea confirmed one new 2,3-digalloyl oregonin (**91**), and two known alnuside A (7-(3,4-dihydroxyphenyl)-5-hydroxy-1-(4-hydroxy-phenyl)-3-heptanone-5-*O*-β-D-xylopyranoside. **38**) and alnuside C (1,7-*bis*-(3,4-dihydroxyphenyl)-5-hydroxy-3-heptanone-5-*O*-[2-(2-methyl-butenoyl)]-β-D-xylopyranoside (**69**) [9] (Figure 21) from 80% acetone extract of leaves of *Alnus sibirica* Fisch. Ex Turcz.

Subsequently, the cytotoxicity test and results of these three diarylheptanoids (**91, 38, 69**) were as follows:

First, regarding 2,2-diphenyl-1-picrylhydrazyl (DPPH. **92**) (Figure 22) radical scavenging activity, each three diarylheptanoids (**91, 38, 69**) were dissolved in absolute ethanol and then added to DPPH solution (0.1 mM in absolute ethanol). Each of the three diarylheptanoids (**91, 38, 69**) in DPPH solution was gently mixed for 30 minutes and then the optical density was measured at 518 nm using a microplate reader. L-Ascorbic acid (**93**) (Figure 22) was used as a positive control.

Second, regarding nitroblue tetrazolium test (NBT)/superoxide anion radical scavenging activities (SOSA), each of the three diarylheptanoids (**91, 38, 69**) was dissolved in 50 mM phosphate buffer (pH 7.5) containing 0.05 mM EDTA, 0.2 mM hypoxanthine, and 0.1 mM NBT. Next, xanthine oxidase (1.2 U /μL) was added to the mixture. The optical density was measured at 612 nm using a microplate reader after gently mixing for 30 minutes. The xanthine oxidase inhibitor allopurinol (**94**) (Figure 22) was used as a positive control.

Third, the DPPH (**92**) radical scavenging activity (μM) and superoxide anion scavenging activity (μM) of the three diarylheptanoids (**91, 38, 69**) were as follows:

2,3-Digalloyl oregonin (**91**): 6.66 ± 0.08 (μM) (for DPPH. **92**) and 8.57 ± 0.36 (μM) (for superoxide); alnuside A (7-(3,4-dihydroxyphenyl)-5-hydroxy-1-(4-hydroxyphenyl)-3-heptanone-5-*O*-β-D-xylopyranoside. **38**): 33.85 ± 0.16 (μM) (DPPH. **92**) and 23.87 ± 0.28 (μM) (superoxide); alnuside C (1,7-*bis*-(3,4-dihydroxyphenyl)-5-hydroxy-3-heptanone-5-*O*-[2-(2-methylbutenoyl)]-β-D-xylopyranoside. **69**): 11.43 ± 0.06 (μM) (DPPH. **92**) and 9.04 ± 0.09 (μM) (superoxide); L-ascorbic acid (**93**): 20.50 ± 0.71 (μM) (for DPPH. **92**) and – (no effect) (μM) (superoxide); allopurinol (**94**): – (no effect) (μM) (DPPH. **92**) and 7.51 ± 0.53 (μM) (superoxide).

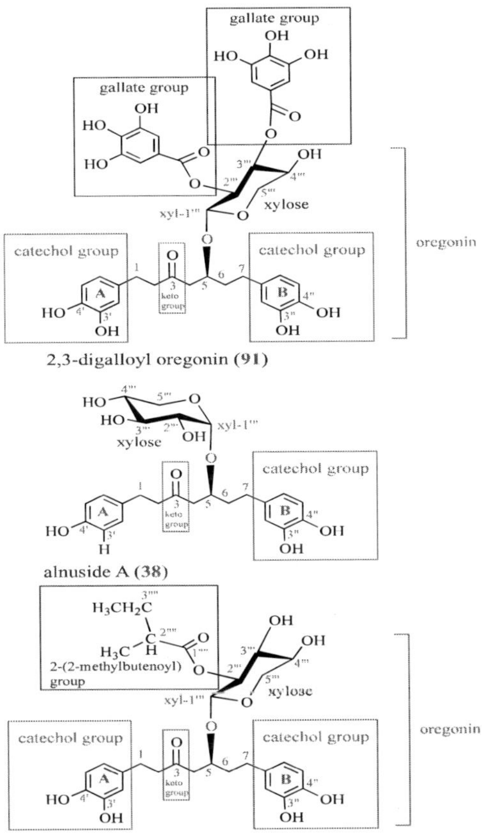

Figure 21. 2,3-Digalloyl oregonin (**91**), alnuside A (7-(3,4-dihydroxyphenyl)-5-hydroxy-1-(4-hydroxyphenyl)-3-heptanone-5-*O*-β-D-xylopyranoside. **38**), and alnuside C (1,7-*bis*-(3,4-dihydroxyphenyl)-5-hydroxy-3-heptanone-5-*O*-[2-(2-methylbutenoyl)]-β-D-xylopyranoside. **69**).

From the above results, three diarylheptanoids (**91, 38, 69**) isolated from leaves of *Alnus sibirica* Fisch. Ex Turcz. showed strong scavenging activity against (DPPH. **92**) radical and NBT / superoxide anion. A novel 2,3-digalloyl oregonin (**91**), a diarylheptanoid having a galloyl group, has stronger antioxidant activity than L-ascorbic acid (**93**), and showed almost the same efficacy when compared to allopurinol (**94**).

In particular, the antioxidant activity of 2,3-digalloyl oregonin (**91**) containing a diarylheptanoid having two galloyl moieties was more potent than the antioxidant activity of alnuside A (**38**) and alnuside C (**69**) whose structure is similar to 2,3-digalloyl oregonin (**92**).

This result suggests that the presence of polyhydroxy group in the diarylheptanoid structure is important to have a stronger antioxidant effect [54].

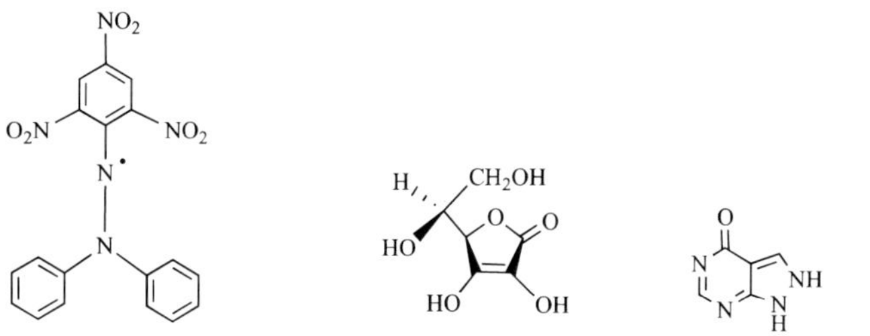

2,2-diphenyl-1-picrylhydrazyl (DPPH. 92) L-ascorbic acid (93) allopurinol (94)

Figure 22. 2,2-Diphenyl-1-picrylhydrazyl (DPPH. 92), L-ascorbic acid (93) and allopurinol (94).

2.2.1.1.9. *Alnus sieboldiana*

2.2.1.1.9.1. *Alnus sieboldiana*/1986

In 1986, Hashimoto *et al.* found five novel diarylheptanoids (**95-99**) of two 1,7-diphenylheptane-3,5-diols (yashabushidiol A (*meso*-1,7-diphenyl-heptane-3,5-diol. **95**), yashabushidiol B (1,7-diphenylheptane-(3*R*),(5*R*)-diol. **96**), yashabushiketodiol A (1,7-diphenylheptane-3-keto-(1*R*),(5*S*)-diol. **97**), yashabushiketodiol B (1,7-diphenylheptane-3-keto-(1*S*),(5*S*)-diol. **98**), and yashabushitriol (1,7-diphenylheptane-(1*R*),(3*R*),(5*S*)-triol. **99**) (Figure 23) from the male fowers of *Alnus sieboldiana* [55].

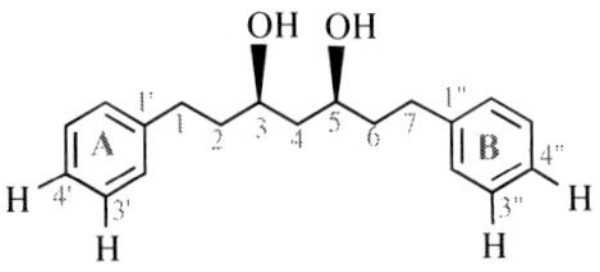

yashabushidiol A (*meso*-1,7-diphenylheptane-3,5-diol. **95**)

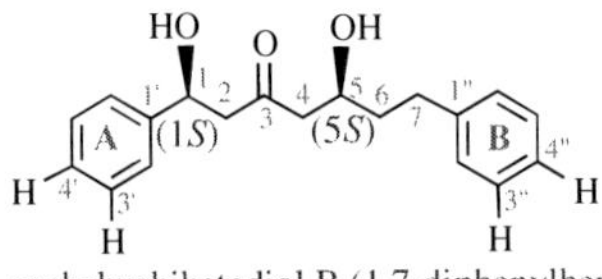

yashabushiketodiol B (1,7-diphenylheptane-3-keto-(1*S*),(5*S*)-diol. **98**)

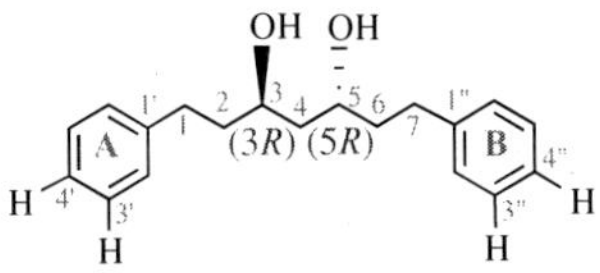

yashabushidiol B (1,7-diphenylheptane-(3*R*),(5*R*)-diol. **96**)

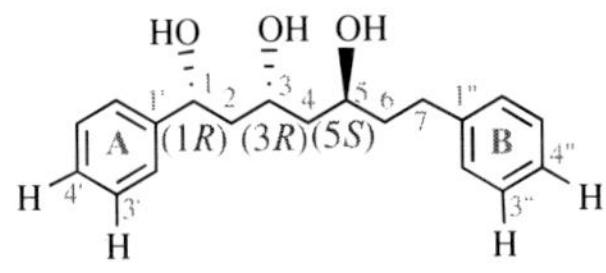

yashabushitriol (1,7-diphenylheptane-(1*R*),(3*R*),(5*S*)-triol. **99**)

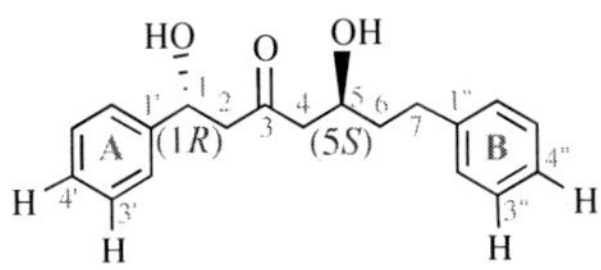

yashabushiketodiol A (1,7-diphenylheptane-3-keto-(1*R*),(5*S*)-diol. **97**)

Figure 23. Five diarylheptanoids (**95-99**) of two 1,7-diphenylheptane-3,5-diols (yashabushidiol A (*meso*-1,7-diphenylheptane-3,5-diol. **95**), yashabushidiol B (1,7-diphenylheptane-(3 *R*),(5*R*)-diol. **96**), yashabushiketodiol A (1,7-diphenylheptane-3-keto-(1 *R*),(5*S*)-diol. **97**), yashabushiketodiol B (1,7-diphenylheptane-3-keto-(1*S*),(5*S*)-diol. **98**), and yashabushitriol (1,7-diphenylheptane-(1*R*),(3*R*),(5*S*)-triol. **99**) from the male fowers of *Alnus sieboldiana*.

2.2.1.1.9.2. *Alnus sieboldiana*/1990

In 1990, Aoki *et al.* isolated and confirmed one diarylheptanoid of dihydroyashabushiketol ((5*S*)-1,7-diphenyl-5-hydroxyheptan-3-one. **15**) [56, 57] (Figure 24) from both the male and female flowers of *Alnus sieboldiana* [39].

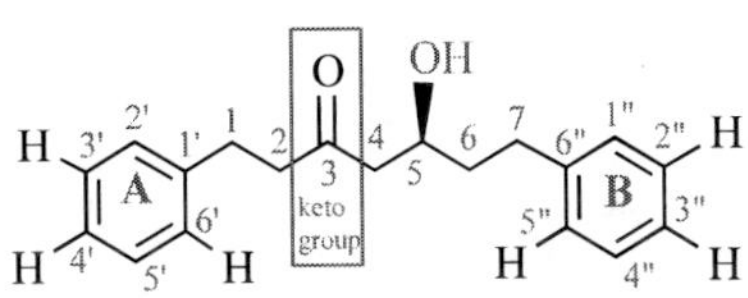

dihydroyashabushiketol ((5*S*)-1,7-diphenyl-5-hydroxyheptan-3-one. **15**)

Figure 24. One diarylheptanoid of dihydroyashabushiketol ((5*S*)-1,7-diphenyl-5-hydroxyheptan-3-one. **15**) from both the male and female flowers of *Alnus sieboldiana*.

2.2.1.1.9.3. *Alnus sieboldiana*/2013

In 2013, Chiba *et al.* confirmed a novel cyclic diarylheptanoid 3,17-dihydroxy-tricyclo[12.3.1.1^{2,6}]-nonadeca-1(18),2,4,6(19),14,16-hexaen-9,11-dione (**100**), and two known cyclic diarylheptanoids alnusone (**101**) [58, 38, 59, 60, 61, 62] and alnusonol (**102**) [58, 38, 59, 60, 61, 62, 63] (Figure 25) from the methanol extracts of the branch wood of *Alnus sieboldiana*.

(a novel cyclic diarylheptanoid)

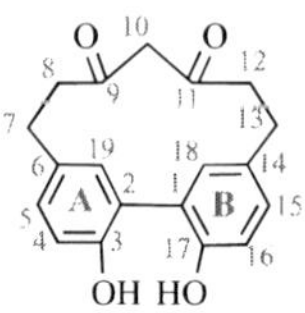

3,17-dihydroxy-tricyclo[12.3.1.1^{2,6}]-nonadeca-1(18),2,4,6(19),14,16-hexaen-9,11-dione (**100**)

(two known cyclic diarylheptanoids)

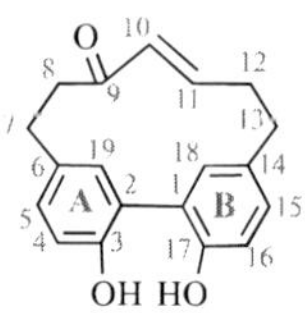

alnusone (**101**)

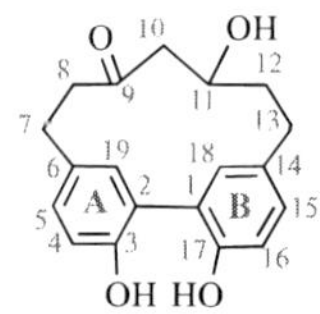

alnusonol (**102**)

(an α-glucosidase inhibitor)

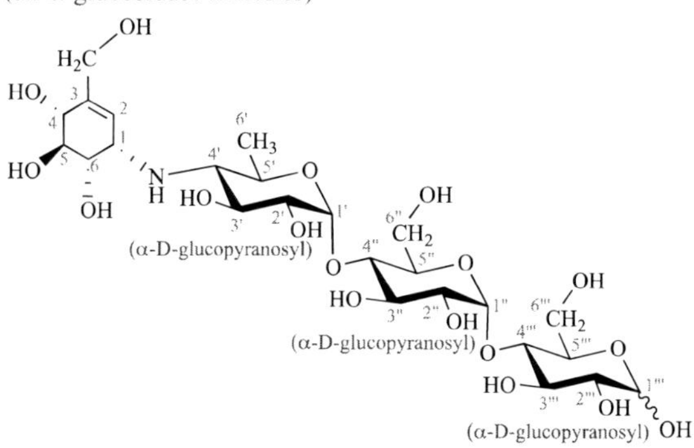

acarbose (*O*-4,6-dideoxy-4-[[(1*S*,4*R*,5*S*,6*S*)-4,5,6-trihydroxy-3-(hydroxymethyl)-2-cyclohexene-1-yl]amino]-α-D-glucopyranosyl-(1→4)-*O*-α-D-glucopyranosyl-(1→4)-D-glucopyranose. **103**)

Figure 25. Three cyclic diarylheptanoids 3,17-Dihydroxy-tricyclo[12.3.1.1^{2,6}]-nonadeca-1(18),2,4,6(19),14,16-hexaen-9,11-dione (**100**), alnusone (**101**) and alnusonol (**102**) from the methanol extracts of the branch wood of *Alnus sieboldiana*. Acarbose (*O*-4,6-dideoxy-4-[[(1*S*,4*R*,5*S*,6*S*)-4,5,6-trihydroxy-3-(hydroxymethyl)-2-cyclohexene-1-yl]amino]-α-D-glucopyranosyl-(1→4)-*O*-α-D-glucopyranosyl-(1→4)-D-glucopyranose. **103**)

The glucose tolerance was as follows: α-glucosidase inhibitory activity of three cyclic diarylheptanoids 3,17-dihydroxy-tricyclo[12.3.1.$1^{2,6}$]-nonadeca-1(18),2,4,6(19),14,16-hexaen-9,11-dione (**100**), alnusone (**101**) and alnusonol (**102**) was examined by the comparison to that (α-glucosidase inhibitory activity) of the α-glucosidase inhibitor acarbose (*O*-4,6-dideoxy-4-[[(1*S*,4*R*,5*S*,6*S*)-4,5,6-trihydroxy-3-(hydroxymethyl)-2-cyclohexene-1-yl]amino]-α-D-glucopyranosyl-(1→4)-*O*-α-D-glucopyranosyl-(1→4)-D-glucopyranose. **103**) (Figure 25) used as a positive control.

As a result, the 50% inhibitory concentration (IC_{50}) value (μg/mL) of three cyclic diarylheptanoids (**100**, **101**, **102**), and acarbose (**103**) for α-glucosidase was 1.35 (relative activity: 334)、8.69 (relative activity: 60), 2.34 (relative activity: 193), and 451 (relative activity: 1), respectively. Here, the IC_{50}) value (μg/mL) of acarbose (**103**), one α-glucosidase inhibitor used as a positive control, was 451.

From the above results, three types of cyclic diarylheptanoids 3,17-dihydroxy-tricyclo[12.3.1.$1^{2,6}$]-nonadeca-1(18),2,4,6(19),14,16-hexaen-9,11-dione (**100**), alnusone (**101**), and alnusonol (**102**) are suggested to be developed as a new type of antidiabetic drug after modification by drug design [64].

2.2.1.2. Betula

2.2.1.2.1. *Betula platyphylla* Sukatchev var. japonica Hara (Shirakamba in Japanese)

In 1984, Terazawa *et al.* isolated a new diarylheptanoid glucoside, platyphylloside (1,7-(4'-hydroxyphenyl)heptan-3-on-5-β-D-glucoside. **19**) (Figure 26) from the green inner-bark of *Betula platyphylla* Sukatchev var. japonica Hara (shirakamba in Japanese) [65].

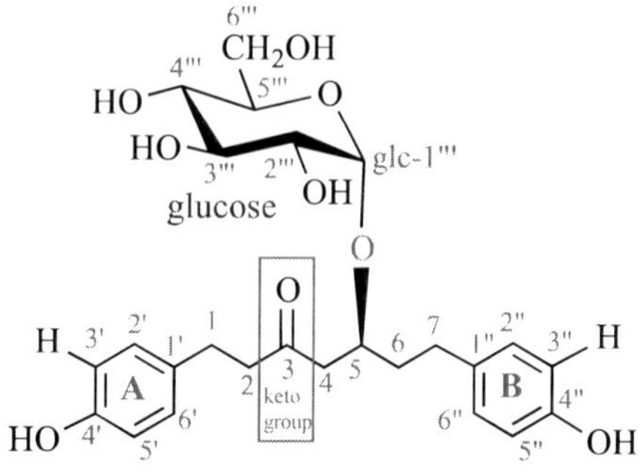

platyphylloside (1,7-(4'-hydroxyphenyl)heptan-3-on-5-β-D-glucoside. **19**)

Figure 26. Platyphylloside (1,7-(4'-hydroxyphenyl)heptan-3-on-5-β-D-glucoside. **19**) from the green inner-bark of *Betula platyphylla* Sukatchev var. japonica Hara (shirakamba in Japanese).

2.2.1.2.2. *Betula papyrifera*

In 2007, Mshvildadze V *et al.* isolated four diarylheptanoid glycosides: a novel papyriferoside A ((*S*)-1,7-*bis*-(4-hydroxyphenyl)-heptan-3-one-5-*O*-α-L-arabinofuranosyl-(1→6)-β-D-glucopyranoside. **104**), 5-*O*-β-D-apiofuranosyl-(1→2)-β-D-glucopyranosyl-1,7-*bis*-(4-hydroxyphenyl)-heptan-3-one (**105**) [12], aceroside VII (**37**) [66], platyphylloside (1,7-(4'-hydroxyphenyl)heptan-3-on-5-β-D-glucoside (original **19**) [12] and one diarylheptanoid: 1,7-*bis*-(4-hydroxyphenyl)-4-hepten-3-one (**106**) [67] (Figure 27) from MeOH extract of the inner bark of *Betula papyrifera*.

On *in vitro* cytotoxicity using the resazurin reduction test for five diarylheptanoids (**104, 105, 37, 19, 106**), first, 50% inhibitory concentration (IC_{50}) (μM) of platyphylloside (1,7-(4'-hydroxyphenyl)heptan-3-on-5-β-D-glucoside. **19**) against human lung cancer (A-549) was the highest 13.8±0.5, followed by 22±1 (1,7-*bis*-(4-hydroxyphenyl)-4-hepten-3-one (**106**)), 30±2 (papyriferoside A ((*S*)-1,7-*bis*-(4-hydroxyphenyl)-heptan-3-one-5-*O*-α-L-arabinofuranosyl-(1→6)-β-D-glucopyranoside. **104**)), 52±4 (5-*O*-β-D-apiofuranosyl-(1→2)-β-D-glucopyranosyl-1,7-*bis*-(4-hydroxyphenyl)-heptan-3-one (**105**)), and >100 (aceroside VII (**37**)), respectively. Two positive controls were 1.0±0.3

against etoposide (**107**) and 24±10 against 5-fluorouracil (**108**) (Figure 27), respectively.

Second, 50% inhibitory concentration (IC_{50}) (μM) of platyphylloside (1,7-(4'-hydroxyphenyl)heptan-3-on-5-β-D-glucoside. **19**) against human colorectal cancer (DLD-1) was the highest 12.6±0.3, followed by 20.8±0.8 (**104**), 21.2±0.9 (**106**), 30±1 (**105**), and >100 (**37**), respectively. Two positive controls were 4±1 against etoposide (**107**) and 23±6 against 5-fluorouracil (**108**) (Figure 27), respectively.

Third, 50% inhibitory concentration (IC_{50}) (μM) of platyphylloside (**19**) against human normal skin fibroblasts (WS1) was the highest 10.3±0.3, followed by 17±2 (**105**), 20±1 (**106**), 20.6±0.7 (**104**), and >100 (**37**), respectively. Two positive controls were not detected (n.d.) against etoposide (**107**) and n.d. against 5-fluorouracil (**108**) (Figure 27), respectively.

Based on the above results, the diarylheptanoid glycoside platyphylloside (**19**) has the strongest cytotoxic activity (IC_{50}) (μM): 10.3 to 13.8) with respect to the antitumor effect of five diarylheptanoids (**104, 105, 37, 19, 106**) against three types of cancer cell lines. In particular, the antitumor activity against human colorectal cancer (DLD-1) cell line was stronger than that of 5-fluorouracil (**108**).

Furthermore, one diarylheptanoid 1,7-*bis*-(4-hydroxyphenyl)-4-hepten-3-one (**106**) cytotoxic activity (IC_{50}) (μM): 20 - 22), and two kinds of diarylheptanoid glycosides: papyriferoside A ((*S*)-1,7-*bis*-(4-hydroxyphenyl)-heptan-3-one-5-*O*-α-L-arabinofuranosyl-(1→6)-β-D-glucopyranoside. **104**) cytotoxic activity (IC_{50}) (μM): 20 - 30) and 5-*O*-β-D-apiofuranosyl-(1→2)-β-D-glucopyranosyl-1,7-*bis*-(4-hydroxyphenyl)-heptan-3-one (**105**) cytotoxic activity (IC_{50}) (μM): 17 - 52) showed moderate cytotoxicity. On the other hand, the cytotoxic activity (IC_{50}) (μM) of aceroside VII (**37**) was inactive (IC_{50}) (μM): >100) against all three cancer cell lines.

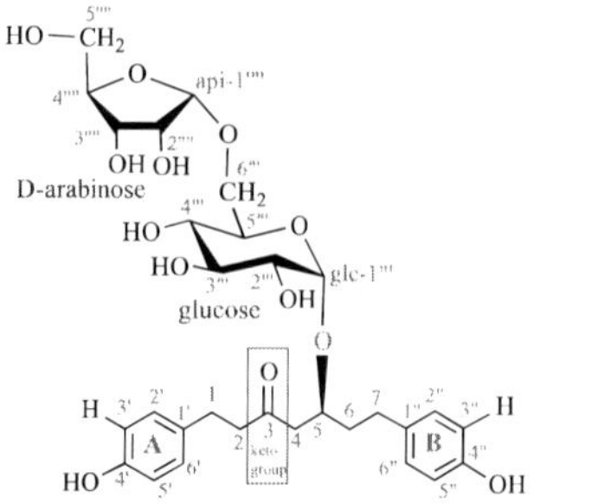

(*S*)-1,7-*bis*-(4-hydroxyphenyl)-heptan-3-one-5-*O*-α-L-arabinofuranosyl-(1→6)-β-D-glucopyranoside (papyriferoside A. **104**)

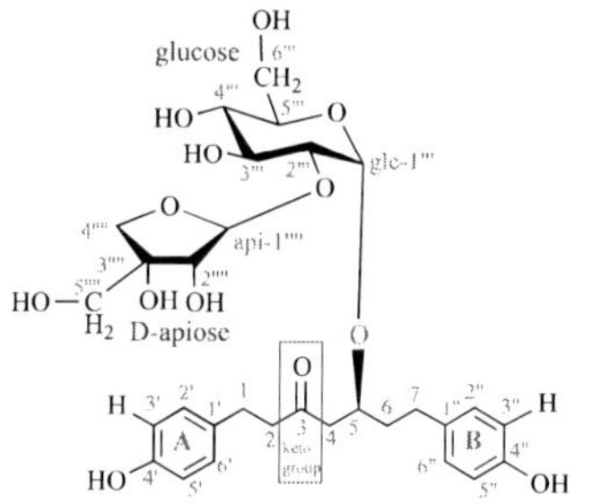

5-*O*-β-D-apiofuranosyl-(1→2)-β-D-glucopyranosyl-1,7-*bis*-(4-hydroxyphenyl)-heptan-3-one (**105**)

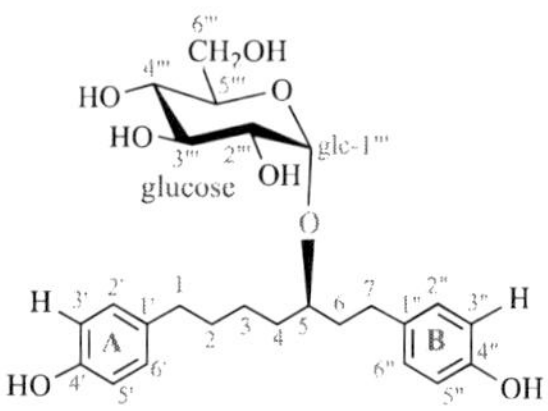

aceroside VII (**37**)

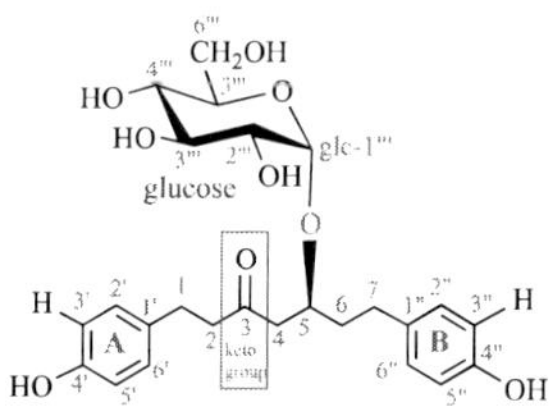

platyphylloside (1,7-(4'-hydroxyphenyl)heptan-3-on-5-β-D-glucoside. **19**)

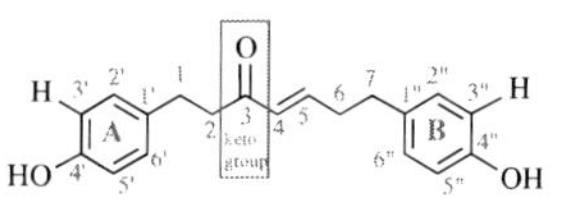

1,7-*bis*-(4-hydroxyphenyl)-4-hepten-3-one (**106**)

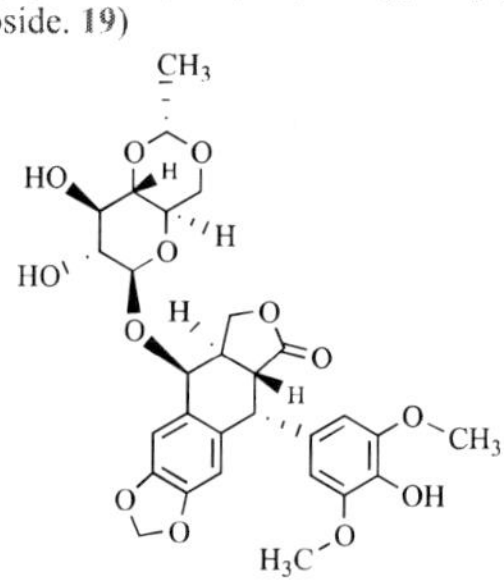

etoposide (**107**)

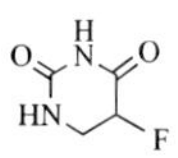

5-fluorouracil (**108**)

Figure 27. Four diarylheptanoid glycosides: a novel (*S*)-1,7-*bis*-(4-hydroxyphenyl)-heptan-3-one-5-*O*-α-L-arabinofuranosyl-(1→6)-β-D-glucopyranoside (papyriferoside A. **104**), 5-*O*-β-D-apiofuranosyl-(1→2)-β-D-glucopyranosyl-1,7-*bis*-(4-hydroxyphenyl)-heptan-3-one (**105**), aceroside VII (**37**), platyphylloside (1,7-(4'-hydroxyphenyl)heptan-3-on-5-β-D-glucoside. **19**), and one diarylheptanoid: 1,7-*bis*-(4-hydroxyphenyl)-4-hepten-3-one (**106**) from MeOH extract of the inner bark of *Betula papyrifera*. Two antineoplastic drug controls were etoposide (**107**) and 5-fluorouracil (**108**), respectively.

These *in vitro* cytotoxicity results suggest that the presence of a ketone at the C-3 position is important for the cytotoxic activity of diarylheptanoids, from a viewpoint of structure-activity relationship (SAR). Furthermore, the β-D-glucopyranose moiety at the C-5 position of a diarylheptanoid glycoside platyphylloside (**19**) appears to have a more beneficial effect on cytotoxic activity when compared to that(β-D-glucopyranose moiety) of two types of diarylheptanoid glycosides: papyriferoside A (**104**) and 5-*O*-β-D-apiofuranosyl-(1→2)-β-D-glucopyranosyl-1,7-*bis*-(4-hydroxyphenyl)-heptan-3-one (**105**).

However, four types of cytotoxic diarylheptanoids (**104**, **105**, **19**, **106**) inhibit the growth of normal and healthy cells and therefore it is important to note that it is not selective for three cancer cell lines [28].

2.2.1.3. Carpinus

2.2.1.3.1. *Carpinus cordata* Blume

2.2.1.3.1.1. *Carpinus cordata* Blume/1988

In 1988, Sawa *et al.* confirmed 11-oxo-3,8,9,17-tetrahydroxy-[7,0]-metacyclophane (Compound I. **109**) (a new diarylheptanoids having the *m, m'- bridged cyclic structure* including the isopropylidene group as a partial structure at the side chain), alnusone (Compound II. **101**), and alnusonol (Compound III. **102**) (Figure 28) from the extractives of sawashiba (*Carpinus cordata* Bl.) wood [61].

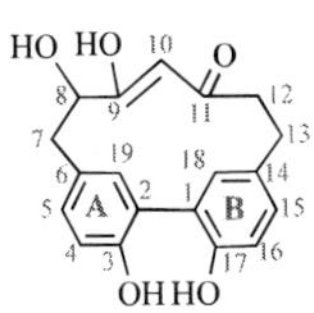

11-oxo-3,8,9,17-tetrahydroxy-[7,0]-metacyclophane (Compound I. **109**)

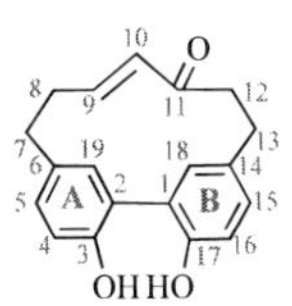

alnusone (Compound II. **101**)

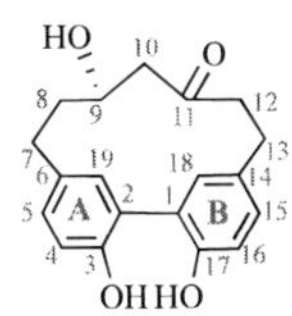

alnusonol (Compound III. **102**)

Figure 28. Three diarylheptanoids with *m, m'-bridged cyclic structures*: 11-oxo-3,8,9,17-tetrahydroxy-[7,0]-metacyclophane (Compound I. **109**), alnusone (Compound II. **#II**), and alnusonol (Compound III.
from the extractives of the wood of sawashiba (*Carpinus cordata* Bl.).

2.2.1.3.1.2. *Carpinus cordata* Blume/1989

In 1989, Sasaya *et al.* confirmed 11-oxo-3,9,12,17-tetrahydroxy-[7,0]-metacyclophane (**I10**) and 11-oxo-3,7,12,13,17-pentahydroxy-[7,0]-

metacyclophane (**111**) (Figure 29) from the extractives of sawashiba, *Carpinus cordata* Bl. [68].

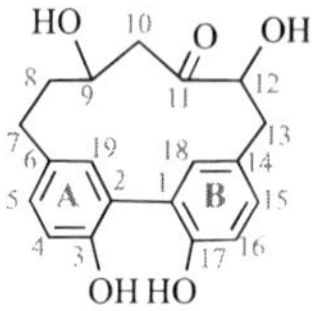

11-oxo-3,9,12,17-tetrahydroxy-[7,0]-metacyclophane (**110**)

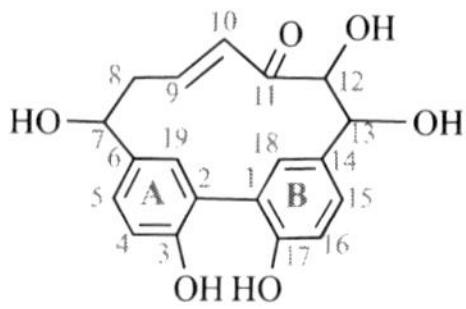

11-oxo-3,7,12,13,17-pentahydroxy-[7,0]-metacyclophane (**111**)

Figure 29. 11-Oxo-3,9,12,17-tetrahydroxy-[7,0]-metacyclophane (**110**) and 11-oxo-3,7,12,13,17-pentahydroxy-[7,0]-metacyclophane (**111**) from the extractives of Sawashiba, *Carpinus cordata* Blume.

2.2.1.4. *Corylus*

2.2.1.4.1. *Corylus sieboldiana* Blume

2.2.1.4.1.1. *Corylus sieboldiana* Blume/1994/1

In 1994, Watanabe *et al.* isolated two novel cyclic diarylheptanoids: 11-oxo-3,12,17-trihydroxy-9-ene-[7,0]-metacyclophane (**112**) and 11-oxo-3,8,12,17-tetrahydroxy-9-ene-[7,0]-metacyclophane (**113**) (Figure 30) from the extractives of the wood of *Corylus sieboldiana* Blume. [69].

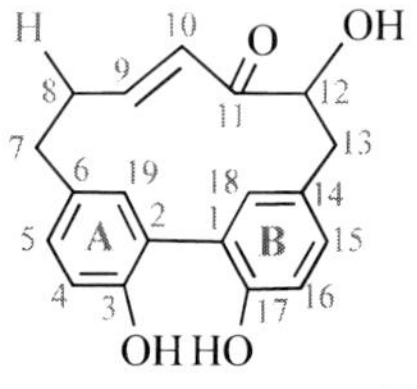

11-oxo-3,12,17-trihydroxy-9-ene-[7,0]-metacyclophane (**112**)

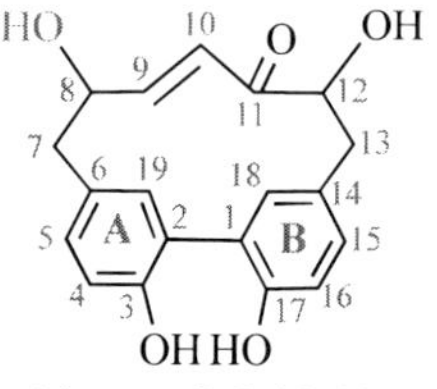

11-oxo-3,8,12,17-tetrahydroxy-9-ene-[7,0]-metacyclophane (**113**)

Figure 30. 11-Oxo-3,12,17-trihydroxy-9-ene-[7,0]-metacyclophane (**112**) and 11-oxo-3,8,12,17-tetrahydroxy-9-ene-[7,0]-metacyclophane (**113** from the extractives of the wood of *Corylus sieboldiana* Blume.

2.2.1.4.1.2. *Corylus sieboldiana* Blume/1994/2

In 1994, Watanabe *et al.* isolated anc confirmed six diarylheptanoids - 11-oxo-3,8,9,17-tetrahydroxy-[7,0]-metacyclophane (**109**), alnusone (**101**), alnusonol (**102**), 11-oxo-3,7,12,13,17-pentahydroxy-[7,0]-metacyclophane (**111**), 11-oxo-3,17-dihydroxy-8,9-isopropylidene-[7,0]-metacyclophane (**114**), platyphyllonol (**115**) (Figure 31) - from the extractives of the wood of *Corylus sieboldiana* Blume. Five diarylheptanoids (**109, 101, 102, 111, 114**) had *m, m'-bridged cyclic structures* except for platyphyllonol (**115**). A diarylheptanoid (**109)** was a novel compound 11-oxo-3,8,9,17-tetrahydroxy-[7,0]-metacyclophane (**109**).

Diarylheptanoids

1. *m, m'-bridged cyclic structures* (five diarylheptanoids)

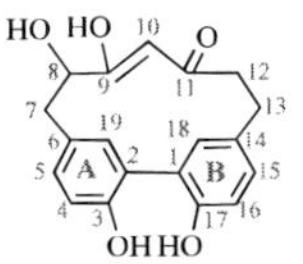

11-oxo-3,8,9,17-tetrahydroxy-[7,0]-metacyclophane (**109**)

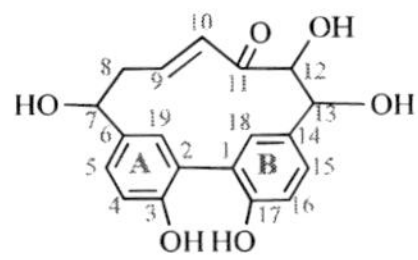

11-oxo-3,7,12,13,17-pentahydroxy-[7,0]-metacyclophane (**111**)

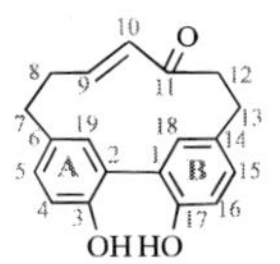

alnusone (**101**)

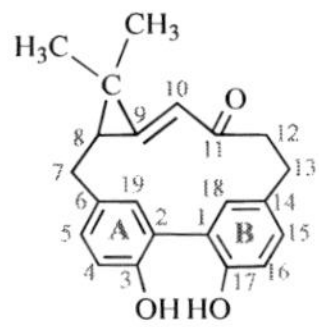

11-oxo-3,17-dihydroxy-8,9-isopropylidene-[7,0]-metacyclophane (**114**)

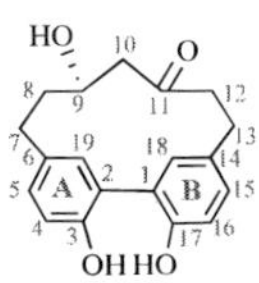

alnusonol (**102**)

2. *acyclic structure* (one diarylheptanoid)

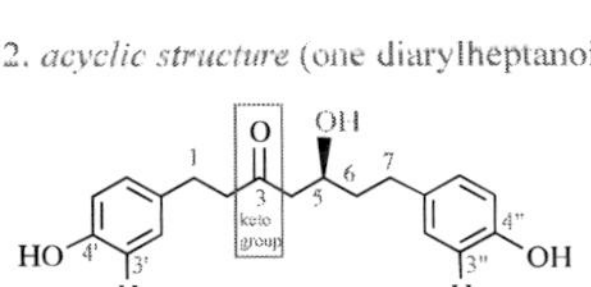

platyphyllonol (**115**)

Figure 31. 11-Oxo-3,8,9,17-tetrahydroxy-[7,0]-metacyclophane (**109**), alnusone (**101**), alnusonol (**102**), 11-oxo-3,7,12,13,17-pentahydroxy-[7,0]metacyclophane (**111**), 11-oxo-3,17-dihydroxy-8,9-isopropylidene-[7,0]-metacyclophane (**114**), and platyphyllonol (**115**) from the extractives of the wood of *Corylus sieboldiana* Blume.

Furthermore, 11-oxo-3,7,12,13,17-pentahydroxy-[7,0]-metacyclophane (**111**) and 11-oxo-3,17-dihydroxy-8,9-isopropylidene-[7,0]-metacyclophane (**114**) had been isolated from the wood of *Carpinus cordata* Blume.

Additionally, **115**, the only *acyclic* diarylheptanoid, was platyphyllonol (**115**). It was shown that most of diaylheptanoids from the wood of *Corylus sieboldiana* are *m, m'-cyclic type*, which corresponds with the diarylheptanoids obtained from the wood of *Carpinus species*. Thus, it is supposed that diarylhetanoids from the wood of the tribe *Coryleae* are mainly *m, m'-cyclic type*. These *m, m'-cyclic diarylheptanoids* are interesting in view of their chemotaxonomy [62].

2.2.1.4.2. *Corylus avellana* L. (Hazelnuts)

2.2.1.4.2.1. *Corylus avellana* L. (Hazelnuts)/2017/1

In 2017, Esposito T *et al.* identified a cyclic diarylheptanoid: carpinontriol B (**116**) (Figure 32) [70] from the shells of *Corylus avellana* L. (hazelnuts).

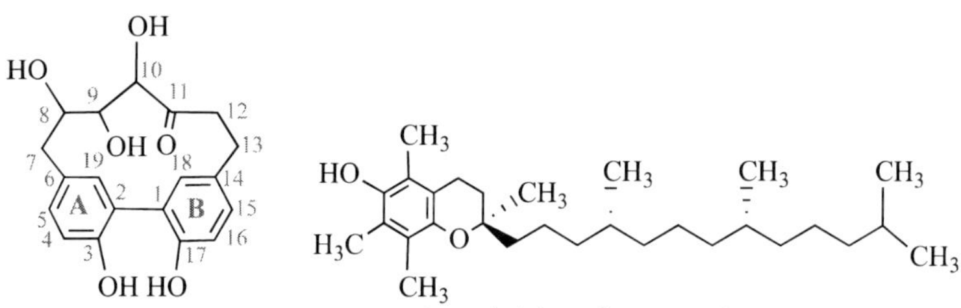

carpinontriol B (**116**) α-tocophenol (vitamin E. **117**)

Figure 32. A cyclic diarylheptanoid: carpinontriol B (**116**) from the shells of *Corylus avellana* L. (hazelnuts). A positive control of the DPPH assay α-tocophenol (vitamin E. **117**).

First, the antioxidant activity (50% effective concentration (EC_{50}))(μg/mL) against free-radical scavenging activity was carpinontriol B (**116**) (EC_{50}: 78.2±2.1) and a positive control of the DPPH assay α-tocophenol (vitamin E. **117**) (EC_{50}: 10.1±1.3) (Figure 32), respectively.

Second, their cytotoxic activity (50% inhibitory concentration (IC_{50})) of carpinontriol B (**116**) against three types of human malignant melanoma (A375) cell line, human melanoma (SK-Mel-28) cell line, and human cervical cancer (HeLa) cell lines was >1000 μM (not active (NA)) [71].

2.2.1.4.2.2. *Corylus avellana* L. (Hazelnuts)/2017/2

In 2017, Singldinger *et al.* confirmed a cyclic diarylheptanoid asadanin (**118**) (Figure 33) as the major inducer of the sporadic bitter off-taste from the hazelnut kernels of *Corylus avellana* L. (hazelnuts) [72].

In 2018, Singldinger *et al.* confirmed two bitter tasting diarylheptanoids asadanin (**118**) and giffonin P (**119**) (Figure 33) from the Cimiciato-infected hazelnuts of *Corylus avellana* L. (hazelnuts).

Asadanin (**118**) is the key contributor to the bitter taste of Cimiciato-infected hazelnuts. Neither the physical damage alone nor a general microbial infection is able to initiate a stress-induced asadanin (**118**) generation. However, most likely either specific Cimiciato-specific microorganisms associated with the bugs or specific chemical stimulants in the bugs' saliva triggered asadanin (**118**) biosynthesis. In addition, germination of hazelnut also enhanced the activation of diarylheptanoid biosynthesis and promoted the production of higher content of bitter phytochemicals and bitter diarylheptanoids [73].

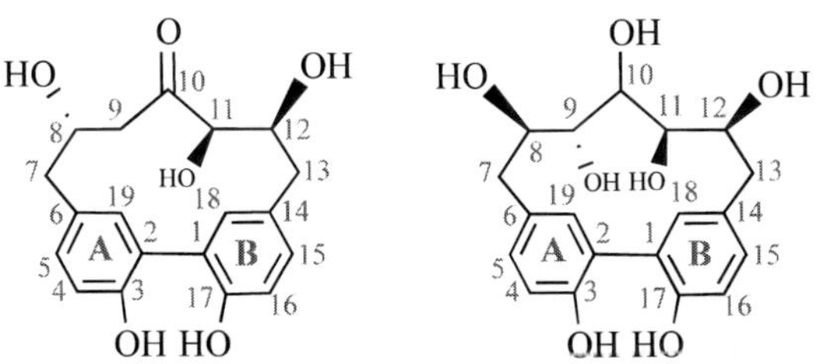

asadanin (8,11-*trans*, 11,12-*cis*. **118**) giffonin P (**119**)

Figure 33. Asadanin (8,11-*trans*, 11,12-*cis*. **118**) and giffonin P (**119**) from the Cimiciato-infected hazelnuts of *Corylus avellana* L. (hazelnuts).

2.2.1.5. Ostrya

2.2.1.5.1. *Ostrya japonica*

2.2.1.5.1.1. *Ostrya japonica*/1965

In 1965, Yasue *et al.* extracted the wood of *Ostrya japonica* SARG. with methanol to give 2% soluble materials. 2% soluble extracts were divided into two parts of *n*-hexane and ether soluble fraction. The phenolic constituents of the ether soluble fraction contained mainly a novel phenolic compound, asadanin (**118**) (Figure 33) $C_{19}H_{20}O_6$, mp. 236-239°C (Figure 33), and its homologues analogue [74].

In 1965, Yasue confirmed that asadanin (**118**) (Figure 33) is colourless needles, $C_{19}H_{20}O_6$, with mp. 236-239°C, $[\alpha]_D^{17}$ + 84°, λ_{max}. C_2H_5OH (ultraviolet (UV) spectrum with absorbtion peaks) at 253 and 302 mμ, and infrared (IR) spectrum with ν_{max}.^{KBr} 3380cm^{-1} (-OH), 1705cm^{-1} (>C=O), 1590, 1510cm^{-1} (aromatic double bonds), 1405cm^{-1} ($-CH_2-\overset{O}{\overset{\|}{C}}-$). Asadanin (**118**) gave violet colour with aqueous $FeCl_3$, red-orange colour with diazotized sulfanilic acid and positive results by FBHLING'S solution and tetrazolium chloride test [75].

In 1965, Yasue confirmed that the skeleton of asadanin (**118**) is a biphenyl structure with a seven carbon atoms between 5 and 5' positions [76, 77].

2.2.1.5.1.2. *Ostrya japonica*/1966

In 1966, Yasue *et al.* confirmed the presence of asadanin (8,11-*trans*,11,12-*cis*. **118**) (Figure 34) and epiasadanol (8,9-*cis*. triciclo [12.3.1.12,6]nonadeca-1(18),2,4,6(19),14,16-hexaene-3,8,9,10,12,17-hexol(8CI,9CI). **120**) (Figure 34) in asada heartwood. The relative arrangement of asadanin (**118**) is 8,11-*trans*,11,12-*cis*, and the relative arrangement of epiasadanol (tricyclo[12.3.1.12,6]nonadeca-1(18),2,4,6 (19),14,16-hexaene-3,8,9,10,12,17-hexol(8CI,9CI). **120**) is 8,9-*cis* [78].

In 1966, Yasue *et al*. confirmed that isoasadanol (tricyclo[12.3.1.12,6]-nonadeca-1(18),2,4,6(19),14,16-hexaene-3,8,9,10,12,17-hexol (7CI,8CI, 9CI). **121**)(Figure 34) from the heartwood of *Ostrya japonica*.

Isoasadanol (**121**) is a diastereoisomer of asadanol (tricyclo-[12.3.1.12,6]nonadeca-1(18),2,4,6(19),14,16-hexaene-3,8,9,10,12,17-hexol(9CI). **122**) (Figure 34) and epiasadanol (tricycle-[12.3.1.12,6] nonadeca-1(18),2,4,6(19),14,16-hexaene-3,8,9,10,12,17-hexol(8CI,9CI). **120**) (Figure 34) [79].

2.2.1.5.1.3. *Ostrya japonica*/1968

In 1968, Yasue found seven diarylheptanoids, asadanin (8,11-*trans*, 11,12-*cis*. **118**)(Figure 34), epiasadanol (8,9-*cis*. **120**) (Figure 34), isoasadanol (all *cis-form*. **121**)(Figure 34), deoxoasadanin (**123**) (Figure 34), trideoxyasadanin-8-ene (**124**) (Figure 34), dideoxyasadanin-8-ene (**125**) (Figure 34) and monodeoxyasadanin (**126**) (Figure 34) from the heartwood of *Ostrya japonica*.

Asadanol (**122**) (Figure 34) is the product formed by chemical treatment of asadanin (8,11-*trans*, 11,12-*cis*. **118**).

Monodeoxyasadanin (**126**) has the same bitter taste as asadanin (8,11-*trans*, 11,12-*cis*. **118**) and is considered to be one of the causative substances of asada wood. There are various functional groups in organic substances that responsible for bitterness, but in the homolog of asadanin (8,11-*trans*, 11,12-*cis*. **118**), the α-ketol structure can be considered to be a bitter functional group. In other words, various derivatives of asadanin (8,11-*trans*, 11,12-*cis*. **118**) that do not have the α-ketol structure do not exhibit bitterness. In addition, the homologous family having only a hydroxyl group in the alicyclic moiety exhibits sweetness, which is consistent with the general concept that polyhydroxy compounds exhibit sweetness [80].

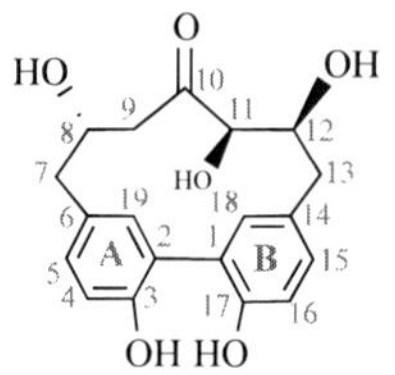

asadanin (8,11-*trans*, 11,12-*cis*. **118**)

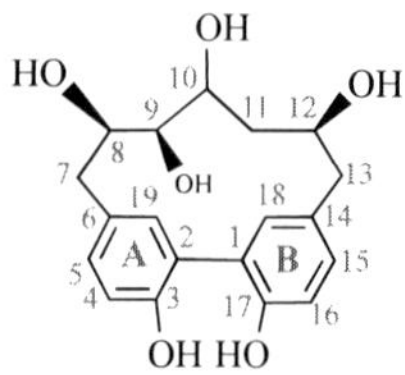

epiasadanol (8,9-*cis*. **120**)

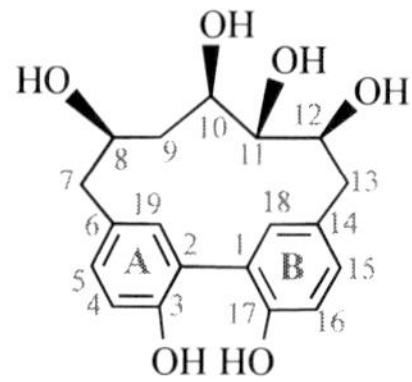

isoasadanol (all *cis*-form. **121**)

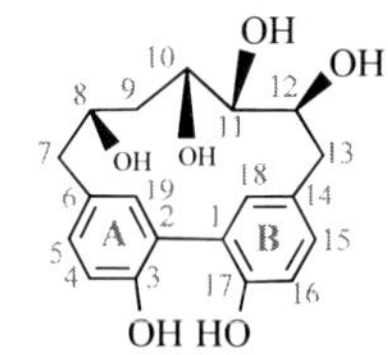

asadanol (**122**)

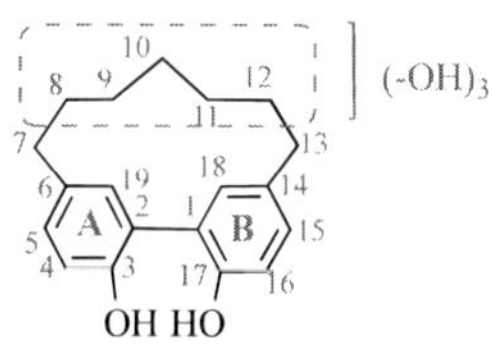

deoxoasadanin (**123**)

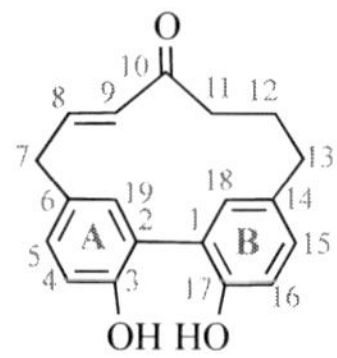

trideoxyasadanin-8-ene (**124**)

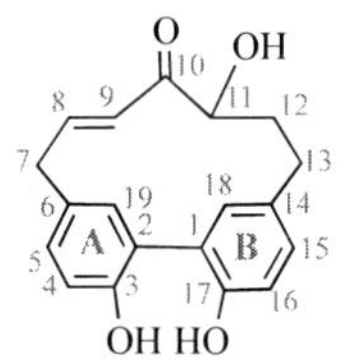

dideoxyasadanin-8-ene (**125**)

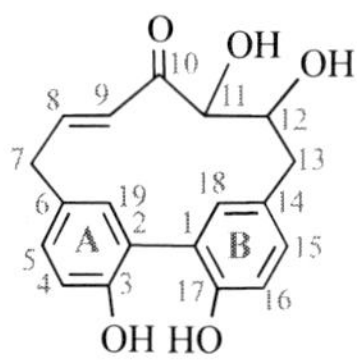

monodeoxyasadanin (**126**)

Figure 34. Asadanin (8,11-*trans*, 11,12-*cis*. **118**), epiasadanol (8,9-*cis*. **120**), isoasadanol (all *cis*-form. **121**), asadanol (**122**), deoxoasadanin (**123**), trideoxyasadanin-8-ene (**124**), dideoxyasadanin-8-ene (**125**), and monodeoxyasadanin (**126**) from the heartwood of asada heartwood. Asadanol (**122**) is the product of chemical treatment from asadanin (8,11-*trans*, 11,12-*cis*. **118**).

2.2.2. Casuarinaceae

2.2.2.1. *Casuarina*

2.2.2.1.1. *Casuarina junghuhniana*

In 1990, Kaneda *et al.* confirmed the presence of two diarylheptanoids of which a novel casuarinondiol (**127**) and alnusdiol (**128**) (Figure 35) were identified from the roots of *Casuarma junghuhniana* Miquel [81].

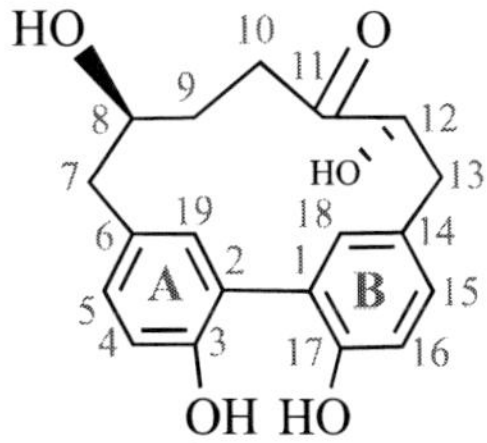

casuarinondiol (**127**)

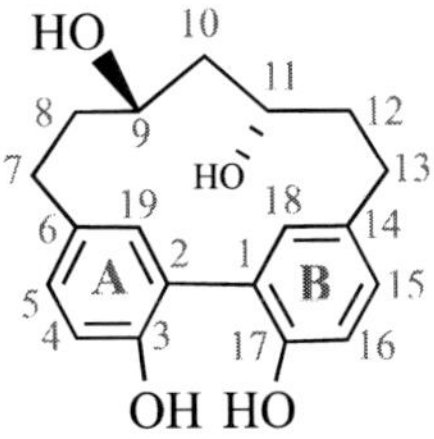

alnusdiol (**128**)

Figure 35. Casuarinondiol (**127**) and alnusdiol (**128**) from the roots of *Casuarma junghuhniana* Miquel.

2.2.3. Myricaceae

2.2.3.1. Morella

2.2.3.1.1. *Morella salicifolia*

Morella salicifolia was named *as Myrica salicifolia* HOCHST. Recently, the genus Myrica has been classified into two genera, the genus Myrica and the genus Morella. *Myrica salicifolia* HOCHST was renamed *Morella salicifolia* as it belongs to the genus *Morella* [82]. In Tanzania folklore medicine, *Morella salicifolia* has been used for the treatment of cough, toothache, decoction, tonic, stomach troubles and skin diseases [83], headache [84], tuberculosis, chronic diarrhea, cryptococcal meningitis, and opportunistic diseases of human immunodeficiency virus such as herpes simplex/acquired immune deficiency syndrome [85]. In addition, in Ethiopian folklore medicine, *Morella salicifolia* has been used to treat skin diseases [86], pain, inflammation, and respiratory diseases [87, 88]. In Uganda folklore medicine, *Morella salicifolia* has been used to treat male sexual dysfunction and erectile dysfunction [89].

In 2017, Makule *et al.* identified six novel cyclic diarylheptanoids from the bark of *Morella salicifolia* along with ten known cyclic diarylheptanoids. The confirmed cyclic diarylheptanoids are as follows:

Six novel cyclic diarylheptanoids: 7-hydroxymyricanol 5-*O*-β-D-glucopyranoside (**129**), juglanin B 3-*O*-β-D-glucopyranoside (**130**), 16-hydroxyjuglanin B 17-*O*-β-D-glucopyranoside (**131**), myricanone 5-*O*-β-

D-glucopranosyl-(1→6)-β-D-glucopyranoside (**132**), neomyricanone 5-*O*-β-D-glucopranosyl-(1→6)-β-D-glucopyranoside (**133**), and myricanone 17-*O*-α-L-arabinofuranosyl-(1→6)-β-D-glucopyranoside (**134**) (Figure 36).

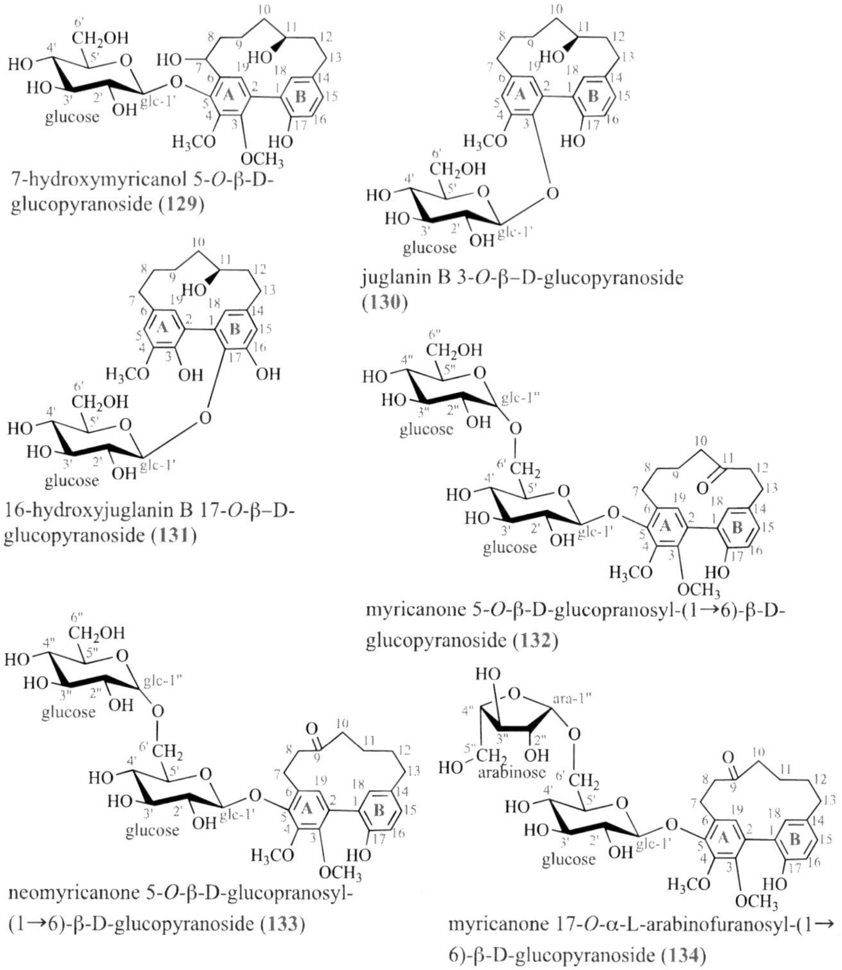

Figure 36. Six novel cyclic diarylheptanoids from the bark of *Morella salicifolia*. 7-hydroxymyricanol 5-*O*-β-D-glucopyranoside (**129**), juglanin B 3-*O*-β-D-glucopyranoside (**130**), 16-hydroxyjuglanin B 17-*O*-β–D-glucopyranoside (**131**), myricanone 5-*O*-β-D-glucopranosyl-(1→6)-β-D-glucopyranoside (**132**), neomyricanone 5-*O*-β-D-glucopranosyl-(1→6)-β-D-glucopyranoside (**133**), and myricanone 17-*O*-α-L-arabinofuranosyl-(1→6)-β-D-glucopyranoside (**134**).

Ten known cyclic diarylheptanoids: juglanin B-sulfate (**135**) [90, 91], myricanol (**136**) [92, 93, 94, 95], myricanone (**79**) [92, 95], myricanol 5-*O*-β-D-glucopyranoside (**137**) [96], myricanone 5-*O*-β-D-glucopyranoside (**81**) [97], myricanol 11-*O*-β-D-xylopyranoside (**138**) [98], myricanol 5-*O*-β-D-(6'-*O*-galloyl)-glucopyranoside (**139**) [99] (Figure 37), myricanone 5-*O*-β-D-(6'-*O*-galloyl)-glucopyranoside (**140**) [91], myricanol 5-*O*-α-L-arabinofuranosyl-(1→6)-β-D-glucopyranoside (**141**) [100], and myricanol gentiobiosidse: myricanol 5-*O*-β-D-glucopranosyl-(1→6)-β-D-glucopyranoside (**142**) [99] (Figure 37(continued 1)) [101].

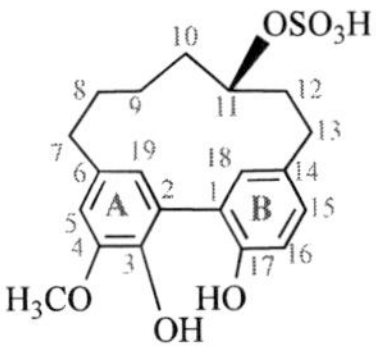

juglanin B-sulfate (**135**)

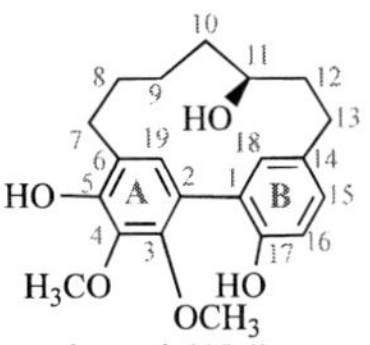

myricanol (**136**)

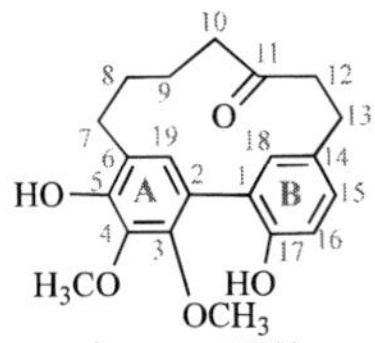

myricanone (**79**)

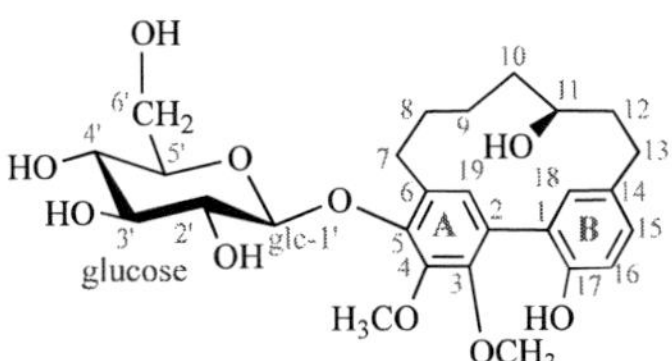

myricanol 5-*O*-β-D-glucopyranoside (**137**)

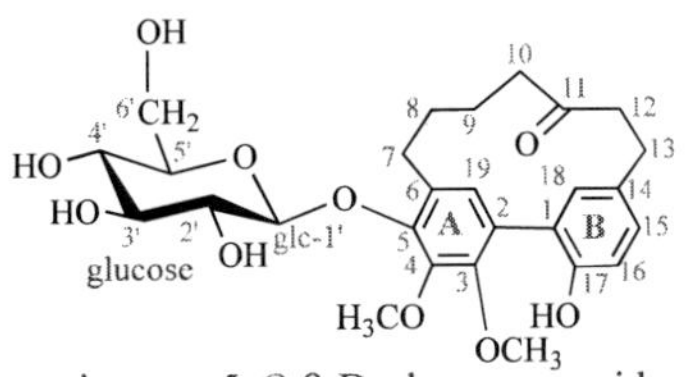

myricanone 5-*O*-β-D-glucopyranoside (**81**)

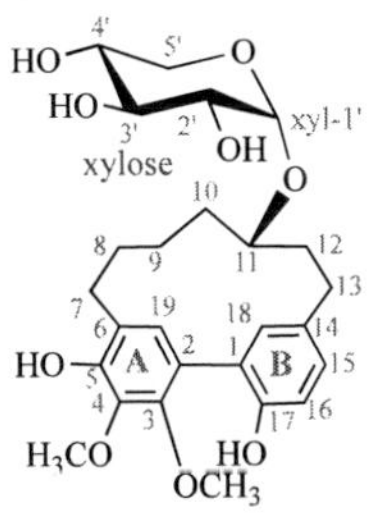

myricanol 11-*O*-β-D-xylopyranoside (**138**)

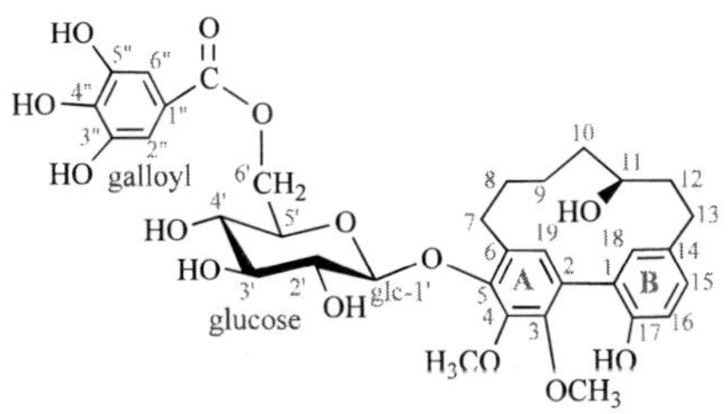

myricanol 5-*O*-β-D-(6'-*O*-galloyl)-glucopyranoside (**139**)

Figure 37. Ten known cyclic diarylheptanoids from the bark of *Morella salicifolia*. juglanin B-sulfate (**135**), myricanol (**136**), myricanone (**79**), myricanol 5-*O*-β-D-glucopyranoside (**137**), myricanone 5-*O*-β-D-glucopyranoside (**81**), myricanol 11-*O*-β-D-xylopyranoside (**138**), and myricanol 5-*O*-β-D-(6'-*O*-galloyl)-glucopyranoside (**139**).

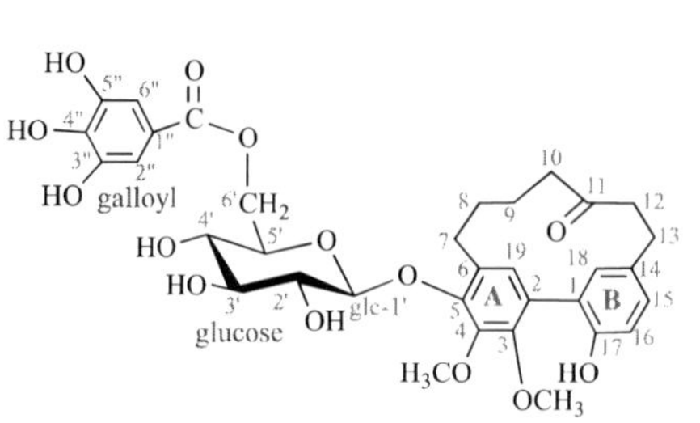

myricanone 5-*O*-β-D-(6'-*O*-galloyl)-glucopyranoside (**140**)

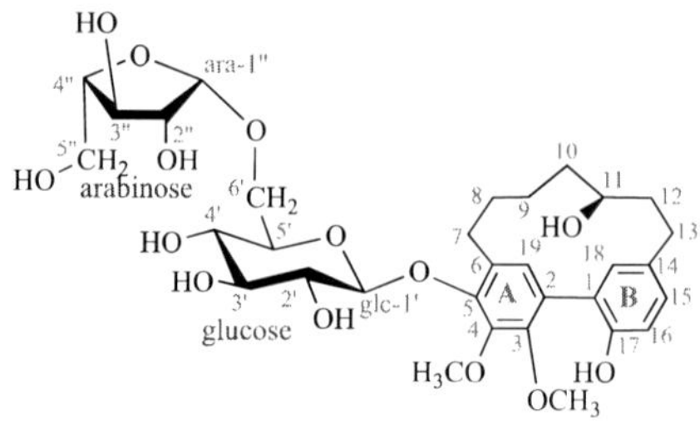

myricanol 5-*O*-α-L-arabinofuranosyl-(1→6)-β-D-glucopyranoside (**141**)

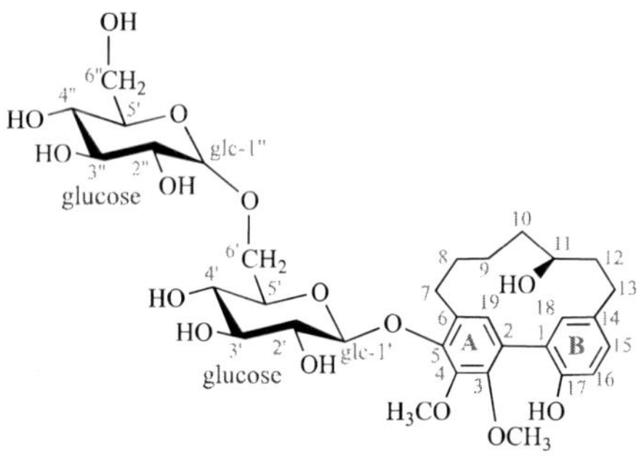

myricanol gentiobiosidse: myricanol 5-*O*-β-D-glucopranosyl-(1→6)-β-D-glucopyranoside (**142**)

Figure 37(continued 1). Ten known cyclic diarylheptanoids from the bark of *Morella salicifolia*. myricanone 5-*O*-β-D-(6'-*O*-galloyl)-glucopyranoside (**140**), myricanol 5-*O*-α-L-arabinofuranosyl-(1→6)-β-D-glucopyranoside (**141**), and myricanol gentiobiosidse: myricanol 5-*O*-β-D-glucopranosyl-(1→6)-β-D-glucopyranoside (**142**).

2.2.3.2. *Myrica*

2.2.3.2.1. *Myrica nagi*

2.2.3.2.1.1. *Myrica nagi* /1971

In 1971, Begley *et al.* confirmed myricanol (**136**) and myricanone (**79**) (Figure 38) from the diethyl ether extract of the stem bark of *Myrica nagi* [95].

2.2.3.2.2. *Myrica gale* L.

2.2.3.2.2.1. *Myrica gale* L. /1976/1

In 1976, Anthonsen *et al.* confirmed porson (**143**) (Figure 38) from the ethyl acetate extract of the stems of *Myrica gale* L. (bog myrtle) [102].

2.2.3.2.2.2. *Myrica gale* L. /1976/2

In 1976, Malterud *et al.* confirmed galeon (**144**) and hydroxygaleon (**145**) (Figure 38) from the ethyl acetate extract of the stems of *Myrica gale* L. [103].

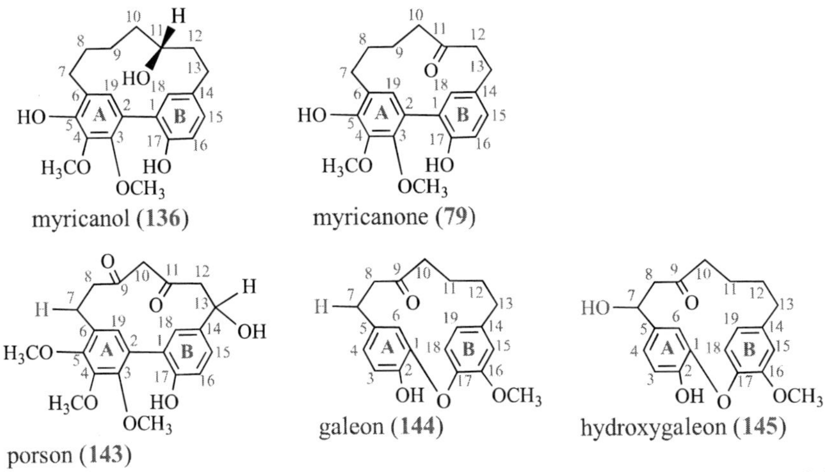

Figure 38. Myricanol (**136**) and myricanone (**79**) from the diethyl ether extract of the stem bark of *Myrica nagi*, and porson (**143**), galeon (**144**) and hydroxygaleon (**145**) from the ethyl acetate extract of the stems of *Myrica gale* L..

2.2.3.2.2.3. *Myrica gale* L. var.tomentosa C. Dc. (Yachi-Yanagi)/1995

In 1995, Nagai *et al.* confirmed two novel diarylheptanoids (12-dehydroporson (**146**)) and 12-hydroxymyricanone (**147**) (Figure 39) together with myricanone (**79**) and porson (**143**) (Figure 39) from the branches of *Myrica gale* L. var.tomentosa C. Dc. (Yachi-yanagi) [104].

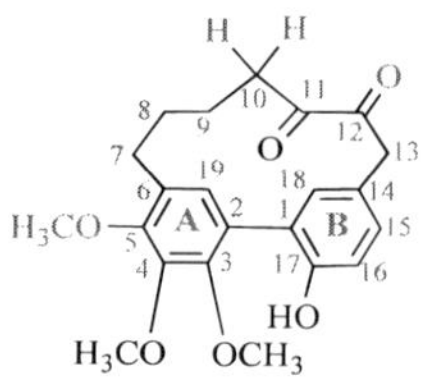

12-dehydroporson (**146**)

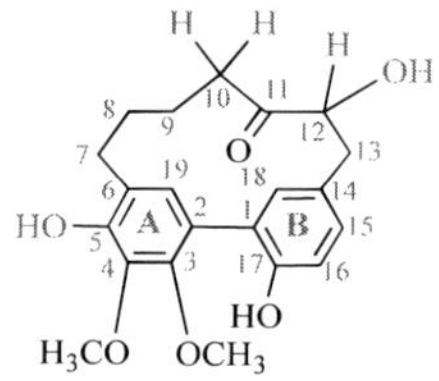

12-hydroxymyricanone (**147**)

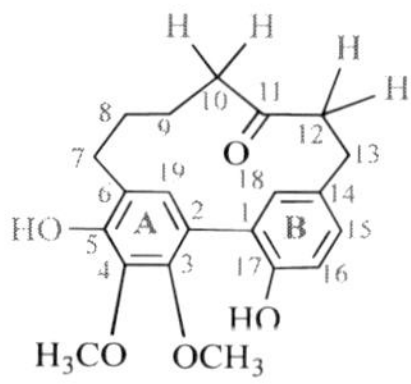

myricanone (**79**)

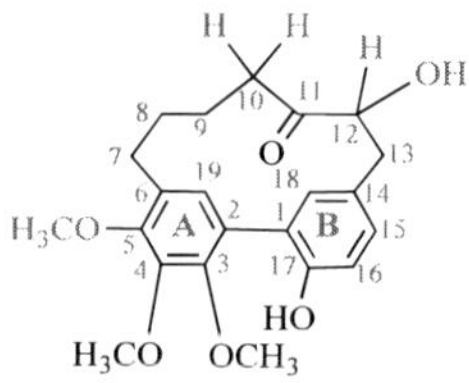

porson (**143**)

Figure 39. 12-Dehydroporson (**146**), 12-hydroxymyricanone (**147**), myricanone (**79**), and porson (**143**) from the branches of *Myrica gale* L. var.tomentosa C. Dc. (Yachi-yanagi).

2.2.3.2.2.4. *Myrica gale* L. var.tomentosa C. Dc. (Yachi-Yanagi)/1997

In 1997, Morihara *et al.* confirmed two novel diarylheptanoids (myricatomentoside I (**148**) and myricatomentoside II (**149**)) together with (+)-galeon (**150**) (Figure 40) from the branches of *Myrica gale* L. var.tomentosa C. Dc. (Yachi-yanagi) [105].

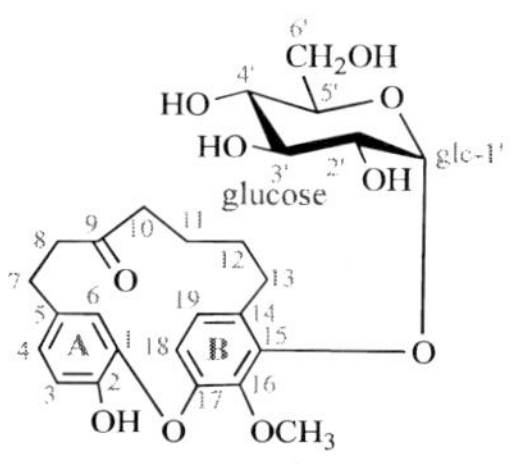

myricatomentoside I (**148**)

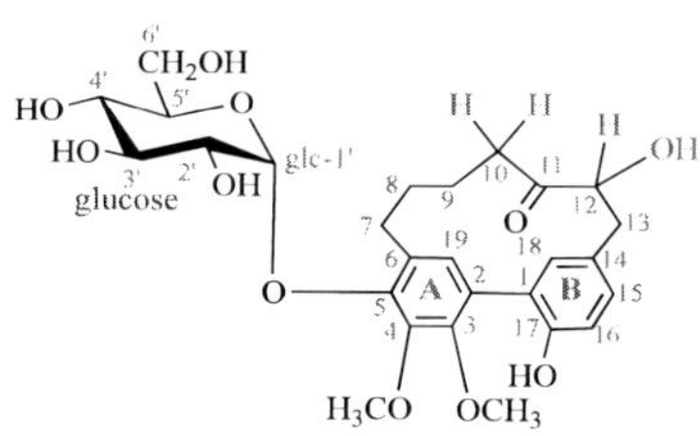

myricatomentoside II (**149**)

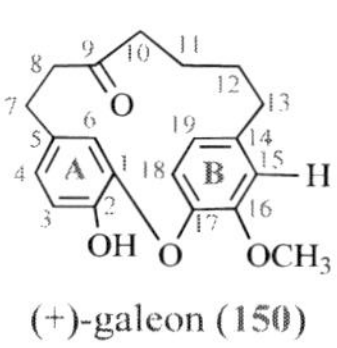

(+)-galeon (**150**)

Figure 40. Myricatomentoside I (**148**), myricatomentoside II (**149**), and (+)-galeon (**150**) from the branches of *Myrica gale* L. var.tomentosa C. Dc. (Yachi-yanagi).

2.2.3.2.3. *Myrica rubra*

2.2.3.2.3.1. *Myrica rubra*/1984, 1988, 1991

In 1984, Inoue *et al.* confirmed myricanol glucoside (**151**) (Figure 41) from the stem bark of *Myrica rubra* SIEB. et ZUCC. (Photos 1-3) [106].

In 1988, Yaguchi *et al.* confirmed myricanol galloylglucoside (**152**) and myricanol gentiobioside (**142**) (Figure 41) from the stem bark of *Myrica rubra* SIEB. et ZUCC. [99].

In 1991, Sakurai *et al.* confirmed myricanol 5-*O*-β-D-glucopyranosyl-(1→3)-β-D-glucopyranoside (**153**) and myricanol 5-*O*-α-L-arabinofuranosyl-(1→6)-β-D-glycopyranoside (**141**) (Figure 41) from the stem bark of *Myrica rubra* SIEB. et ZUCC. [100].

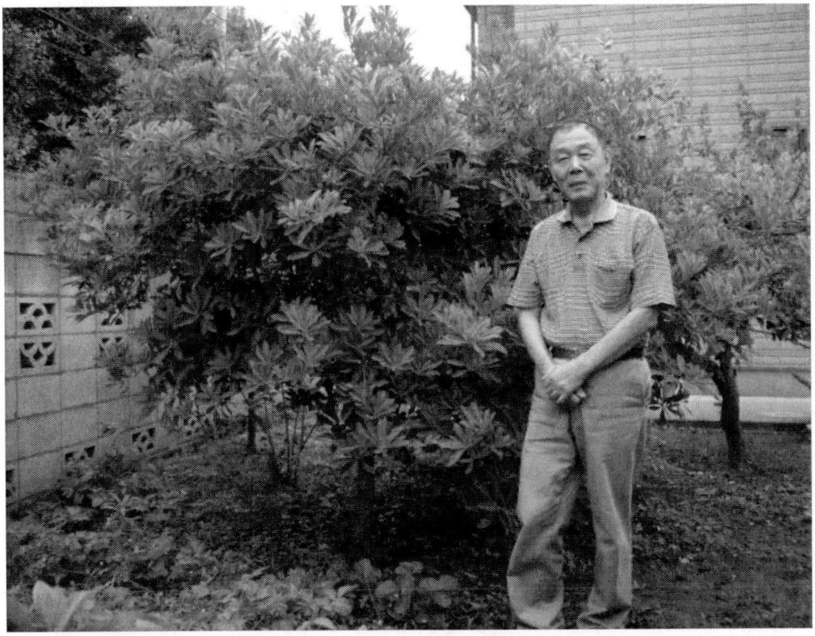

Photo 1. Whole tree of *Myrica rubra* SIEB. et ZUCC. (bayberry) at home garden of author Noboru Motohashi in Tokyo, Japan. Photographed by Noboru Motohashi. 6/24/2007 Sun.

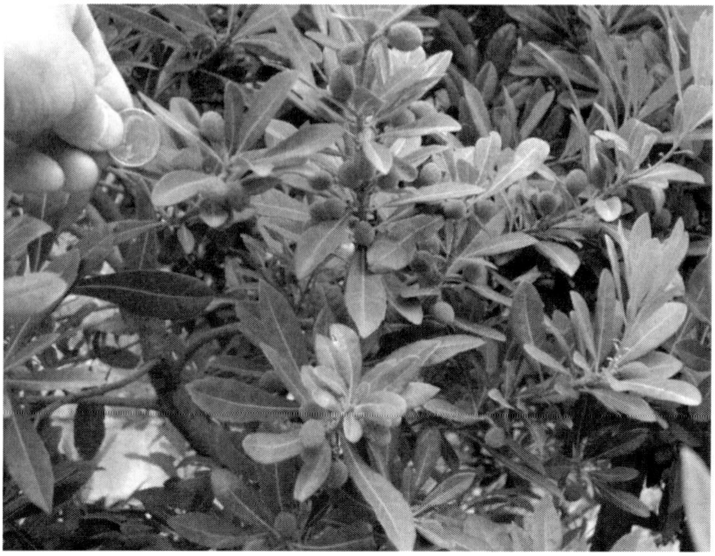

Photo 2. Bayberry tree with young fruits at home garden of author Noboru Motohashi in Tokyo, Japan. Photographed by Noboru Motohashi. 5/13/2007 Sun.

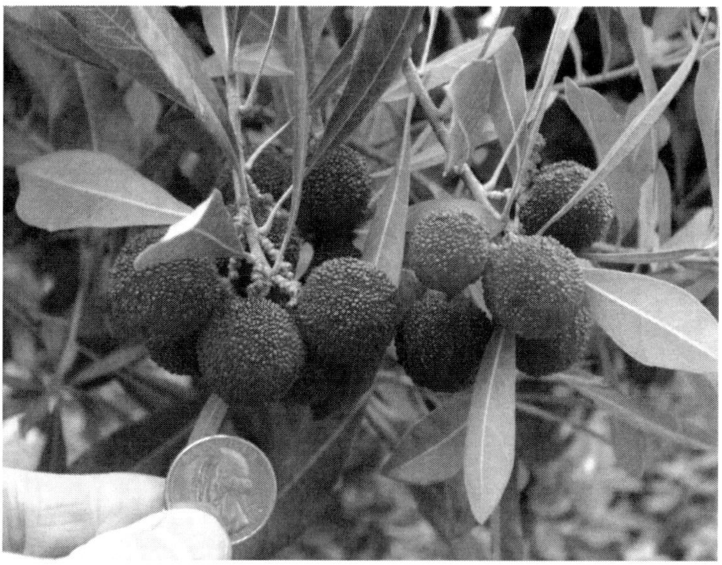

Photo 3. Ripe bayberries at home garden of author Noboru Motohashi in Tokyo, Japan. Photographed by Noboru Motohashi. 6/24/2007 Sun.

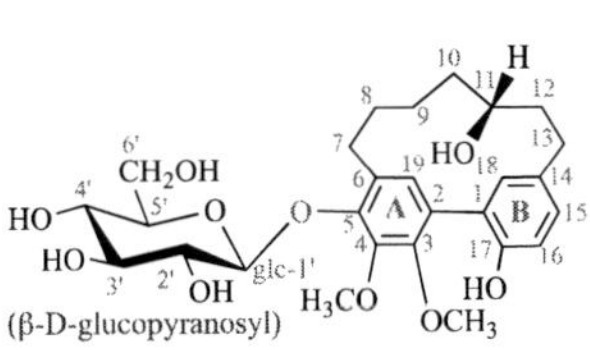

myricanol glucoside (**151**)

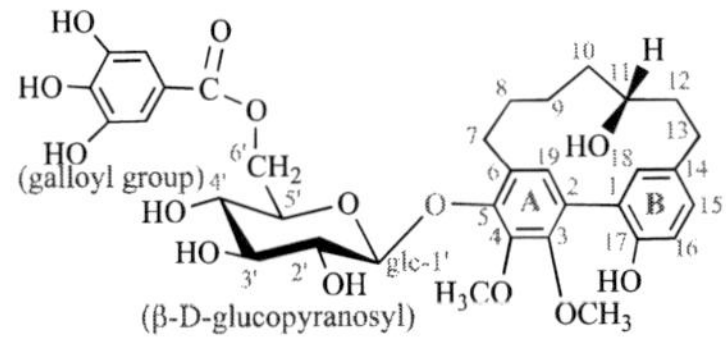

myricanol galloylglucoside (**152**)

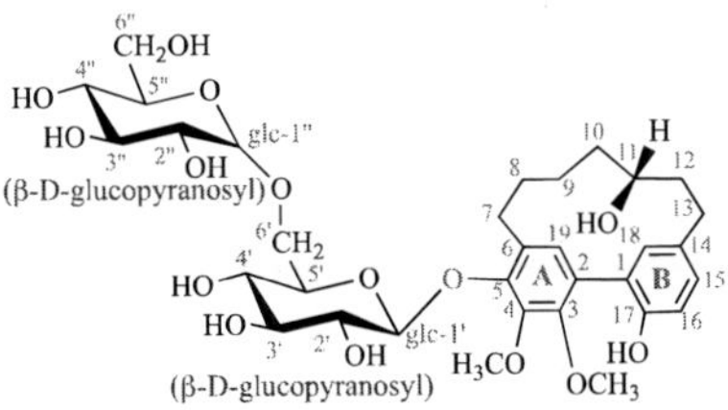

myricanol gentiobioside (**142**)

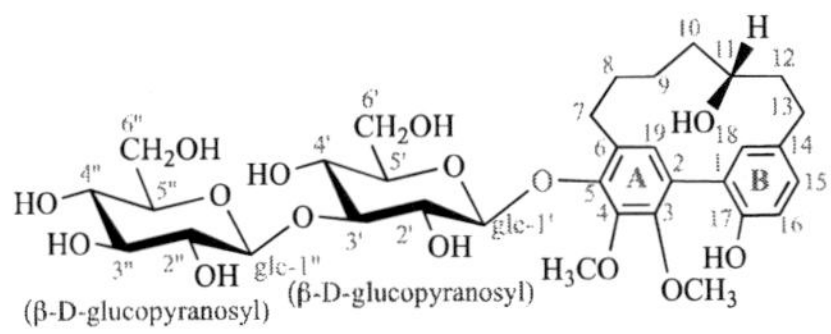

myricanol 5-*O*-β′-D-glucopyranosyl-(1→3)-β-D-glucopyranoside (**153**)

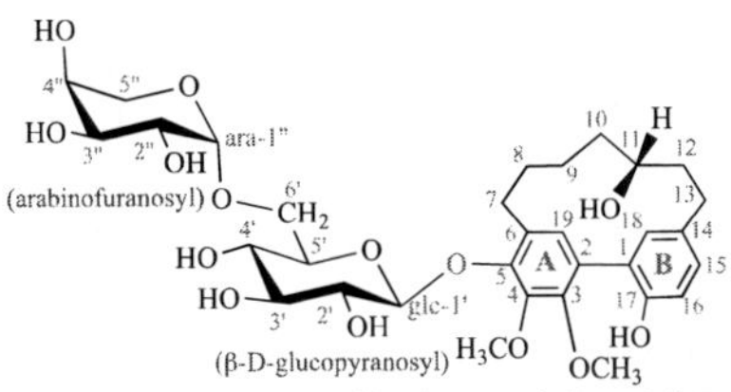

myricanol 5-*O*-β-L-arabinofuranosyl-(1→6)-β-D-glycopyranoside (**141**)

Figure 41. Myricanol glucoside (**151**), myricanol galloylglucoside (**152**), myricanol gentiobioside (**142**), myricanol 5-*O*-β′-D-glucopyranosyl-(1→3)-β-D-glucopyranoside (**153**), and myricanol 5-*O*-β-L-arabinofuranosyl-(1→6)-β-D-glycopyranoside (**141**) from the stem bark of *Myrica rubra* SIEB. et ZUCC..

2.2.3.2.3.2. *Myrica rubra* Sieb. et Zucc./2002/1

The bark of *Myrica rubra* Sieb. Et Zucc. has been used in Japan as an astringent, antidote and anti-diarrheal agent, and in China it has also been used as an external preparation for the treatment of burns and skin diseases.

In 2002, Tao *et al.* confirmed three new biphenyl type diarylheptanoid glycosides of myricanol 11-*O*-β-D-glucopyranoside (**154**), myricanone 5-*O*-β-D-glucopyranoside (**81**), and neomyricanone 5-*O*-β-D-glucopyranoside (**155**) together with ten known biphenyl type diarylheptanoids of (+)-

S-myricanol 5-*O*-β-D-glucopyranoside (11α-OH. **82**), myricanol glucoside (11β-OH. **156**), (+)-*S*-myricanol (11α-OH. **80**), myricanol (11β-OH. **136**), myricanone (11-O. **79**) (Figure 42), myricanene A 5-*O*-α-L-arabinofuranosyl-(1→6)-β-D-glucopyranoside (**157**), myricanene A (**158**), myricanene B 5-*O*-α–L-arabinofuranosyl-(1→6)-β-D-glucopyranoside (**159**), myricanene B (**160**) and myricanane (**161**) (Figure 42(continued 1)) from the bark of Chinese *Myrica rubra*. However, (+)-*S*-myricanol (11α-OH. **80**), myricanene A (**158**), myricanene B (**160**), and myricanane (**161**) are each aglycone (non-sugar part) of biphenyl type diarylheptanoids.

First, these several types of biphenyl type diarylheptanoids were investigated for their inhibitory effects on NO production in lipopolysaccharide (LPS)-activated mouse peritoneal macrophages. N^G-monomethyl-L-arginine, monoacetate salt (L-NMMA. **162**) (Figure 43), a cell-permeable competitive NOS inhibitor, was used as a control.

Among these biphenyl-type diarylheptanoids, 50% inhibitory concentration (IC_{50}) of six biphenyl-type diarylheptanoids ((+)-*S*-myricanol (11α-OH. **80**), myricanol (11β-OH. **136**), myricanone (11-O. **79**), myricanene A (**158**), myricanene B (**160**), myricanane (**161**)) was a 19-30 μM, and IC_{50} of L-NMMA (**162**) was 28 μM. Therefore, the six biphenyl-type diarylheptanoids showed significant inhibitory effects on NO production.

Their NO production inhibitory activity (IC_{50}: 19-30 μM) was almost equivalent to the NO production inhibitory activity of non-selective NOS inhibitor N^G-monomethyl-L-arginine, monoacetate salt (L-NMMA. **162**) (IC_{50}: 28 μM). However, the NO production inhibitory activity of their corresponding glycosides (myricanone 5-*O*-β-D-glucopyranoside (**81**), (+)-*S*-myricanol 5-*O*-β-D-glucopyranoside (11α-OH. **82**), myricanol glucoside (11β-OH. **156**), myricanene A 5-*O*-α-L-arabinofuranosyl-(1→6)-β-D-glucopyranoside (**157**) showed weak or no activity. The reason for this is speculated to be as follows: Their glycosides (**81, 82, 156**、 **157**) cannot reach the active site because the glycosides (**81, 82, 156, 157**) hardly penetrate the cell membrane.

Second, these several types of biphenyl type diarylheptanoids were investigated for their inhibitory effects on the induction of inducible nitric oxide synthase (iNOS) in lipopolysaccharide (LPS)-activated mouse peritoneal macrophages.

(three novel biphenyl type diarylheptanoid glycosides)

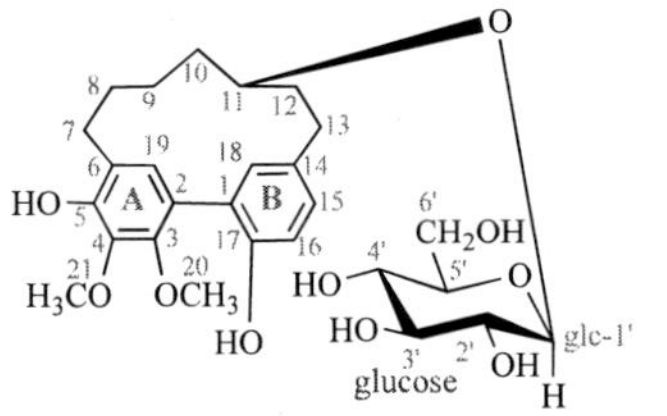

myricanol 11-*O*-β-D-glucopyranoside (**154**)

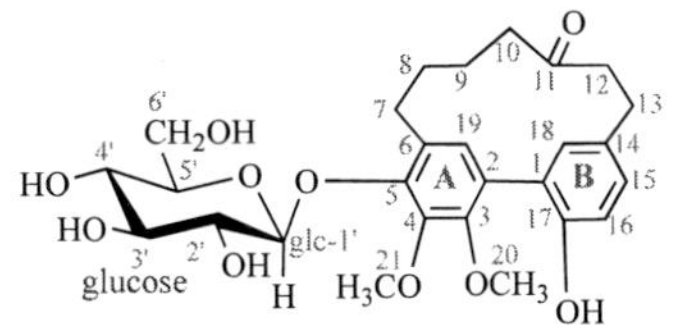

myricanone 5-*O*-β-D-glucopyranoside (**81**)

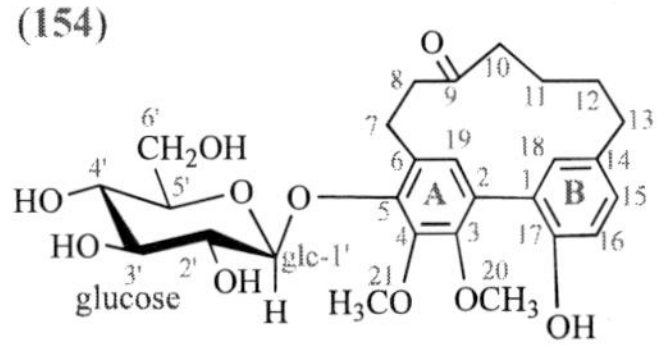

neomyricanone 5-*O*-β-D-glucopyranoside (**155**)

(ten known biphenyl type diarylheptanoids)

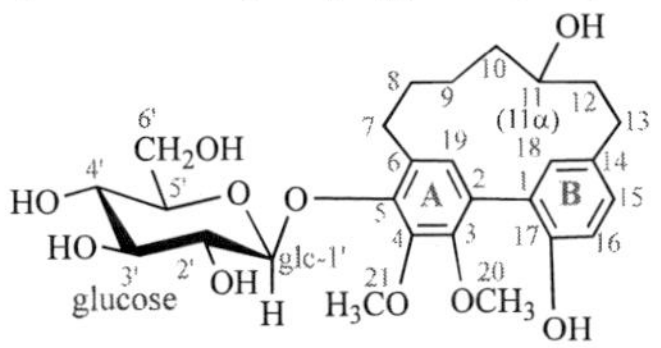

(+)-*S*-myricanol 5-*O*-β-D-glucopyranoside (11α-OH. **82**)

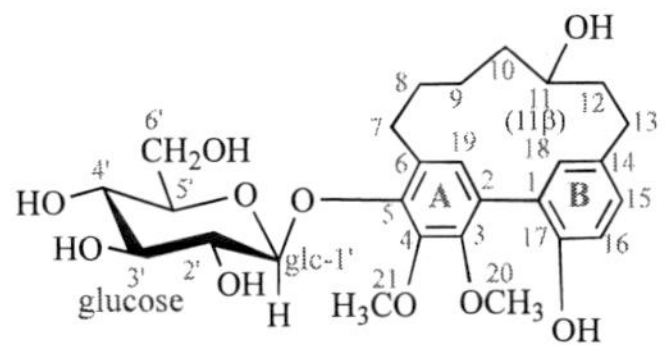

myricanol glucoside (11β-OH. **156**)

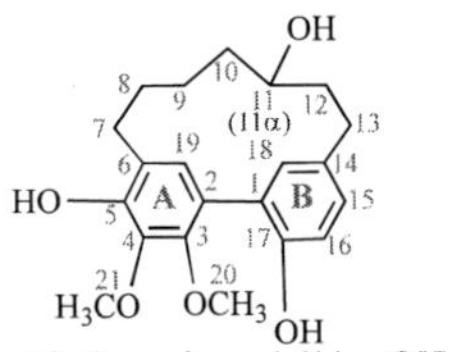

(+)-*S*-myricanol (11α-OH. **80**)

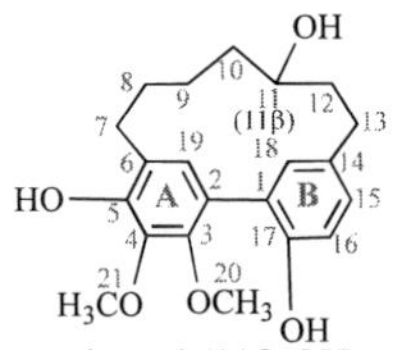

myricanol (11β-OH. **136**)

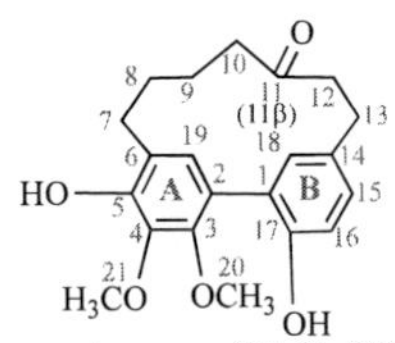

myricanone (11-O. **79**)

Figure 42. Three new biphenyl type diarylheptanoid glycosides of myricanol 11-*O*-β-D-glucopyranoside (**154**), myricanone 5-*O*-β-D-glucopyranoside (**81**), and neomyricanone 5-*O*-β-D-glucopyranoside (**155**) together with ten known biphenyl type diarylheptanoids of (+)-*S*-myricanol 5-*O*-β-D-glucopyranoside (11α-OH. **82**), myricanol glucoside (11β-OH. **156**), (+)-*S*-myricanol (11α-OH. **80**), myricanol (11β-OH. **136**), and myricanone (11-O. **79**) from the bark of Chinese *Myrica rubra*.

(ten known biphenyl type diarylheptanoids)(continued)

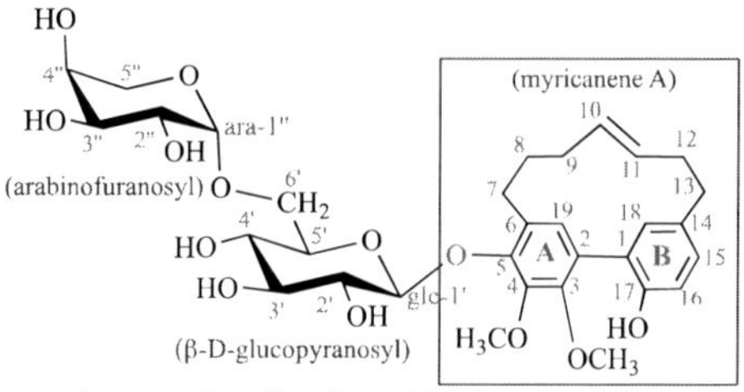

myricanene A 5-*O*-α-L-arabinofuranosyl-(1→6)-β-D-glucopyranoside (**157**)

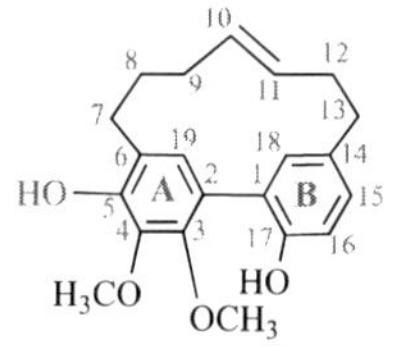

myricanene A (**158**)

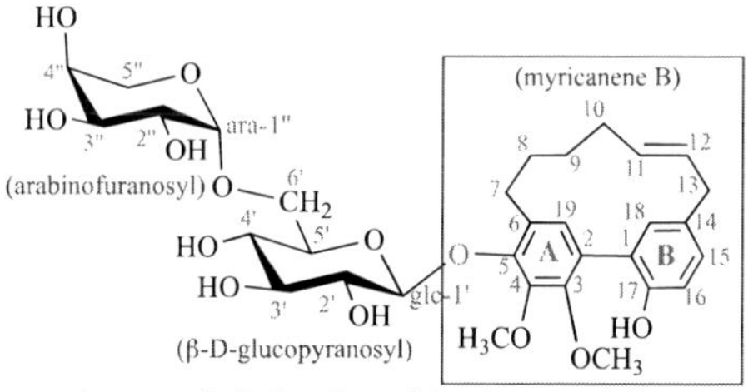

myricanene B 5-*O*-α-L-arabinofuranosyl-(1→6)-β-D-glucopyranoside (**159**)

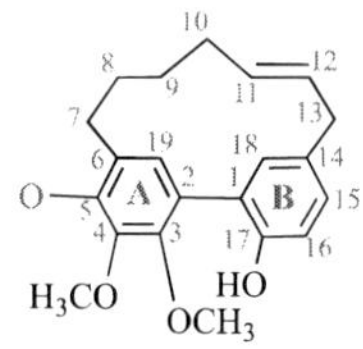

myricanene B (**160**)

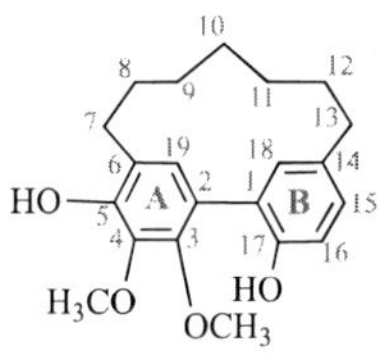

myricanane (**161**)

Figure 42(continued 1). Ten known biphenyl type diarylheptanoids of myricanene A 5-*O*-α-L-arabinofuranosyl-(1→6)-β-D-glucopyranoside (**157**), myricanene A (**158**), myricanene B 5-*O*-α-L-arabinofuranosyl-(1→6)-β-D-glucopyranoside (**159**), myricanene B (**160**) and myricanane (**161**) from the bark of Chinese *Myrica rubra*.

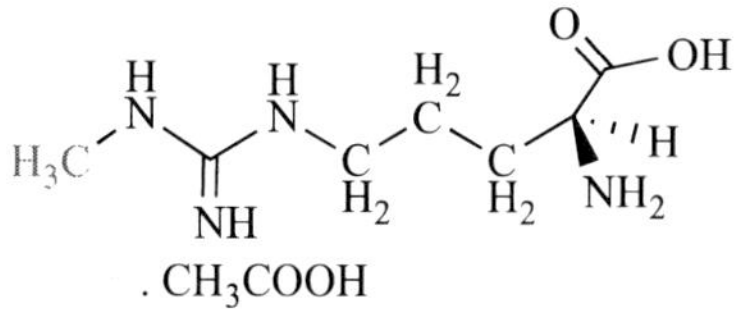

N^G-monomethyl-L-arginine, monoacetate salt (L-NMMA. **162**)

Figure 43. N^G-monomethyl-L-arginine, monoacetate salt (L-NMMA. **162**).

The effects of two biphenyl-type diarylheptanoid components (myricanol (11β-OH. **136**) and myricanone (11-O. **79**) on inducible nitric oxide synthase (iNOS) induction in lipopolysaccharide (LPS)-activated mouse peritoneal macrophages are closely related to NO inhibition.

Since there is a high correlation between NO production inhibition and iNOS induction inhibition by biphenyl type diarylheptanoid components (**136, 79**), two biphenyl-type diarylheptanoid components (**136** and **79**) inhibited iNOS induction mainly on LPS-activated mouse peritoneal macrophages. As a result, it suggests that the NO production was also inhibited.

The inhibitory activity of these biphenyl-type diarylheptanoids on NO production in LPS-activated macrophages appeared to demonstrate the effect of an old folklore traditional medicine for the treatment of inflammation [98].

2.2.3.2.3.3. *Myrica rubra*/2002/2

In 2002, Matsuda *et al.* identified three novel diarylheptanoid glycosides - (+)-*S*-myricanol 5-*O*-β-D-glucopyranoside (**163**), myricanene A 5-*O*-α-L-arabinofuranosyl(1→6)-β-D-glucopyranoside (**164**), and myricanene B 5-*O*-α-L-arabinofuranosyl(1→6)-β-D-glucopyranoside (**165**) together with three known diarylheptanoid glycosides - myricanol (**136**) [106, 107], myricanol glucoside (**151**) [106], and myricanone (**79**) [106, 107] from the bark of *Myrica rubra* (Figure 44).

Second, for the purpose of searching for antiallergic components from natural sources, β-hexosaminidase release prevention effect by *Myrica rubra* bark components was tested for β-hexosaminidase release induced by dinitrophenylated bovine serum albumin (DNP-BSA) from rat basophilic leukemia (RBL-2H3) cells sensitized with anti-DNP IgE. Because, regarding antigen-immunoglobulin E (IgE) response, this IgE has been known as substances causing immediate allergic phenomena.

Then, their inhibitory effects of these six diarylheptanoids from *Myrica rubra* bark on the release of intragranular enzyme β-hexosaminidase in RBL-2H3 cells were studied.

As a result, the 50% inhibitory concentration (IC_{50}) (μM) was highest in myricanone (**79**) (IC_{50}: 46 μM), followed by myricanol (**136**) (IC_{50}: 63 μM). Thus at these concentrations, an antigen-immunoglobulin E (IgE antibody. IgE) response was not induced 50% in the presence of cell extracts.

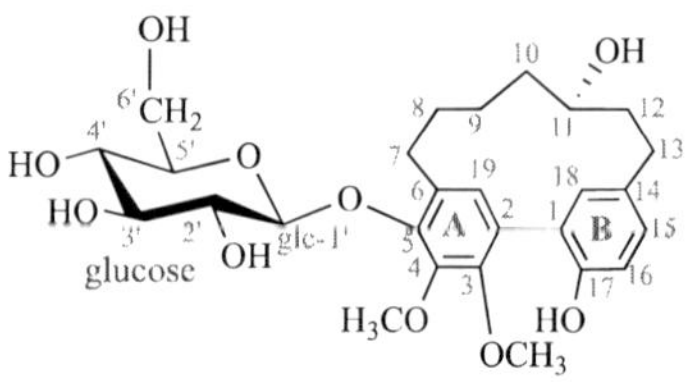

(+)-*S*-myricanol 5-*O*-β-D-glucopyranoside (**163**)

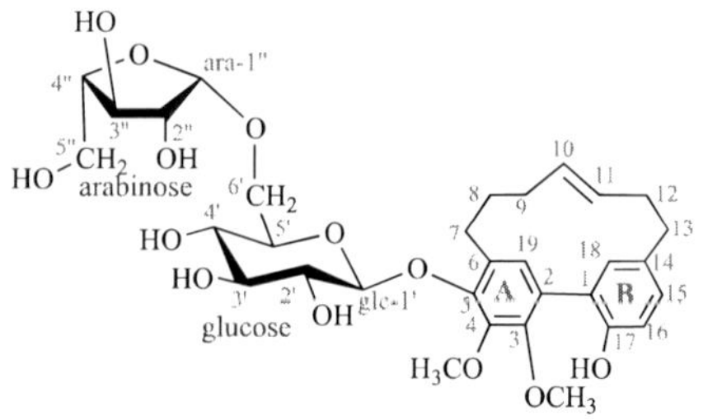

myricanene A 5-*O*-α-L-arabinofuranosyl(1→6)-β-D-glucopyranoside (**164**)

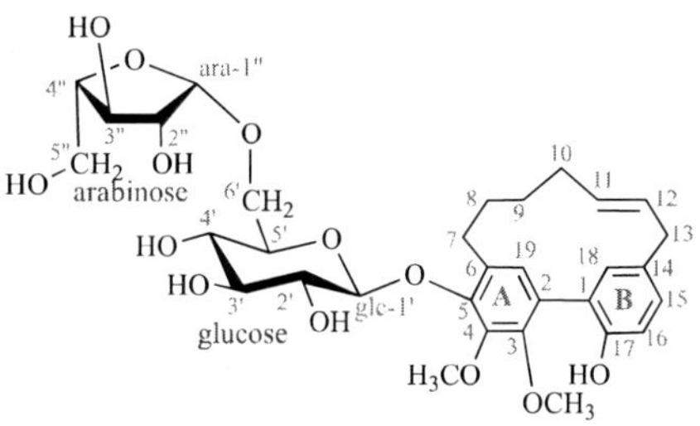

myricanene B 5-*O*-α-L-arabinofuranosyl(1→6)-β-D-glucopyranoside (**165**)

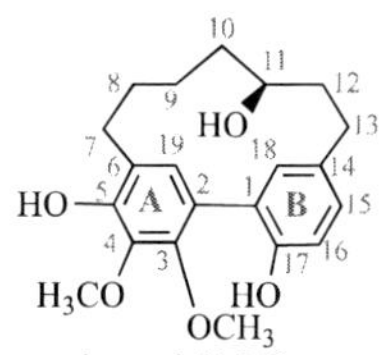

myricanol (**136**)

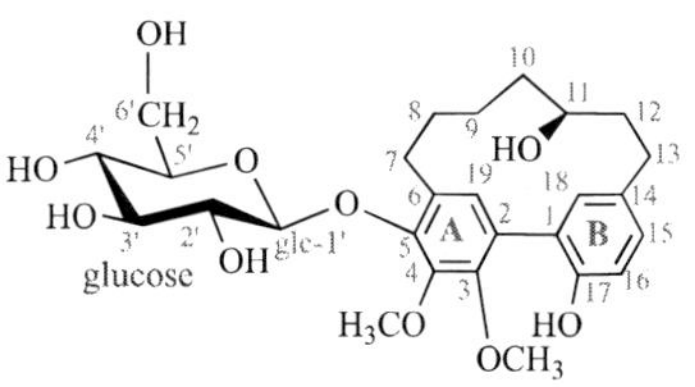

myricanol glucoside (**151**)

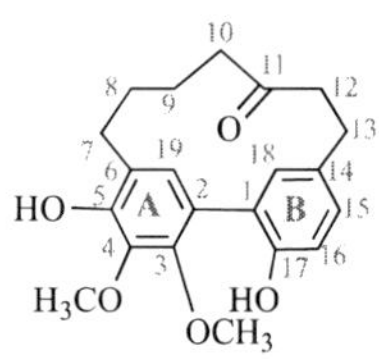

myricanone (**79**)

Figure 44. Three novel diarylheptanoid glycosides - (+)-*S*-myricanol 5-*O*-β-D-glucopyranoside (**163**), myricanene A 5-*O*-α-L-arabinofuranosyl(1→6)-β-D-glucopyranoside (**164**), and myricanene B 5-*O*-α-L-arabinofuranosyl(1→6)-β-D-glucopyranoside (**165**) together with three known diarylheptanoid glycosides - myricanol (**136**), myricanol glucoside (**151**), and myricanone (**79**) from the bark of *Myrica rubra*.

On the other hand, he other four types of biphenyl type diarylheptanoid glycosides ((+)-*S*-myricanol 5-*O*-β-D-glucopyranoside (**163**), myricanene A 5-*O*-α-L-arabinofuranosyl(1→6)-β-D-glucopyranoside (**164**), myricanene B 5-*O*-α-L-arabinofuranosyl(1→6)-β-D-glucopyranoside (**165**), myricanol glucoside (**151**)) did not show the significant effect of inhibiting β-hexosaminidase release.

Furthermore, regarding the release inhibitory effect of diarylheptanoids on β-hexosaminidase enzyme activity, it was investigated whether the β-hexosaminidase release inhibitory effect was due to inhibition of enzyme activity or inhibition of degranulation. As a result, these active diarylheptanoids ((+)-*S*-myricanol 5-*O*-β-D-glucopyranoside (**163**), myricanene A 5-*O*-α-L-arabinofuranosyl(1→6)-β-D-glucopyranoside (**164**), myricanene B 5-*O*-α-L-arabinofuranosyl(1→6)-β-D-glucopyrano-side (**165**), myricanol (**136**), myricanone (**79**)) did not affect the enzyme activity of β-hexosaminidase. That is, effects on inhibiting β-hexosaminidase release of these five kinds of active diarylheptanoids (**163**, **164**, **165**, **136**, and **79**) were found to be due to degranulation inhibitory activity of biphenyl type diarylheptanoid. This degranulation inhibitory activity of biphenyl diarylheptanoid is the first report of degranulation inhibitory activity of biphenyl diarylheptanoids [96].

2.3. Order Dioscoreales

2.3.1. Dioscoreaceae

2.3.1.1. Dioscorea

The gemus Dioscorea found in Japan is *Dioscorea batatas* Decaisne (Photos 4 and 5).

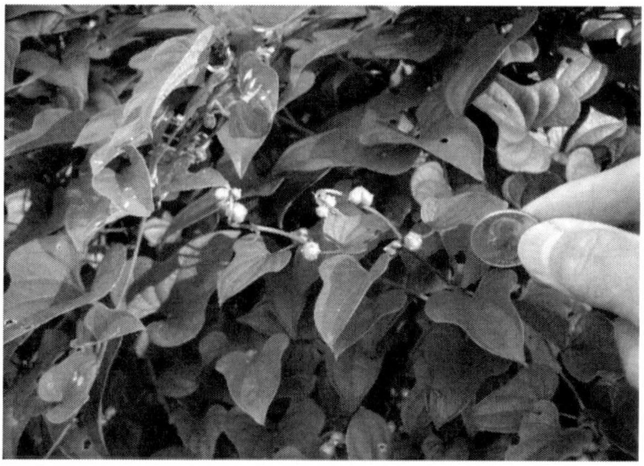

Photo 4. Tree of *Dioscorea batatas* Decaisne with fruits of yam found in Japan. Photographed by Noboru Motohashi at Tokyo Metropolitan Medicinal Garden, Tokyo, Japan. 8/1/2007 Wed.

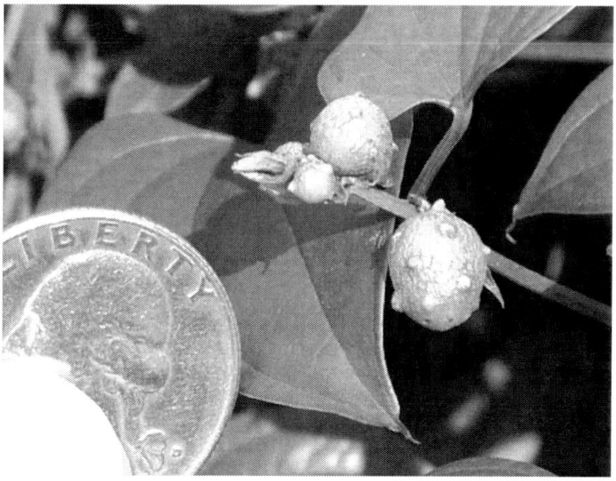

Photo 5. (Macrophoto) Fruits of *Dioscorea batatas* Decaisne of yam found in Japan. Photographed by Noboru Motohashi at Tokyo Metropolitan Medicinal Garden, Tokyo, Japan. 8/1/2007 Wed.

2.3.1.1.1. *Dioscorea septemloba*

In 2017, Zhang *et al.* confirmed *three novel diarylheptanoids*, dioscorol A (**166**), dioscoroside E1 (**167**), and dioscoroside E2 (**168**) (Figure 45), together with *five known diarylheptanoids,* 1,7-*bis*(4-hydroxyphenyl)-hepta-4*E*,6*E*-dien-3-one (**169**) [109], 1,7-*bis*(4-hydroxyphenyl)-1,4,6-heptatrien-3-one (**170**) [110], 3,5-dihydroxy-1,7-

bis(4-hydroxyphenyl)heptane (**171**) [111], (3*R*,5*R*)-3,5-dihydroxy-1,7-*bis*(4-hydroxyphenyl)heptane 3-*O*-β-D-glucopyranoside (**172**) [111], and (3*R*,5*R*)-3,5-dihydroxy-1,7-*bis*(4-hydroxy-3-methoxyphenyl)-heptane 3-*O*-β-D-glucopyranoside (**173**) [111] (Figure 45) from the 70% ethanol-water extract of *Dioscorea septemloba* rhizomes [108].

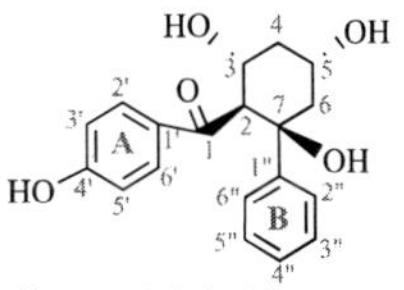
dioscorol A (**166**)

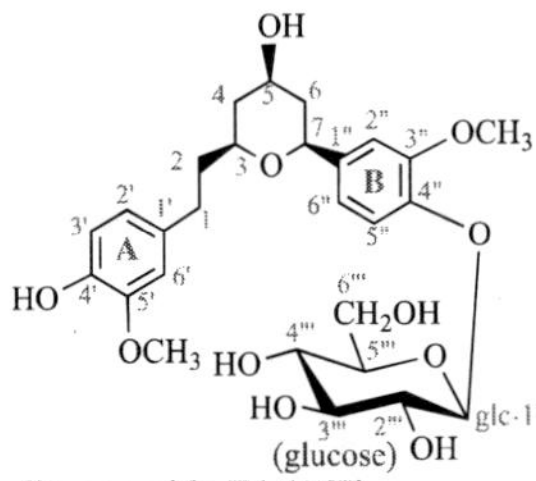
dioscoroside E1 (**167**)

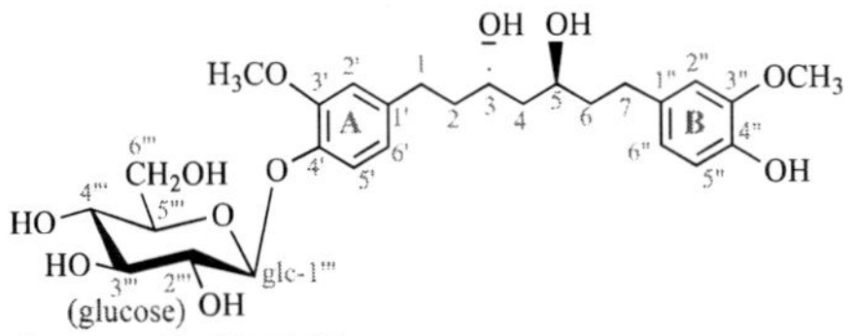
dioscoroside E2 (**168**)

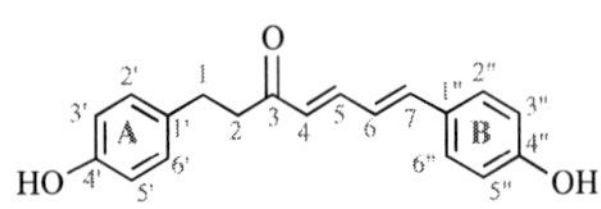
1,7-*bis*(4-hydroxyphenyl)-hepta-4*E*,6*E*-dien-3-one (**169**)

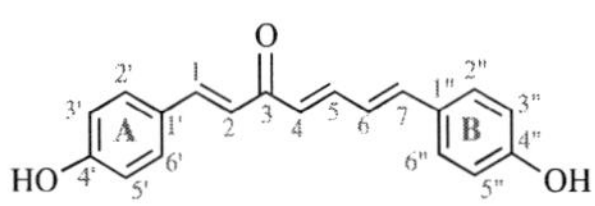
1,7-*bis*(4-hydroxyphenyl)-1,4,6-heptatrien-3-one (**170**)

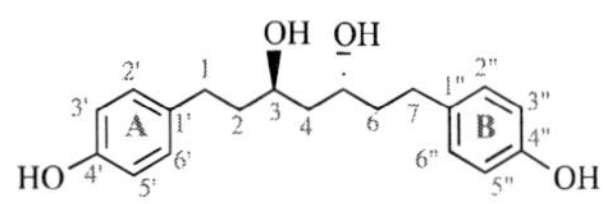
3,5-dihydroxy-1,7-*bis*(4-hydroxyphenyl)heptane (**171**)

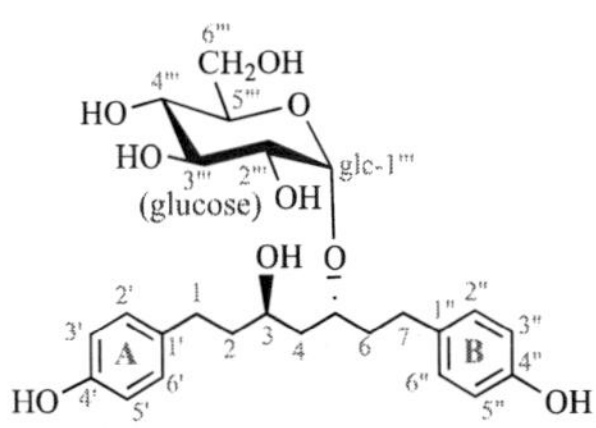
(3*R*,5*R*)-3,5-dihydroxy-1,7-*bis*(4-hydroxyphenyl)heptane 3-*O*-β-D-glucopyranoside (**172**)

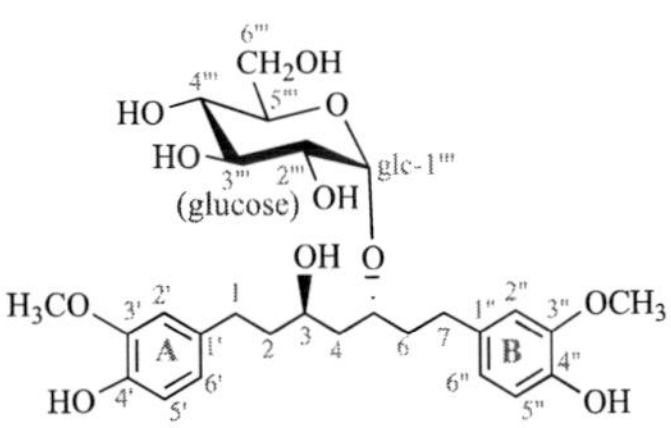
(3*R*,5*R*)-3,5-dihydroxy-1,7-*bis*(4-hydroxy-3-methoxyphenyl)-heptane 3-*O*-β-D-glucopyranoside (**173**)

Figure 45. Three novel diarylheptanoids, dioscorol A (**166**), dioscoroside E1 (**167**), dioscoroside E2 (**168**), and five known diarylheptanoids, 1,7-*bis*(4-hydroxyphenyl)-hepta-4*E*,6*E*-dien-3-one (**169**), 1,7-*bis*(4-hydroxyphenyl)-1,4,6-heptatrien-3-one (**170**), 3,5-dihydroxy-1,7-*bis*(4-hydroxyphenyl)heptane (**171**), (3*R*,5*R*)-3,5-dihydroxy-1,7-*bis*(4-hydroxyphenyl)heptane 3-*O*-β-D-glucopyranoside (**172**), and (3*R*,5*R*)-3,5-dihydroxy-1,7-*bis*(4-hydroxy-3-methoxyphenyl)-heptane 3-*O*-β-D-glucopyranoside (**173**) from the 70% ethanol-water extract of *Dioscorea septemloba* rhizomes.

2.3.1.1.2. *Dioscorea villos*

In 2012, Dong *et al.* identified five new diarylheptanoids (**174** – **178**) (Figure 46) having tetrahydropyrano core skeleton, along with nine known diarylheptanoids (**179** – **187**) (Figure 46(continued 1)) from the ethyl acetate partition of the methanol extract of *Dioscorea villos* roots/rhizomes.

Each diarylheptanoid was as follows:

Five novel diarylheptanoids (**174** – **178**): (1*S*,3*S*,5*R*,6*E*)-1,7-*bis*(4-hydroxyphenyl)-1,5-epoxy-3-hydroxyhept-6-ene (**174**), ((1*S*,3*S*,5*S*)-1,7-*bis*(4-hydroxyphenyl)-1,5-epoxy-3-hydroxyheptane (**175**), (1*R*,3*R*,5*R*)-1,7-*bis*(4-hydroxyphenyl)-1,5-epoxy-3-hydroxyheptane (**176**), (1*S*,3*R*,5*S*)-1,7-*bis*(4-hydroxyphenyl)-1,5-epoxy-3-hydroxyheptane (**177**), (1*R*,3*S*,5*R*)-1,7-*bis*(4-hydroxyphenyl)-1,5-epoxy-3-hydroxyheptane (**178**) (Figure 46).

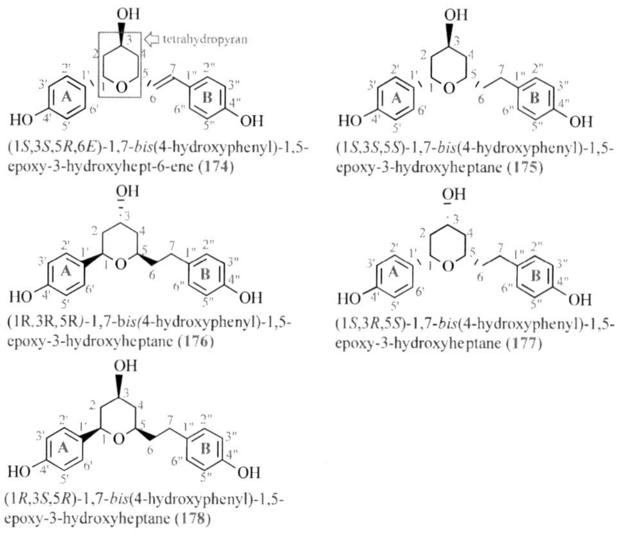

Figure 46. Five novel diarylheptanoids (174 – 178): (1*S*,3*S*,5*R*,6*E*)-1,7-*bis*(4-Hydroxyphenyl)-1,5-epoxy-3-hydroxyhept-6-ene (174), (1*S*,3*S*,5*S*)-1,7-*bis*(4-hydroxyphenyl)-1,5-epoxy-3-hydroxyheptane (175), (1*R*,3*R*,5*R*)-1,7-*bis*(4-hydroxyphenyl)-1,5-epoxy-3-hydroxyheptane (176), (1*S*,3*R*,5*S*)-1,7-*bis*(4-hydroxyphenyl)-1,5-epoxy-3-hydroxyheptane (177), and (1*R*,3*S*,5*R*)-1,7-*bis*(4-hydroxyphenyl)-1,5-epoxy-3-hydroxyheptane (178) from the ethyl acetate partition of the methanol extract of *Dioscorea villos* roots/rhizomes.

Nine known diarylheptanoids (**179** – **187**): (5*R*,1*E*)-1,7-*bis*(4-hydroxyphenyl)-5-hydroxyhept-1-en-3-one (**179**), (5*R*,1*E*)-1,7-*bis*(4-hydroxyphenyl)-5-hydroxyhept-1-en-3-one (**180**), Compound **8** (**181**), Compound **9** (**182**), Compound **10** (**183**), Compound **11** (**184**), Compound

12 (**185**), Compound **13** (**186**), and Compound **14** (**187**) (Figure 46(continued 1)) [112].

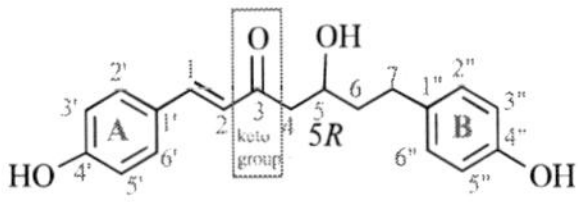

(5*R*,1*E*)-1,7-*bis*(4-hydroxyphenyl)-5-hydroxyhept-1-en-3-one (**179**)

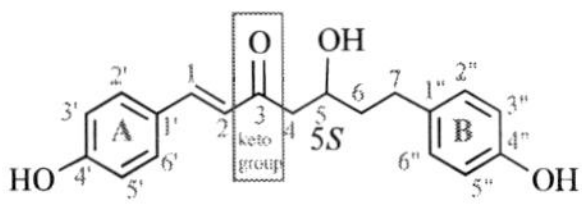

(5*R*,1*E*)-1,7-*bis*(4-hydroxyphenyl)-5-hydroxyhept-1-en-3-one (**180**)

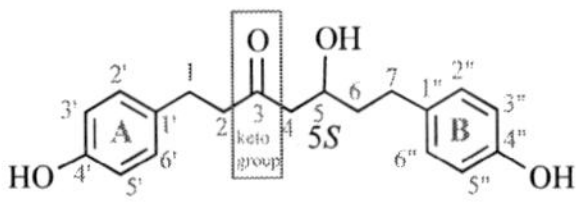

Compound **8** (**181**)

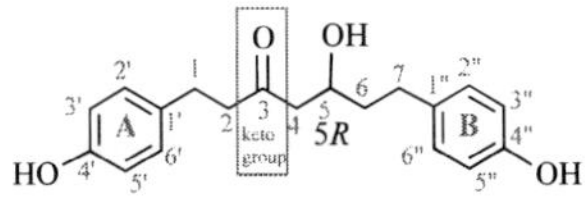

Compound **9** (**182**)

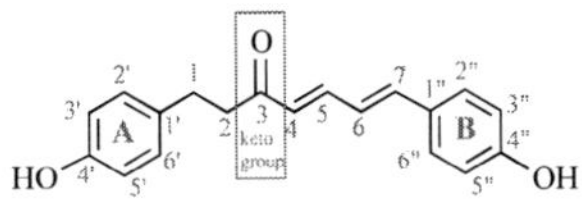

Compound **10** (**183**)

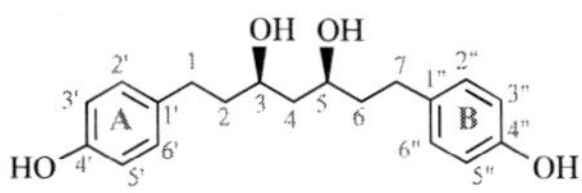

Compound **11** (**184**)

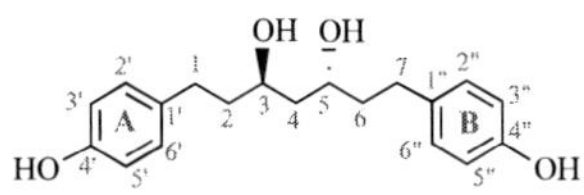

Compound **12** (**185**)

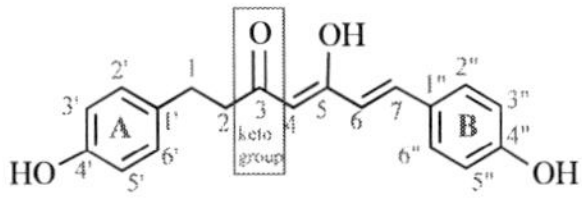

Compound **13** (**186**)

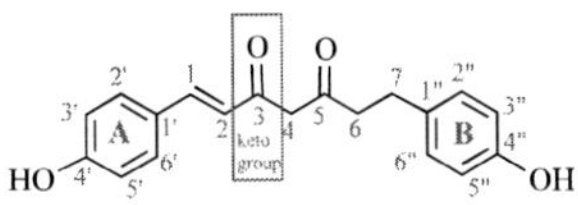

Compound **14** (**187**)

Figure 46(continued 1). Nine known diarylheptanoids (**179** – **187**): (5*R*,1*E*)-1,7-*bis*(4-hydroxyphenyl)-5-hydroxyhept-1-en-3-one (**179**), (5*R*,1*E*)-1,7-*bis*(4-hydroxyphenyl)-5-hydroxyhept-1-en-3-one (**180**), Compound **8** (**181**), Compound **9** (**182**), Compound **10** (**183**), Compound **11** (**184**), and Compound **12** (**185**), Compound **13** (**186**), and Compound **14** (**187**) from the ethyl acetate partition of the methanol extract of *Dioscorea villos* roots/rhizomes.

2.3.1.2. *Tacca*

2.3.1.2.1. *Tacca chantrieri*

In 2002, Yokosuka A *et al.* identified two novel diarylheptanoids: (3*R*,5*R*)-3,5-dihydroxy-1-(3,4-dihydroxyphenyl)-7-(4-hydroxyphenyl)-heptane (**188**) and (3*R*,5*R*)-3,5-dihydroxy-1,7-*bis*-(3,4-dihydroxy-phenyl)heptane (**189**), and seven novel diarylheptanoid glucosides: (3*R*,5*R*)-3,5-dihydroxy-1-(3,4-dihydroxyphenyl)-7-(4-hydroxyphenyl)-heptane 3-*O*-β-D-glucopyranoside (**190**), (3*R*,5*R*)-3,5-dihydroxy-1-(3,4-dihydroxyphenyl)-7-(4-hydroxyphenyl)heptane 5-*O*-β-D-glucopyranoside

(**191**), (3*R*,5*R*)-3,5-dihydroxy-1-(4-hydroxy-3-methoxyphenyl)-7-(4-hydroxyphenyl)heptane 3-*O*-β-D-glucopyranoside (**192**), (3*R*,5*R*)-3,5-dihydroxy-1,7-*bis*(3,4-dihydroxyphenyl)heptane 3-*O*-β-D-glucopyranoside (**193**) (Figure 47), (3*R*,5*R*)-3,5-dihydroxy-1-(4-hydroxy-3-methoxyphenyl)-7-(3,4-dihydroxyphenyl)heptane 3-*O*-β-D-glucopyranoside (**194**), (3*R*,5*R*)-3,5-dihydroxy-1,7-*bis*(4-hydroxy-3-methoxyphenyl)-heptane 3-*O*-β-D-glucopyranoside (**195**) and (3*R*,5*R*)-3,5-dihydroxy-1,7-*bis*(4-hydroxyphenyl)heptane 3-*O*-β-D-glucopyranoside (**196**) (Figure 47 (continued 1)) from the rhizomes of *Tacca chantrieri*.

(two novel diarylheptanoids)

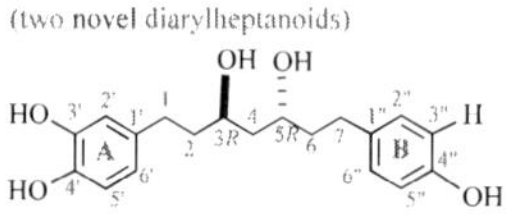

(3*R*,5*R*)-3,5-dihydroxy-1-(3,4-dihydroxyphenyl)-7- (4-hydroxyphenyl)heptane (**188**)

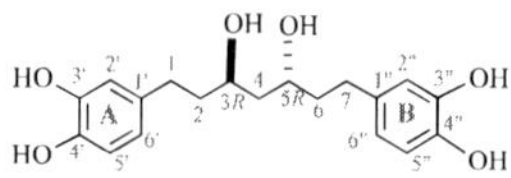

(3*R*,5*R*)-3,5-dihydroxy-1,7-*bis*-(3,4-dihydroxyphenyl)heptane (**189**)

(seven novel diarylheptanoid glucosides)

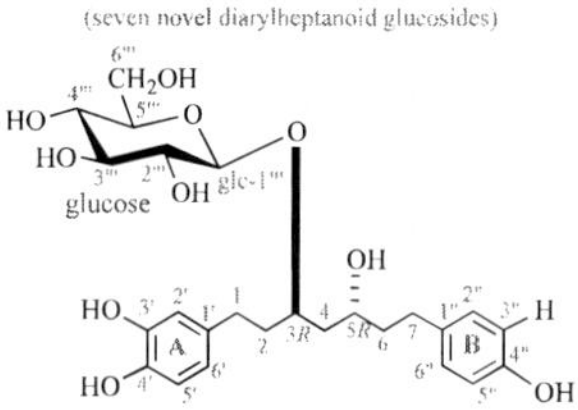

(3*R*,5*R*)-3,5-dihydroxy-1-(3,4-dihydroxyphenyl)-7-(4-hydroxyphenyl)-heptane 3-*O*-β-D-glucopyranoside (**190**)

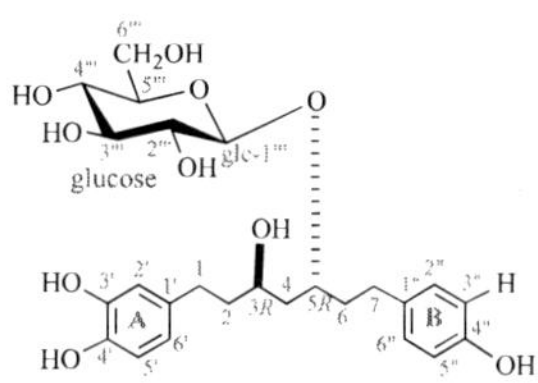

(3*R*,5*R*)-3,5-dihydroxy-1-(3,4-dihydroxyphenyl)-7-(4-hydroxyphenyl)heptane 5-*O*-β-D-glucopyranoside (**191**)

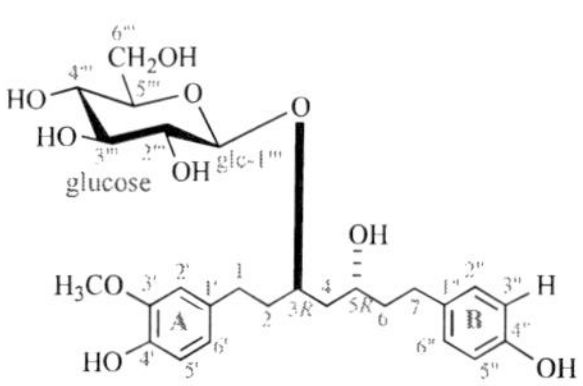

(3*R*,5*R*)-3,5-dihydroxy-1-(4-hydroxy-3-methoxyphenyl)-7-(4-hydroxyphenyl)heptane 3-*O*-β-D-glucopyranoside (**192**)

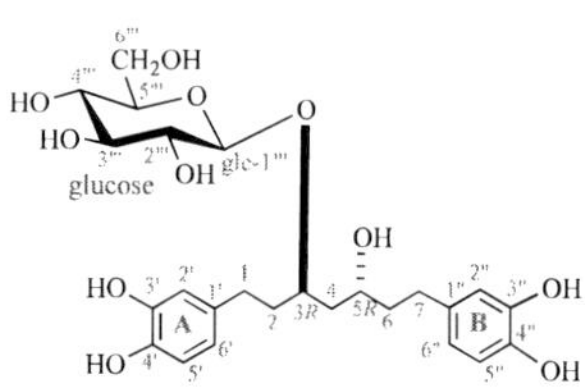

(3*R*,5*R*)-3,5-dihydroxy-1,7-*bis*(3,4-dihydroxyphenyl)heptane 3-*O*-β-D-glucopyranoside (**193**)

Figure 47. Two novel diarylheptanoids: (3*R*,5*R*)-3,5-dihydroxy-1-(3,4-dihydroxyphenyl)-7- (4-hydroxyphenyl)heptane (**188**) and (3*R*,5*R*)-3,5-dihydroxy-1,7-*bis*-(3,4-dihydroxyphenyl)heptane (**189**), and seven novel diarylheptanoid glucosides: (3*R*,5*R*)-3,5-dihydroxy-1-(3,4-dihydroxyphenyl)-7-(4-hydroxyphenyl)-heptane 3-*O*-β-D-glucopyranoside (**190**), (3*R*,5*R*)-3,5-dihydroxy-1-(3,4-dihydroxyphenyl)-7-(4-hydroxyphenyl)heptane 5-*O*-β-D-glucopyranoside (**191**), (3*R*,5*R*)-3,5-dihydroxy-1-(4-hydroxy-3-methoxyphenyl)-7-(4-hydroxyphenyl)heptane 3-*O*-β-D-glucopyranoside (**192**) and (3*R*,5*R*)-3,5-dihydroxy-1,7-*bis*(3,4-dihydroxyphenyl)heptane 3-*O*-β-D-glucopyranoside (**193**) from the rhizomes of *Tacca chantrieri*.

(continued) (seven novel diarylheptanoid glucosides)

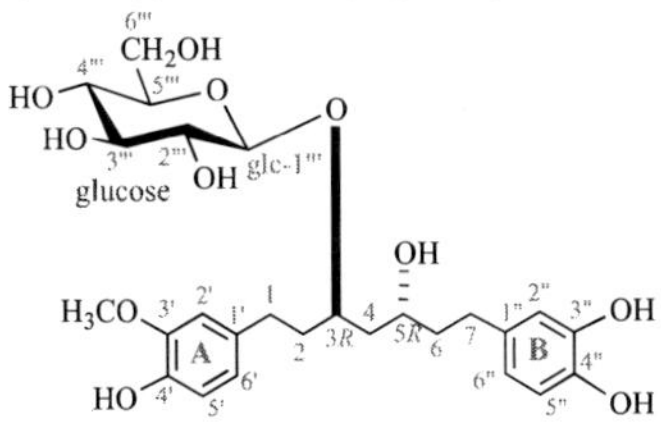

(3*R*,5*R*)-3,5-dihydroxy-1-(4-hydroxy-3-methoxyphenyl)-7-(3,4-dihydroxyphenyl)heptane 3-*O*-β-D-glucopyranoside (**194**)

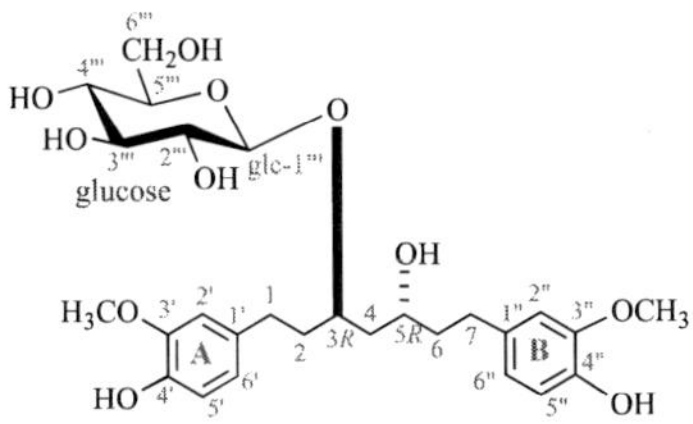

(3*R*,5*R*)-3,5-dihydroxy-1,7-*bis*(4-hydroxy-3-methoxyphenyl)-heptane 3-*O*-β-D-glucopyranoside (**195**)

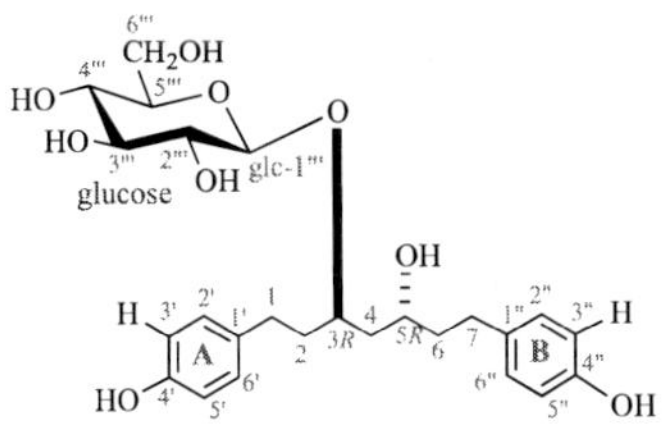

(3*R*,5*R*)-3,5-dihydroxy-1,7-*bis*(4-hydroxyphenyl)heptane 3-*O*-β-D-glucopyranoside (**196**)

Figure 47(continued 1). Seven novel diarylheptanoid glucosides: (3*R*,5*R*)-3,5-dihydroxy-1-(4-hydroxy-3-methoxyphenyl)-7-(3,4-dihydroxyphenyl)heptane 3-*O*-β-D-glucopyranoside (**194**), (3*R*,5*R*)-3,5-dihydroxy-1,7-*bis*(4-hydroxy-3-methoxyphenyl)-heptane 3-*O*-β-D-glucopyranoside (**195**) and (3*R*,5*R*)-3,5-dihydroxy-1,7-*bis*(4-hydroxyphenyl)heptane 3-*O*-β-D-glucopyranoside (**196**) from the rhizomes of *Tacca chantrieri*.

On their cytotoxic activities using a modified methylthiazole tetrazolium (MTT) assay method of novel diarylheptanoids (**188** - **196**) and a positive control etoposide (a type of topoisomerase inhibitor) against human promyelocytic leukemia cells (HL-60), human oral squamous carcinoma cells (HSC-2) and normal human gingival fibroblasts (HGF), two diarylheptanoids (**188** and **189**), and four diarylheptanoid glucosides (**190**, **191**, **193** and **194**) having each three or four phenolic hydroxyl groups showed moderate cytotoxic activity (IC_{50}: 1.8-6.4 μg/mL) against only HL-60 cells.

On the other hand, three diarylheptanoid glucosides (**192**, **195** and **196**) having two phenolic hydroxyl groups did not exhibit apparent cytotoxic activity even at a sample concentration of 10 μg/mL.

These results suggest that the cytotoxicity of diarylheptanoids contributes to the high number of phenolic hydroxyl groups [111].

2.4. Order Ericale

2.4.1. Actinidiaceae

2.4.1.1. Clematoclethra

2.4.1.1.1. *Clematoclethra actinidioides*

In 2006, Guo *et al.* isolated a novel diarylheptanoid actinidione (**197**) (Figure 48) from the 95% ethanol extracts of leaves and twigs of *Clematoclethra actinidioides* Maxim (the family: Actinidiaceae; the genus: Clematoclethra).

Their 50% growth inhibitions (GI_{50} values) (μg/mL) of actinidione (**197**) (Figure 48)/positive control irinotecan (**198**) (Figure 48) of topoisomerase I inhibition were 31.82 μg/mL(**197**)/0.83 μg/mL(**198**) for human lung cancer (Lu-06 cell line), 15.02/0.70 for human neuroma (N-04 cell line), and 26.67/1.58 for human breast cancer (Bre-04 cell line), respectively [113].

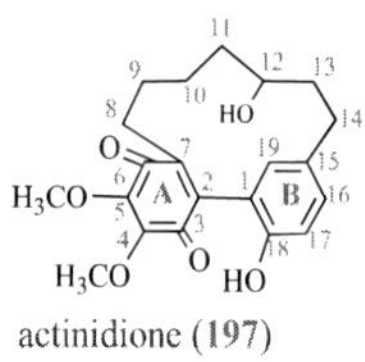
actinidione (**197**)

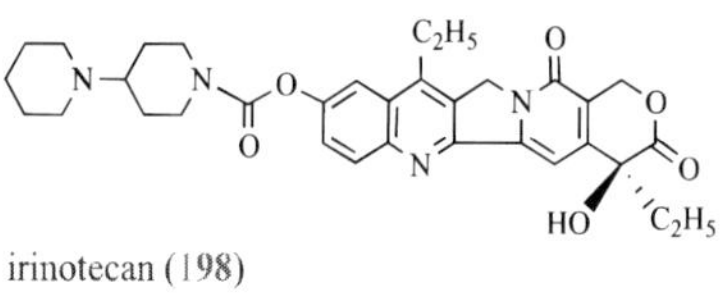
irinotecan (**198**)

Figure 48. Actinidione (**197**) from the 95% ethanol extracts of leaves and twigs of *Clematoclethra actinidioides* Maxim. Positive control irinotecan (**198**) of Topoisomerase I inhibition.

2.5. Order Gentiales

2.5.1 Rubiaceae

2.5.1.1. Pyrostria

2.5.1.1.1. *Pyrostria major* (A. Rich & DC.) Cavaco [Syn. *Canthium major* (A. Rich & DC.)] Cavaco

In 2012, Beniddir MA *et al.* identified eight novel diarylheptanoid glucosides: (3*S*,5*S*)-3,5-dihydroxy-1,7-*bis*(4-methoxyphenyl)heptyl 3-*O*-β-

D-glucopyranoside (**199**), (3*S*,5*S*)-3,5-dihydroxy-1-(3-hydroxy-4-methoxyphenyl)-7-(4-methoxyphenyl)heptyl 3-*O*-β-D-glucopyranoside (**200**), (3*S*,5*S*)-1-(3,4-dihydroxyphenyl)-3,5-dihydroxy-7-(4-methoxy-phenyl)heptyl 3-*O*-β-D-glucopyranoside (**201**), (3*S*,5*S*)-3,5-dihydroxy-1,7-*bis*(3,4-dihydroxyphenyl)heptyl 3-*O*-β-D-glucopyranoside (**202**) (Figure 49), (3*S*,5*S*)-3,5-dihydroxy-7-(3-hydroxy-4-methoxyphenyl)-1-(4-methy-oxyphenyl)heptyl 3-*O*-β-D-glucopyranoside (**203**), 1-(3,4-dihydro-xyphenyl)-3,5-dihydroxy-7-(3-hydroxy-4-methoxyphenyl)heptyl 3-*O*-β-D-glucopyranoside (**204**), 1-(3,4-dihydroxyphenyl)-5-formyl-3-hydroxy-7-(4-methoxyphenyl)heptyl 3-*O*-β-D-glucopyranoside (**205**), and 1,7-*bis*(3,4-dihydroxyphenyl)-5-formyl-3-hydroxyheptyl 3-*O*-β-D-glucopyranoside (**206**) (Figure 49(continued 1)) from the leaves of *Pyrostria major* (A. Rich & DC.) Cavaco [syn. *Canthium major* (A. Rich & DC.)] Cavaco.

Regarding antiplasmodial activity against malaria parasites that infects humans and animals and causes malaria to develop and destroy in erythrocytes, antileishmanial activity and antitrypanosomal activity on eight naturally occuring novel diarylheptanoid glucosides (**199** - **206**), eight naturally occurring novel diarylheptanoid glucosides (**199** - **206**) were estimated on their antiprotozoal activity against *three types of protozoa*: *Plasmodium falciparum* strain FcB1 (erythrocytic stage) chloroquine (**207**) (Figure 50)-resistant strain of *Plasmodium falciparum*), visceral leishmaniasis (VL. kala-azar) pathogen *Leishmania donovani* (MHOM/ET/67/HU3) line (called LV9. intramacroph-age amastigotes, amastigote form) and tropical parasites of tropical Africa causing nagana (nagana pest) in horses *etc.* by transmission of tsetse flies *Trypanosoma brucei* (trypomastigote) CMP strain, minimum effective concentration (MEC), and on their *in vitro* cytotoxic activity against *three types of tumor cell lines*: human promyelocytic leukemia celllines (HL-60), human mouth epidermoid carcinoma HeLa-KB cell (KB cell lines) and Medical Research Council cell strain 5 (MRC-5 cell lines) of diploid human cell culture system composed of fibroblasts from lung tissue of a 14-week-old aborted Caucasian male fetus.

Here, the positive controls for three types of protozoa were a malaria specific drug chloroquine (**207**), pentamidine (**208**) (Figure 50) for a treatment for carinii pneumonia, and an antifungal agent amphotericin B (**209**) (Figure 50). Furthermore, docetaxel (DTX. TXT. **210**) (Figure 50) was used as a positive control for three types of tumor cell lines (HL-60, KB, MRC-5 cell lines).

First, antiplasmodial activity (50% inhibitory concentration (IC_{50}: μM)) against *Plasmodium falciparum* strain FcB1 (erythrocytic stage) was the highest chloroquine (**207**) (0.05 ± 0.02), followed by eight naturally occurring novel diarylheptanoid glucosides (**199** - **206**)) (>20), and pentamidine (**208**) and amphotericin B (**209**) (each not done (n.d.)), respectively.

Second, antileishmanial activity (IC_{50}: μM) against *Leishmania donovani* (MHOM/ET/67/HU3) line. called LV9. intramacroph-age amastigotes (amastigote form) was the highest amphotericin B (**209**) (0.10 ± 0.02), followed by pentamidine (**208**) (11.2 ± 1.3), (3*S*,5*S*)-3,5-dihydroxy-1-(3-hydroxy-4-methoxyphenyl)-7-(4-methoxyphenyl)heptyl 3-*O*-β-D-glucopyranoside (**200**) (31.2 ± 2.5), 1-(3,4-dihydroxyphenyl)-5-formyl-3-hydroxy-7-(4-methoxyphenyl)heptyl 3-*O*-β-D-glucopyranoside (**205**) (33.0 ± 2.6), (3*S*,5*S*)-1-(3,4-dihydroxyphenyl)-3,5-dihydroxy-7-(4-methoxyphenyl)heptyl 3-*O*-β-D-glucopyranoside (**201**) (33.2 ± 2.6), (3*S*,5*S*)-3,5-dihydroxy-1,7-*bis*(3,4-dihydroxyphenyl)heptyl 3-*O*-β-D-glucopyranoside (**202**) (33.3 ± 2.6), 1,7-*bis*(3,4-dihydroxyphenyl)-5-formyl-3-hydroxyheptyl 3-*O*-β-D-glucopyranoside (**206**) (34.6 ± 2.7), (3*S*,5*S*)-3,5-dihydroxy-1,7-*bis*(4-methoxyphenyl)heptyl 3-*O*-β-D-glucopyranoside (**199**) (39.7 ± 3.2), (3*S*,5*S*)-3,5-dihydroxy-7-(3-hydroxy-4-methoxyphenyl)-1-(4-methyoxyphenyl)heptyl 3-*O*-β-D-glucopyranoside (**203**) (41.4 ± 3.3), 1-(3,4-dihydroxyphenyl)-3,5-dihydroxy-7-(3-hydroxy-4-methoxyphenyl)heptyl 3-*O*-β-D-glucopyranoside (**204**) (>100), and chloroquine (**207**) (n.d.), respectively.

Third, antitrypanosomal activity (IC_{50}: μM) was the highest pentamidine (**208**) (3.1), followed by 1-(3,4-dihydroxyphenyl)-3,5-dihydroxy-7-(3-hydroxy-4-methoxyphenyl)heptyl 3-*O*-β-D-glucopyranoside (**204**) (12.5), (3*S*,5*S*)-3,5-dihydroxy-1,7-*bis*(3,4-dihydroxyphenyl)heptyl 3-*O*-β-D-glucopyranoside (**202**), 1-(3,4-dihydroxyphenyl)-5-formyl-3-hydroxy-7-(4-methoxyphenyl)heptyl 3-*O*-β-D-glucopyranoside

(**205**) and 1,7-*bis*(3,4-dihydroxyphenyl)-5-formyl-3-hydroxyheptyl 3-*O*-β-D-glucopyranoside (**206**) (each 25), (3*S*,5*S*)-3,5-dihydroxy-1,7-*bis*(4-methoxyphenyl)heptyl 3-*O*-β-D-glucopyranoside (**199**), (3*S*,5*S*)-3,5-dihydroxy-1-(3-hydroxy-4-methoxyphenyl)-7-(4-metho-xyphenyl)heptyl 3-*O*-β-D-glucopyranoside (**200**), (3*S*,5*S*)-1-(3,4-dihydroxyphenyl)-3,5-dihydroxy-7-(4-methoxyphenyl)heptyl 3-*O*-β-D-glucopyranoside (**201**) and (3*S*,5*S*)-3,5-dihydroxy-7-(3-hydroxy-4-methoxyphenyl)-1-(4-methy-oxyphenyl)heptyl 3-*O*-β-D-glucopyranoside (**203**) (each >100), and chloroquine (**207**) and amphotericin B (**209**) (each n.d.), respectively.

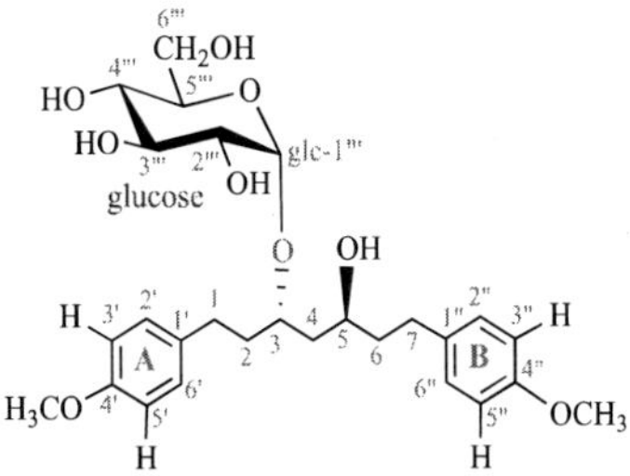

(3*S*,5*S*)-3,5-dihydroxy-1,7-*bis*(4-methoxyphenyl)heptyl 3-*O*-β-D-glucopyranoside (**199**)

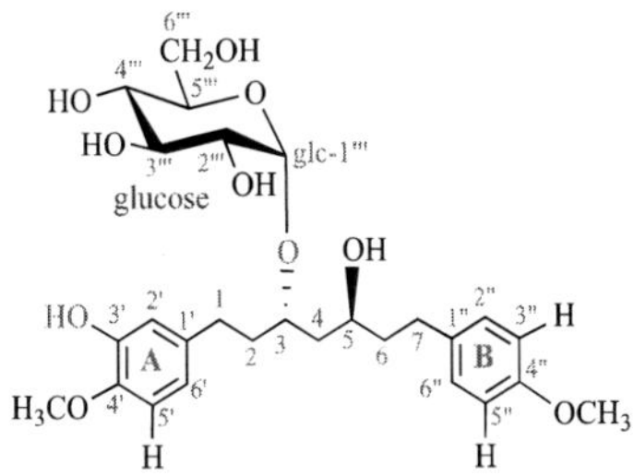

(3*S*,5*S*)-3,5-dihydroxy-1-(3-hydroxy-4-methoxyphenyl)-7-(4-methoxyphenyl)heptyl 3-*O*-β-D-glucopyranoside (**200**)

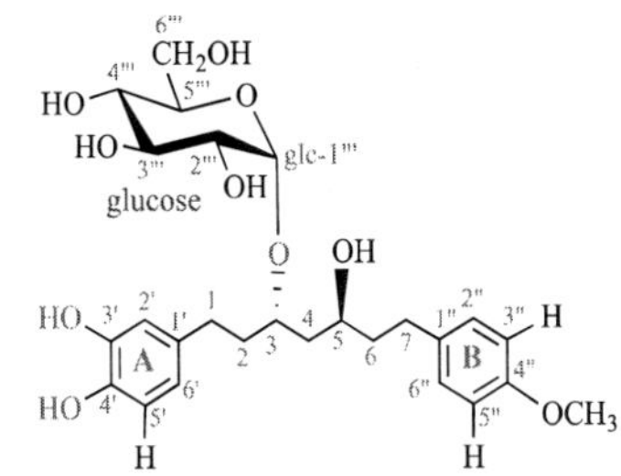

(3*S*,5*S*)-1-(3,4-dihydroxyphenyl)-3,5-dihydroxy-7-(4-methoxyphenyl)heptyl 3-*O*-β-D-glucopyranoside (**201**)

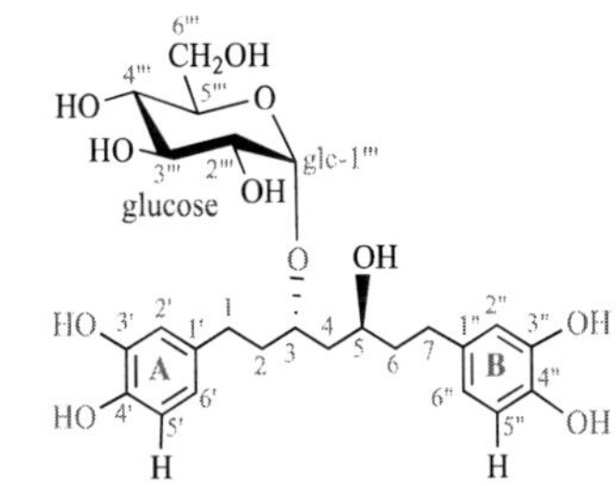

(3*S*,5*S*)-3,5-dihydroxy-1,7-*bis*(3,4-dihydroxyphenyl)heptyl 3-*O*-β-D-glucopyranoside (**202**)

Figure 49. Eight novel diarylheptanoid glucosides: (3*S*,5*S*)-3,5-dihydroxy-1,7-*bis*(4-methoxyphenyl)heptyl 3-*O*-β-D-glucopyranoside (**199**), (3*S*,5*S*)-3,5-dihydroxy-1-(3-hydroxy-4-methoxyphenyl)-7-(4-methoxyphenyl)heptyl 3-*O*-β-D-glucopyranoside (**200**), (3*S*,5*S*)-1-(3,4-dihydroxyphenyl)-3,5-dihydroxy-7-(4-methoxyphenyl)heptyl 3-*O*-β-D-glucopyranoside (**201**), and (3*S*,5*S*)-3,5-dihydroxy-1,7-*bis*(3,4-dihydroxyphenyl)heptyl 3-*O*-β-D-glucopyranoside (**202**) from the leaves of *Pyrostria major* (A. Rich & DC.) Cavaco [syn. *Canthium major* (A. Rich & DC.)] Cavaco).

From the above results, among eight naturally occurring novel diarylheptanoid glucosides (**199 - 206**), 1-(3,4-dihydroxyphenyl)-3,5-dihydroxy-7-(3-hydroxy-4-methoxyphenyl)heptyl 3-*O*-β-D-glucopyranoside (**204**) showed a significant antitrypanosomal activity against *Trypanosoma brucei* (trypomastigote) CMP strain.

Eight naturally occurring novel diarylheptanoid glucosides (**199 - 206**) showed no cytotoxic activity for three any tumor cell lines (HL-60, KB, and MRC-5 cell lines) [114].

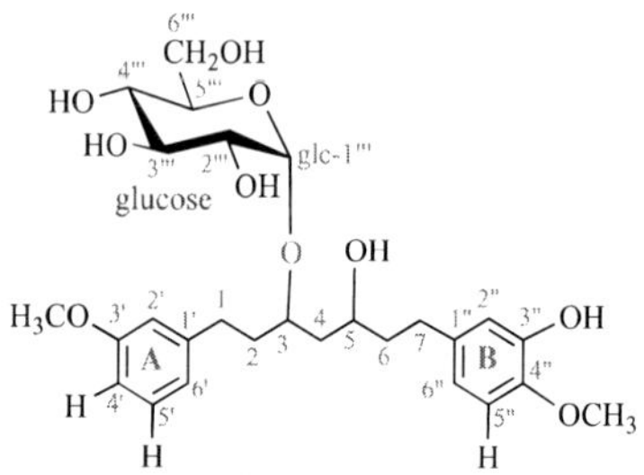

(3*S*,5*S*)-3,5-dihydroxy-7-(3-hydroxy-4-methoxyphenyl)-1-(4-methyoxyphenyl)heptyl 3-*O*-β-D-glucopyranoside (**203**)

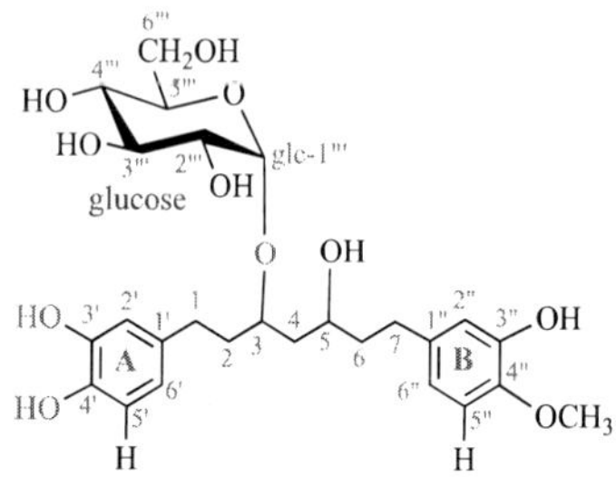

1-(3,4-dihydroxyphenyl)-3,5-dihydroxy-7-(3-hydroxy-4-methoxyphenyl)heptyl 3-*O*-β-D-glucopyranoside (**204**)

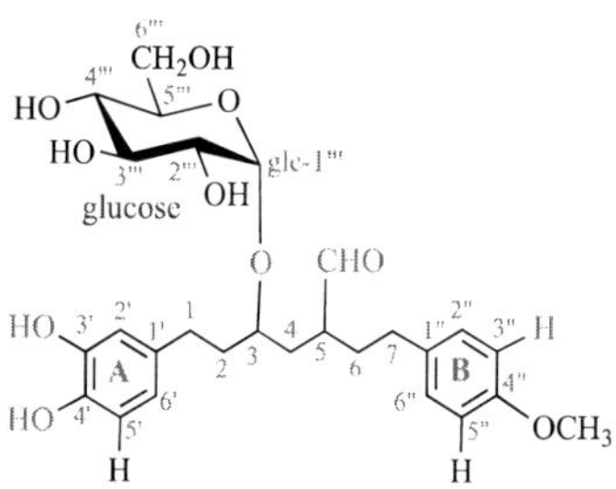

1-(3,4-dihydroxyphenyl)-5-formyl-3-hydroxy-7-(4-methoxyphenyl)heptyl 3-*O*-β-D-glucopyranoside (**205**)

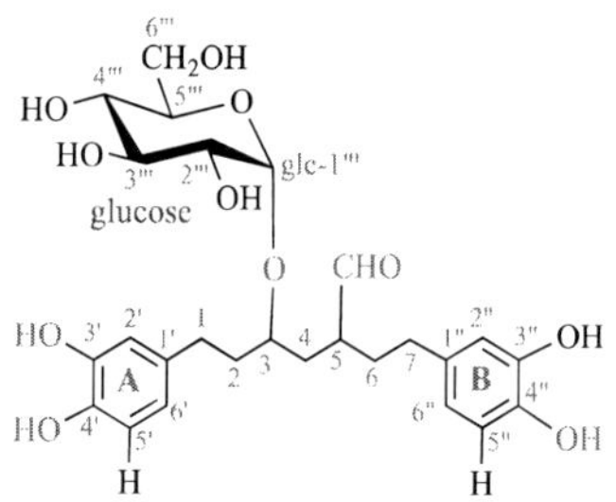

1,7-*bis*(3,4-dihydroxyphenyl)-5-formyl-3-hydroxyheptyl 3-*O*-β-D-glucopyranoside (**206**)

Figure 49(continued 1). Eight novel diarylheptanoid glucosides: (3*S*,5*S*)-3,5-dihydroxy-7-(3-hydroxy-4-methoxyphenyl)-1-(4-methyoxyphenyl)heptyl 3-*O*-β-D-glucopyranoside (**203**), 1-(3,4-dihydroxyphenyl)-3,5-dihydroxy-7-(3-hydroxy-4-methoxyphenyl)heptyl 3-*O*-β-D-glucopyranoside (**204**), 1-(3,4-dihydroxyphenyl)-5-formyl-3-hydroxy-7-(4-methoxyphenyl)heptyl 3-*O*-β-D-glucopyranoside (**205**), and 1,7-*bis*(3,4-dihydroxyphenyl)-5-formyl-3-hydroxyheptyl 3-*O*-β-D-glucopyranoside (**206**) from the leaves of *Pyrostria major* (A. Rich & DC.) Cavaco [syn. *Canthium major* (A. Rich & DC.)] Cavaco).

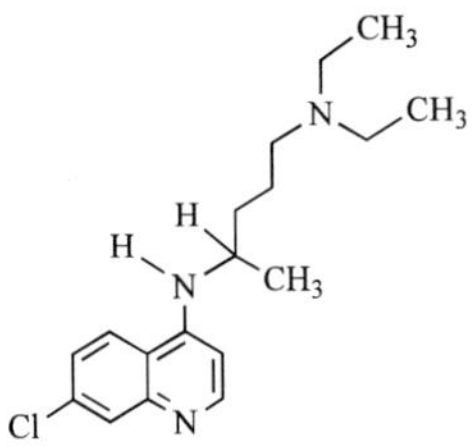

chloroquine (**207**)

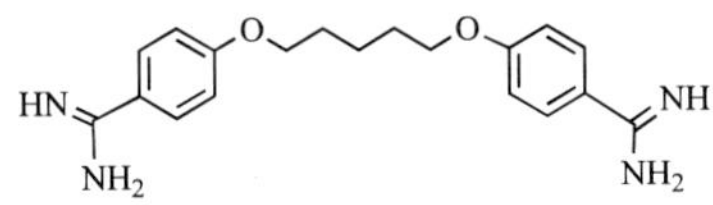

pentamidine (**208**)

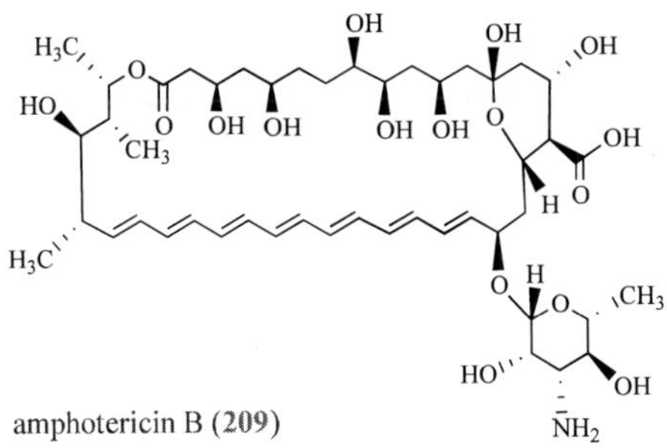

amphotericin B (**209**)

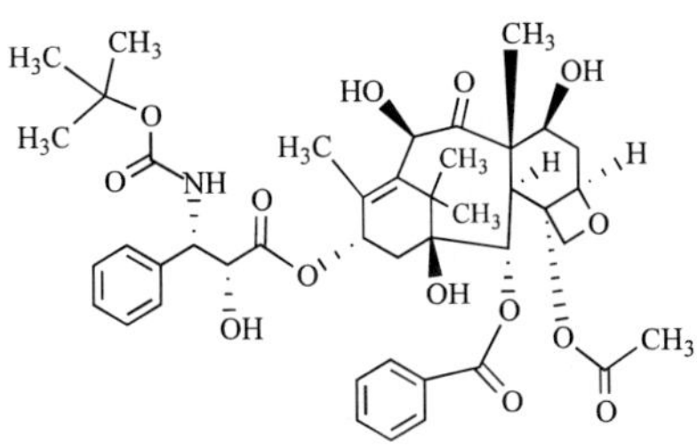

docetaxel (DTX. TXT. **210**)

Figure 50. Positive controls: chloroquine (**207**), pentamidine (**208**), amphotericin B (**209**), and docetaxel (DTX. TXT. **210**).

2.6. Order Juglandales

2.6.1. Juglandaceae

2.6.1.1. Juglans

The genus Juglans found in Japan is *Juglans mandshurica* Maxim. var. sieboldiana Makino (walnut) (Photos 6 and 7).

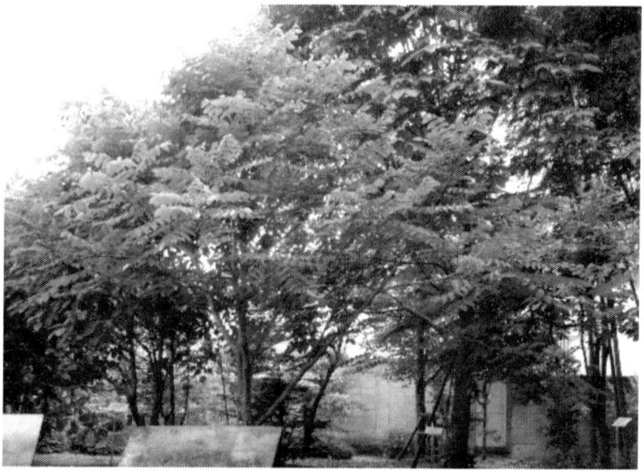

Photo 6. Whole plants of *Juglans mandshurica* Maxim. var. sieboldiana Makino (walnut) of walnut found in Japan. Photographed by Noboru Motohashi at Tokyo Metropolitan Medicinal Garden, Tokyo, Japan. 6/10/2008 Tue.

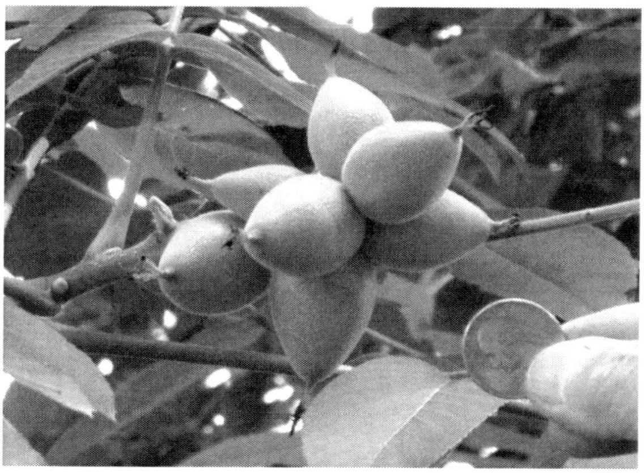

Photo 7. Walnut tree with young fruits. Photographed by Noboru Motohashi at Tokyo Metropolitan Medicinal Garden, Tokyo, Japan. 6/10/2008 Tue.

2.6.1.1.1. *Juglans regia*

In 2008, Liu J *et al.* identified four diarylheptanoids: juglanin A (JA. **211**, rhoiptelol (RH. **212**), juglanin C (JC. **213**) and juglanin B (JB. **214**) (Figure 51) in methanol extracts from the husks of *Juglans regia* L. (green walnut) [115].

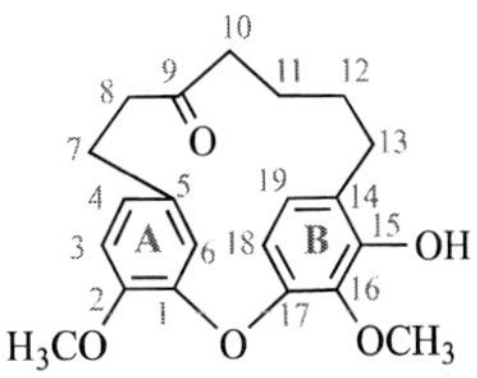

juglanin A (JA. **211**)

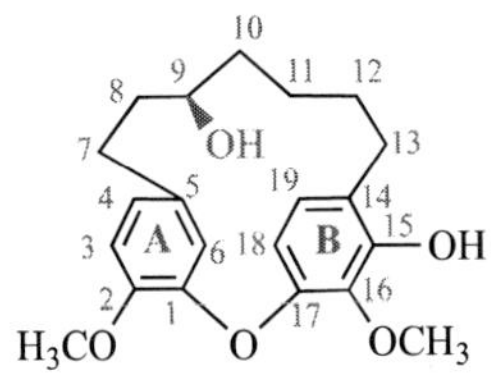

rhoiptelol (RH. **212**)

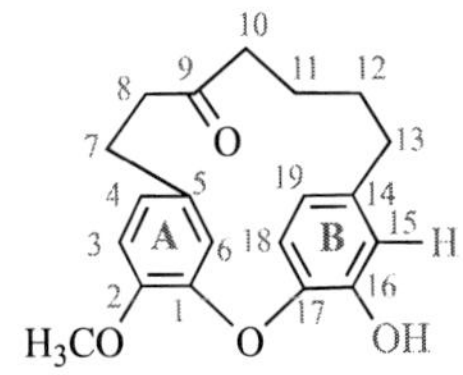

juglanin C (JC. **213**)

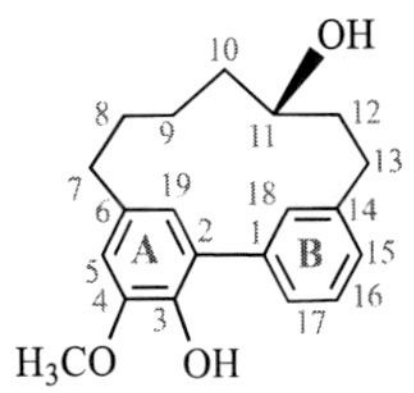

juglanin B (JB. **214**)

Figure 51. Four diarylheptanoids: juglanin A (JA. **211**), rhoiptelol (RH. **212**), juglanin C (JC. **213**) and juglanin B (JB. **214**) in methanol extracts from the husks of *Juglans regia* L. (green walnut).

2.6.1.2. *Platycarya*

2.6.1.2.1. *Platycarya strobilacea*

In 1998, Tanaka *et al.* identified a novel diphenylether-type diarylheptanoid platycarynol (**215**) (Figure 52) from the heartwood of *Platycarya strobilacea* [116].

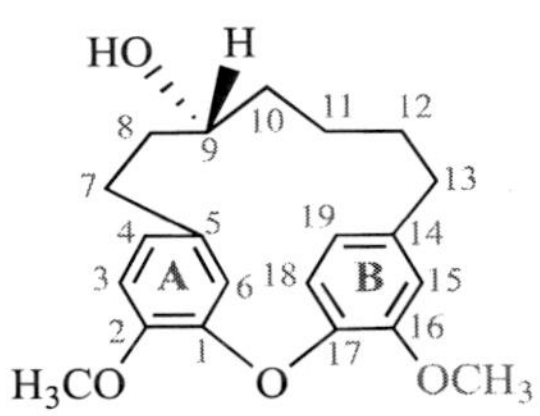

platycarynol (**215**)

Figure 52. A novel diphenylether-type diarylheptanoid platycarynol (**215**) from the heartwood of *Platycarya strobilacea*.

2.6.1.3. Pterocarya

2.6.1.3.1. *Pterocarya tonkinesis* (Franch.) Dode

In 2005, Liu *et al.* confirmed a novel diarylheptanoid pterocarine (**216**) (Figure 53) with kown diarylheptanoid myricatomentogenin ((+)-3',4"-epoxy-1-(4'-hydroxylphenyl)-7-(3"-hydroxyphenyl)heptane-3-one. **217**) (Figure 53) from the air-dried stems and barks of *Pterocarya tonkinesis* (Franch.) Dode.

Pterocarine (**216**) showed the growth inhibitory effects against the cell cycle in tsFT210 cells (a mouse temperature-sensitive mutant tsFT210 cells isolated from the mouse mammary carcinoma cell line FM3A, and tsFT210 cells lack the necessary cdc2 kinase for triggering mitosis in the cdc2 gene) (inhibition rate: 20.2±2.4%), HCT-15 cells (inhibition rate: 23.8±2.4%) and K562 cells (chronic myelogenous leukemia cells) (inhibition rate: 50.5±1.2%) at the concentration of 100 μg/mL pterocarine (**216**), respectively.

Furthermore, pterocarine (**216**) inhibited the cell cycle of mainly the F_0/G_1 phase against tsFT210 cells, HCT-15 cells and K562 cells and, also induced apoptosis against HCT-15 cells (apoptosis rate: 19%) and K562 cells (apoptosis rate: 11%) at the concentration of 100 μg/mL pterocarine (**216**), respectively.

So far, the biological activities of several diarylheptanoids have been known [105, 117, 118]. However, pterocarine (**216**) is a novel member of diarylheptanoids and provided the first report of diarylheptanoids having the biological activities of both the inhibition of cell cycle and apoptosis induction [119].

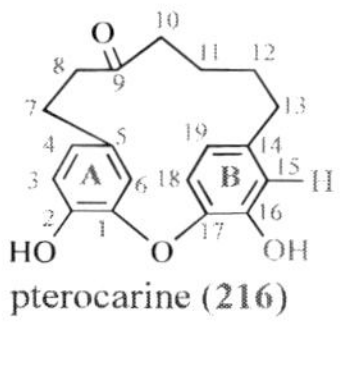

pterocarine (**216**)

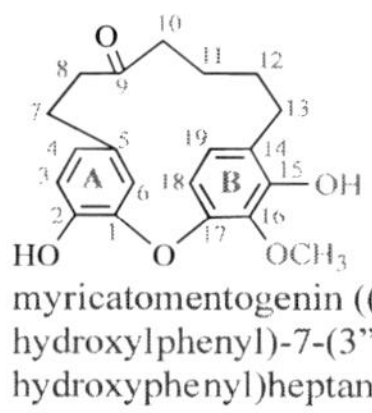

myricatomentogenin ((+)-3',4"-epoxy-1-(4'-hydroxylphenyl)-7-(3"-hydroxyphenyl)heptane-3-one. **217**)

Figure 53. Pterocarine (**216**) and myricatomentogenin ((+)-3',4"-epoxy-1-(4'-hydroxylphenyl)-7-(3"-hydroxyphenyl)heptane-3-one. **217**) from the air-dried stems and barks of *Pterocarya tonkinesis* (Franch.) Dode..

2.6.2. Rhoipteleaceae

2.6.2.1. Rhoiptelea

2.6.2.1.1. *Rhoiptelea chiliantha*

In 1996, Jiang *et al.* isolated three novel diarylheptanoids rhoiptelol A (**218**) from the leaves, and rhoiptelol B (**219**) and rhoiptelol C (**220**) (Figure 54) from the fruits of *Rhoiptelea chiliantha*, respectively [120].

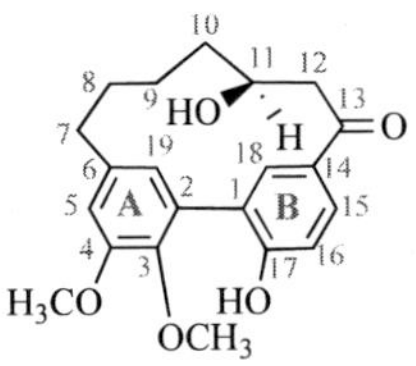

rhoiptelol A (**218**)

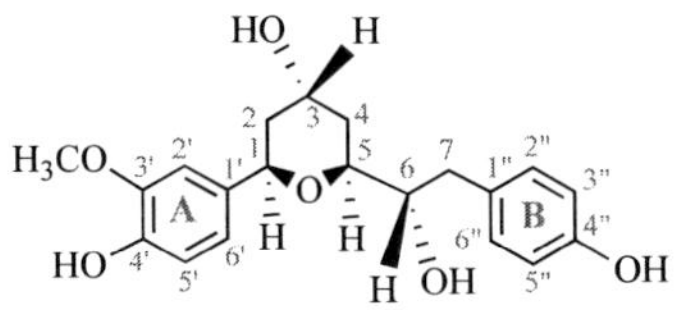

rhoiptelol B (**219**)

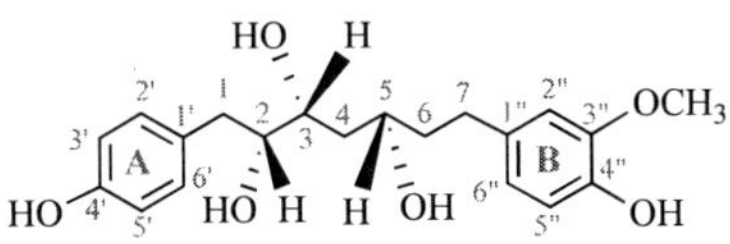

rhoiptelol C (**220**)

Figure 54. Three novel diarylheptanods - rhoiptelol A (**218**) from the leaves, and rhoiptelol B (**219**) and rhoiptelol C (**220**) from the fruits of *Rhoiptelea chiliantha*.

2.7. Order Santalales

2.7.1. Santalaceae (Old Name: Viscaceae)

2.7.1.1. Viscum

2.7.1.1.1. *Viscum cruciatum*

2.7.1.1.1.1. *Viscum cruciatum*/2001

In 2001, Martín-Cordero *et al.* isolated a linear-diarylheptanoid, hirsutanone (1,7-di-(3',4'-dihydroxyphenyl)-4-hepten-3-one. **221**) (Figure

55) from the methanolic extract of the aerial parts of *Viscum cruciatum* (old name: Viscaceae family).

Subsequently, the cytotoxicity of hirsutanone (1,7-di-(3',4'-dihydroxyphenyl)-4-hepten-3-one. **221**) was examined:

First, 50% growth-inhibitory concentration (GI_{50} value) of positive control etoposide (VP-16. **222**) (semi-synthetic antineoplastic agent based on *Podophyllum peltatum* or *Podophyllum emodi* root-derived podophyllotoxin) (Figure 55) was human renal cell carcinoma cell line TK-10 cell (GI_{50} value: 8.1 μg/mL), breast cancer cell line MCF-7 cell (GI_{50} value: 0.33 μg/mL) and melanoma (malignant melanoma) UACC-62 cells (GI_{50} value: 0.97 μg/mL), respectively.

Next, hirsutanone (1,7-di-(3',4'-dihydroxyphenyl)-4-hepten-3-one. **221**) was used for three types of tumor cell lines - human renal cell carcinoma cell line TK-10 cells (50% growth-inhibitory concentration (GI_{50} value): 6.8 μg/mL), breast cancer cell line MCF-7 cells (GI_{50} value: 1.9 □g/mL) and melanoma (melanoma) UACC-62 cells (GI_{50} value: 4.8 μg/mL).

From the above results, hirsutanone (1,7-di-(3',4'-dihydroxyphenyl)-4-hepten-3-one. **221**) exhibited high antitumor activity against these three types of tumor cell lines.

Here, hirsutanone (1,7-di-(3',4'-dihydroxyphenyl)-4-hepten-3-one. **221**) is a diarylheptanoid similar to the structures of three cytotoxic diarylheptanoids - curcumin I (curcumin. diferuloylmethane. 1,7-*bis*-4-hydroxy-3-methoxyphenyl-1,6-heptadiene-3,5-dione. **223**), curcumin II (demethoxycurcumin. (1*E*,6*E*)-1-(4-hydroxy-3-methoxyphenyl)-7-(4-hydroxyphenyl)hepta-1,6-diene-3,5-dione. **224**), and, curcumin III (bis-demethoxycurcumin. (1*E*,6*E*)-1,7-*bis*(4-hydroxyphenyl)hepta-1,6-diene-3,5-dione. **225**) (Figure 55) - from *Curcuma longa* (Ginger family). Therefore, hirsutanone (1,7-di-(3',4'-dihydroxyphenyl)-4-hepten-3-one. **221**) can also be cytotoxic [121, 122, 123, 124].

In addition, curcumin I (curcumin. diferuloylmethane. 1,7-*bis*-4-hydroxy-3-methoxyphenyl-1,6-heptadiene-3,5-dione. **223**) showed higher cytotoxic activity when compared to that (cytotoxic activity) of the other two diarylheptanoids (curcumin II (demethoxycurcumin. (1*E*,6*E*)-1-(4-

hydroxy-3-methoxyphenyl)-7-(4-hydroxyphenyl)hepta-1,6-diene-3,5-dione. **224**) and curcumin III (bisdemethoxycurcumin. (1*E*,6*E*)-1,7-*bis*(4-hydroxyphenyl)hepta-1,6-diene-3,5-dione. **225**)) [124]. The structural difference between curcumin I (curcumin. diferuloylmethane. 1,7-*bis*-4-hydroxy-3-methoxyphenyl-1,6-heptadiene-3,5-dione. **223**) and hirsutanone (1,7-di-(3',4'-dihydroxyphenyl)-4-hepten-3-one. **221**) is the difference in the substituents of C-3' and C-3" on two aromatic rings (A ring and B ring), and the number and position of double bonds and the presence or absence of ketone at C-5 on the aliphatic chain.

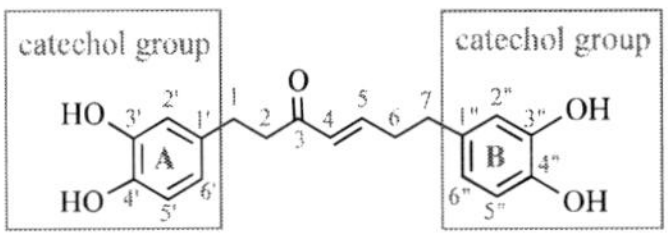

hirsutanone (1,7-di-(3',4'-dihydroxyphenyl)-4-hepten-3-one. **221**)

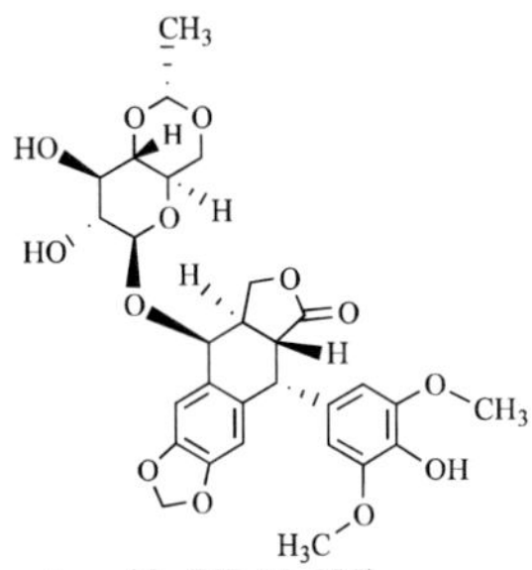

etoposide (VP-16. **222**)

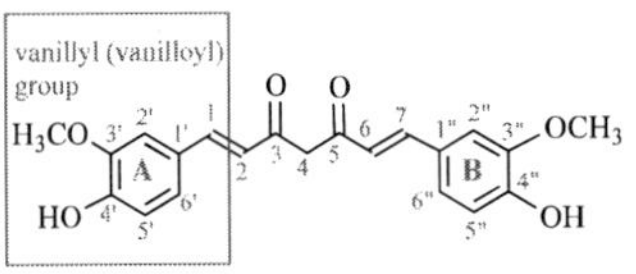

curcumin I (curcumin. diferuloylmethane. 1,7-*bis*-4-hydroxy-3-methoxyphenyl-1,6-heptadiene-3,5-dione. **223**)

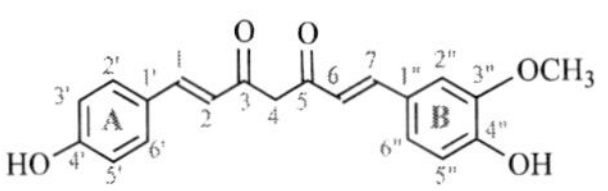

curcumin II (demethoxycurcumin. (1*E*,6*E*)-1-(4-hydroxy-3-methoxyphenyl)-7-(4-hydroxyphenyl)hepta-1,6-diene-3,5-dione. **224**)

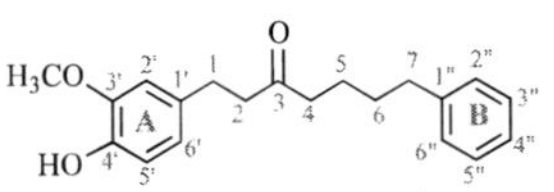

yakuchinone A (1-[4'-hydroxy-3'-methoxy-phenyl]-7-phenylhept-3-one. **226**)

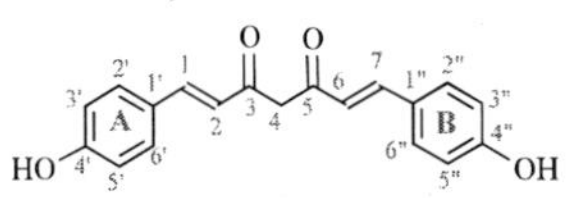

curcumin III (bisdemethoxycurcumin. (1*E*,6*E*)-1,7-*bis*(4-hydroxyphenyl)hepta-1,6-diene-3,5-dione. **225**)

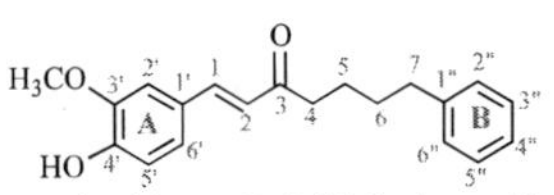

yakuchinone B (1-[4'-hydroxy-3'-methoxyphenyl]-7-phenylhept-1-en-3-one. **227**)

Figure 55. Hirsutanone (1,7-di-(3',4'-dihydroxyphenyl)-4-hepten-3-one. **221**) from the methanolic extract of the aerial parts of *Viscum cruciatum*. Curcumin I (curcumin. diferuloylmethane. 1,7-*bis*-4-hydroxy-3-methoxyphenyl-1,6-heptadiene-3,5-dione. **223**), curcumin II (demethoxycurcumin. (1*E*,6*E*)-1-(4-hydroxy-3-methoxyphenyl)-7-(4-hydroxyphenyl)hepta-1,6-diene-3,5-dione. **224**), and curcumin III (bisdemethoxycurcumin. (1*E*,6*E*)-1,7-*bis*(4-hydroxyphenyl)hepta-1,6-diene-3,5-dione. **225**), yakuchinone A (1-[4'-hydroxy-3'-methoxy-phenyl]-7-phenylhept-3-one. **226**), and yakuchinone B (1-[4'-hydroxy-3'-methoxyphenyl]-7-phenylhept-1-en-3-one. **227**). Positive control: etoposide (VP-16. **222**).

Additionally, diarylheptanoids such as yakuchinone A (1-[4'-hydroxy-3'-methoxy-phenyl]-7-phenylhept-3-one. **226**), and yakuchinone B (1-[4'-hydroxy-3'-methoxyphenyl]-7-phenylhept-1-en-3-one. **227**) (Figure 55) have the ability to suppress the growth of human cancer cells through induction of apoptosis [125]. This result suggests that diarylheptanoid, an active component of cancer cytotoxicity from *Viscum cruciatum*, may be a starting material for the development of anticancer drugs.

So far, open-chain diarylheptanoids have been identified from the Amaryllidaceae, Birchaceae, Ginger and Legumes [126]. Hirsutanone (1,7-di-(3',4'-dihydroxyphenyl)-4-hepten-3-one. **221**) is the first open-chain diarylheptanoid isolated from Santalaceae (old name: Viscaceae) and Viscum [127].

2.7.1.1.1.2. *Viscum coloratum*/2012

In 2012, Zhao *et al.* identified a diarylheptanoid, 1,7-*bis*(4-hydroxyphenyl)-1,4-heptadien-3-one (**228**) (Figure 56) from the stems and leaves of *Viscum coloratum*.

Subsequently, the cytotoxicity of 1,7-*bis*(4-hydroxyphenyl)-1,4-heptadien-3-one (**228**) was examined against 4 types of tumor cell lines – human uterine carcinoma (HeLa cells), human gastric cancer cell line (SGC-7901 cell line), human breast cancer cell line (MCF-7 cells), and human glioma (U251 cell lines) - as the control antineoplastic agent cisplatin (**229**) (Figure 56).

The cytotoxicity (50% inhibitory concentration (IC_{50}) (μM)) was HeLa cells: 1,7-*bis*(4-hydroxyphenyl)-1,4-heptadien-3-one (**228**) (12.08 ± 0.16) and cisplatin (**229**) (17.65 ± 1.52); SGC-7901 cell line: 1,7-*bis*(4-hydroxyphenyl)-1,4-heptadien-3-one (**228**) (44.69 ± 3.23) and cisplatin (**229**) (4.35 ± 0.12); MCF-7 cells: 1,7-*bis*(4-hydroxyphenyl)-1,4-heptadien-3-one (**228**) (13.13 ± 0.41) and cisplatin (**229**) (19.12 ± 2.38); and U251 cell lines: 1,7-*bis*(4-hydroxyphenyl)-1,4-heptadien-3-one (**228**)(> 100) and cisplatin (**229**) (59.21 ± 5.36), respectively.

As a result, among these four types of tumor cells, 50% inhibitory concentration (IC_{50}) (μM) of 1,7-*bis*(4-hydroxyphenyl)-1,4-heptadien-3-

one (**228**) showed higher selective antitumor activity against HeLa cells and MCF-7 cells than cisplatin (**229**) [128].

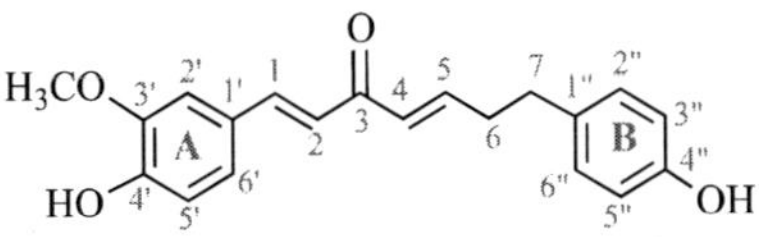

1,7-*bis*(4-hydroxyphenyl)-1,4-heptadien-3-one (**228**)

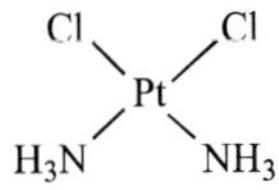

cisplatin (**229**)

Figure 56. A diarylheptanoid, 1,7-*bis*(4-hydroxyphenyl)-1,4-heptadien-3-one (**228**) from the stems and leaves of *Viscum coloratum*. A control antineoplastic agent cisplatin (**229**).

2.8. Order Sapindales

2.8.1. Burseraceae

2.8.1.1. Boswellia

2.8.1.1.1. *Boswellia ovalifoliolata*

In 2003, Lakshmi *et al.* identified two novel macrocyclic diarylheptanoids - ovalifoliolatin A (**230**) and ovalifoliolatin B (**231**) - together with one known macrocyclic diarylheptanoid - acerogenin C (**232**) (Figure 57) from the stems of *Boswellia ovalifoliolata* BAL. & HENRY [129].

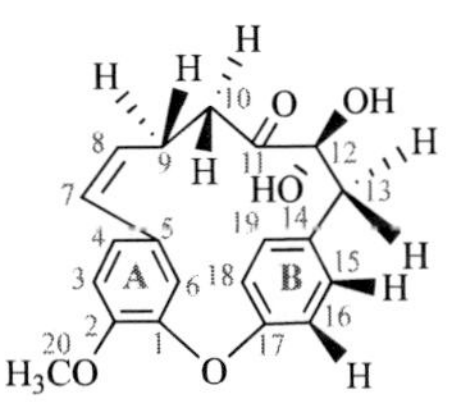

ovalifoliolatin A (**230**)

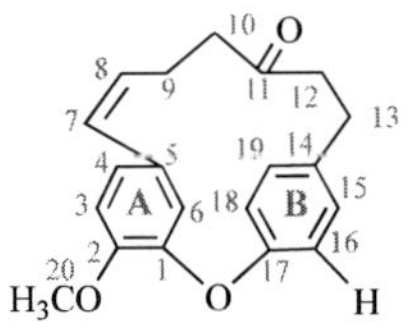

ovalifoliolatin B (**231**)

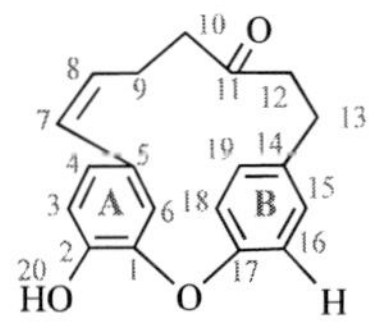

acerogenin C (**232**)

Figure 57. Two novel macrocyclic diarylheptanoids - ovalifoliolatin A (**230**) and ovalifoliolatin B (**231**) together with one known macrocyclic diarylheptanoid- acerogenin C (**232**) from the stems of *Boswellia ovalifoliolata* BAL. & HENRY.

2.8.1.2. Garuga

2.8.1.2.1. *Garuga gamblei* King

In 1989, Kalchhauser *et al.* confirmed two novel diarylpentanoids, garugamblin-1 (**233**) and garugamblin-2 (**234**) (Figure 58), together with a known diarylpentanoid garuganin I (**235**) (Figure 58) from the bark of *Guruga gamblei* King [130, 131].

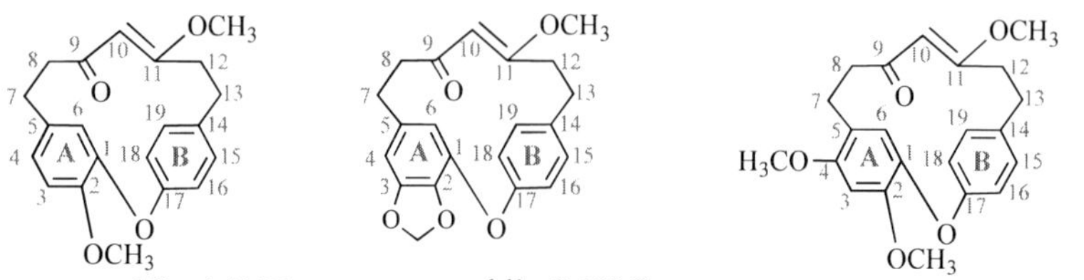

garugamblin-1 (**233**) garugamblin-2 (**234**) garuganin I (**235**)

Figure 58. Garugamblin-1 (**233**), garugamblin-2 (**234**), and garuganin I (**235**) from the bark extract of *Garuga gamblei* King.

2.8.1.2.2. *Garuga pinnata*

2.8.1.2.2.1. *Garuga pinnata*/1985

In 1985, Meena *et al.* isolated a novel diarylpentanoid garuganin I (**235**) (Figure 59) from the leaves and stem bark of *Garuga pinnata* [132].

Subsequently, in 1985, Mishra *et al.* of the same group confirmed the presence of a novel diarylpentanoid garuganin III (**236**) (Figure 59), together with a known diarylpentanoid garuganin I (**235**) (Figure 59) from the *n*-hexane extract of *Garuga pinnata* leaves [133].

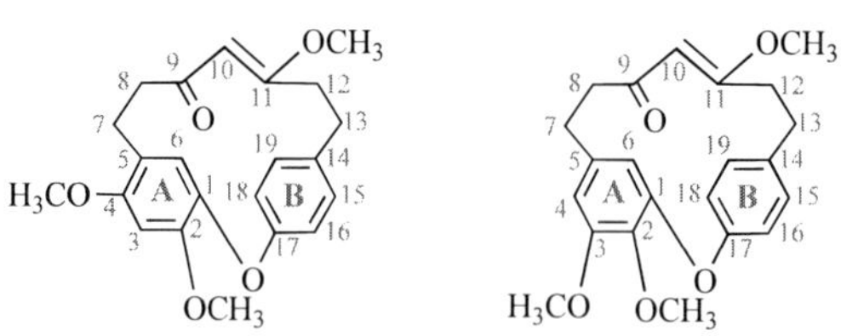

garuganin I (**235**) garuganin III (**236**)

Figure 59. Garuganin I (**235**), and garuganin III (**236**) from the *n*-hexane extract of *Garuga pinnata* leaves.

2.8.1.2.2.2. *Garuga pinnata*/2006

In 2006, Ara *et al*. confirmed three macrocyclic diarylheptanoids, 16-hydroxygaruganin V (**237**), 11-desmethylgarugamblin I (**238**) and 2,11-didesmethylgaruganin III (**239**) (Figure 60) from the petroleum ether and dichloromethane extracts of the stem bark of *Garuga pinnata* [134].

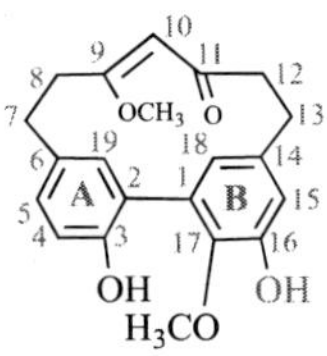

16-hydroxygaruganin V (**237**)

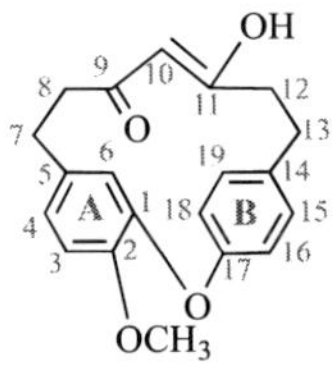

11-desmethylgarugamblin I (**238**)

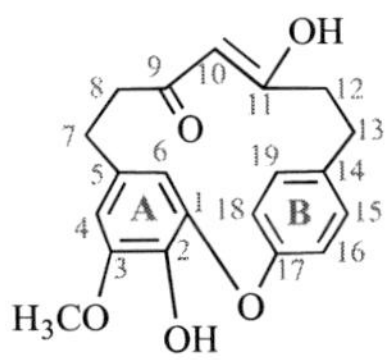

2,11-didesmethylgaruganin III (**239**)

Figure 60. 16-Hydroxygaruganin V (**237**), 11-desmethylgarugamblin I (**238**) and 2,11-didesmethylgaruganin III (**293**) from the petroleum ether and dichloromethane extracts of the stem bark of *Garuga pinnata*.

2.8.1.2.2.3. *Garuga pinnata*/2012

In 2012, *Ara et al.* in the same group as above identified one novel diarylheptanoid: 1-desmethylgaruganin III (**240**) (Figure 61) from petroleum ether and dichloromethane extracts of the stem bark of *Garuga pinnata* Roxb. [135].

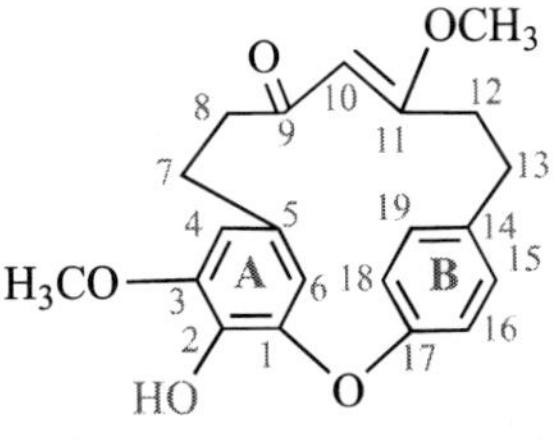

1-desmethylgaruganin III (**240**)

Figure 61. One novel diarylheptanoid: 1-desmethylgaruganin III (**240**) from the stem bark of *Garuga pinnata* Roxb..

2.8.2. Sapindaceae

2.8.2.1. Acer

2.8.2.1.1. *Acer nikoense* Maxim.

2.8.2.1.1.1. *Acer nikoense* Maxim./1976

In 1976, Nagai *et al.* isolated a diaryl ether-type diarylheptanoid acerogenin A (**241**) (Figure 62) from the stem bark of *Acer nikoense* MAXIM. (Photos 8 and 9) [136].

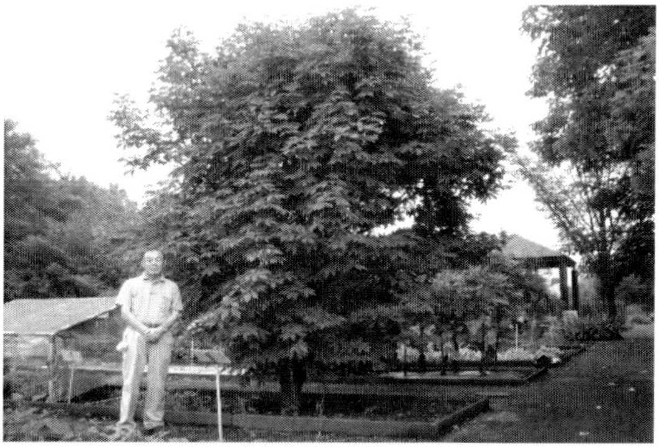

Photo 8. Whole tree of Acer nikoense Maxim. (nikko maple). Photographed by Noboru Motohashi at Tokyo Metropolitan Medicinal Garden, Tokyo, Japan. 7/13/2007 Fri.

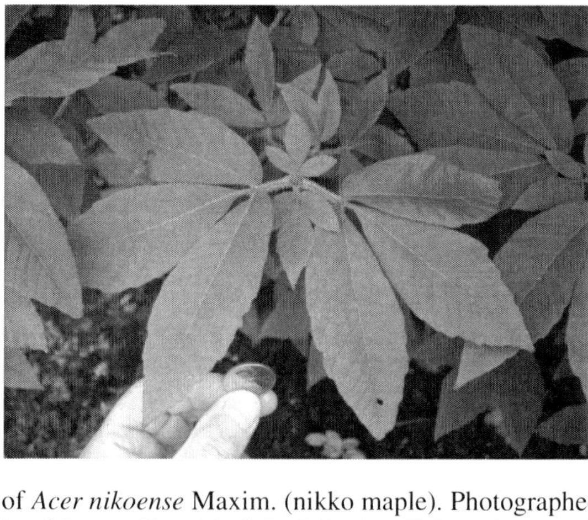

Photo 9. Leaves of *Acer nikoense* Maxim. (nikko maple). Photographed by Noboru Motohashi at Tokyo Metropolitan Medicinal Garden, Tokyo, Japan. 7/13/2007 Fri.

2.8.2.1.1.2. *Acer nikoense* Maxim./1978

In 1978, Nagai *et al.* isolated a monoglucoside of acerogenin A (**241**) of *m-,p'*-bridged diphenyl ether-type diarylheptanoid aceroside I (acerogenin A β-D-glucopyranoside. **242**) (Figure 62) from the stem bark of *Acer nikoense* MAXIM. [137].

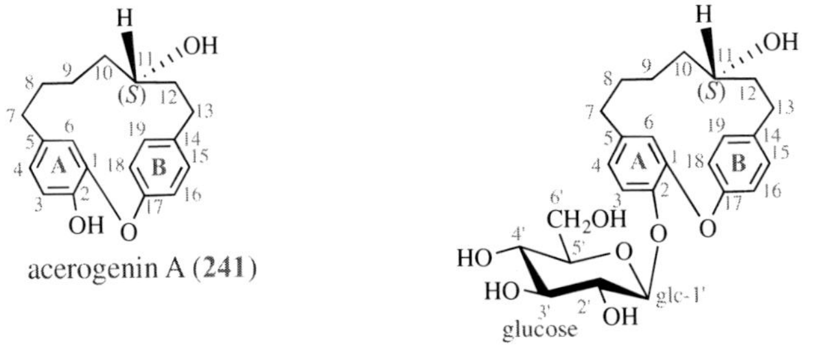
acerogenin A (**241**)

aceroside I (acerogenin A β–D-glucopyranoside. **242**)

Figure 62. Acerogenin A (**241**) and aceroside I (acerogenin A β–D-glucopyranoside. **242**) from the stem bark of *Acer nikoense* MAXIM.

2.8.2.1.1.3. *Acer nikoense* Maxim./2003

The plant *Acer nikoense* is unique to Japan and has been used as a folklore medicine for liver and eye diseases.

In 2003, first, Morikawa *et al.* confirmed *three novel diarylheptanoids* of aceroside B1 (**243**), aceroside B2 (**244**) (the 9-isomer of acerosides B1 (**243**)) and aceroketoside (**245**) (Figure 63) having a 3-ketohexopyranosyl part together with *five known diarylheptanoids* of acerogenin A (**246**, 0.0078%) [137, 138], acerogenin B (**247**, 0.0035%) [139], acerogenin E (**248**, 0.0005%) [140], acerogenin K (**249**, 0.0012%) [141] (Figure 63), and (-)-centrolobol (**3**, 0.0025%) [138] (Figure 63) from the methanolic extract of *Acer nikoense* Maxim. stem bark.

Here, inorganic free radical NO is widely involved in physiological and pathological processes such as vasodilation, nonspecific host defense, ischemia-reperfusion injury, chronic or acute inflammation [142]. Inorganic free radical NO is produced by oxidation of L-arginine (**250**) (Figure 63) by nitric oxide synthase (NOS). That is, NOS is a family of enzymes that catalyze the production of nitric oxide (NO) from L-arginine

(**250**), inducible NOS in particular is involved in the pathological overproduction of NO. Inducible nitric oxide synthase (iNOS) is expressed in a variety of cell types, including macrophages, endothelial cells, and smooth muscle cells, in response to pro-inflammatory substances such as interleukin-1β, tumor necrosis factor-α, and LPS.

Additionaly, it is known that some diarylheptanoids showed the inhibitions of nitric oxide (NO) production [98].

Second, based on the above facts, *first*, all five known diarylheptanoids (**246** - **249**, **3**) did not show cytotoxicity by MTT assay.

Second, on the inhibition effects of NO production by five known diarylheptanoids (**246** - **249**, **3**) against nitric oxide synthase (NOS), one nonselective nitric oxide synthase (NOS) inhibitor (cell-permeable competitive NOS inhibitor) N^G-monomethyl-L-arginine, monoacetate salt (L-NMMA. **162**) (Figure 63) is used as a positive control.

As a result, the inhibition effect of NO production in lipopolysaccharide (LPS)-activated mouse peritoneal macrophages by five known diarylheptanoids (**246** - **249**, **3**) was as follows:

Five known diarylheptanoids (**246** - **249**, **3**) showed 50% inhibitory concentration (IC_{50}) 24-88 μM.

Among these (**246** - **249**, **3**), 50% inhibition concentration (IC_{50}) of acerogenin E (**248**) (IC_{50}: 24 μM) is the highest, followed by acerogenin K (**249**) (IC_{50}: 25 μM), N^G-monomethyl-L-arginine, monoacetate salt (L-NMMA. **162**) (IC_{50}: 28 μM), (-)-centrolobol (**3**) (IC_{50}: 73 μM), acerogenin A (**246**), (IC_{50}: 74 μM), and acerogenin B (**247**) (IC_{50}: 88 μM).

The 50% inhibitory concentration (IC_{50}) of acerogenin E (**248**) (IC_{50}: 24 μM) and acerogenin K (**249**) (IC_{50}: 25 μM) is almost equivalent value when compared to that (50% inhibitory concentration (IC_{50})) of the non-selective NOS inhibitor N^G-monomethyl-L-arginine, monoacetate salt (L-NMMA. **162**) (IC_{50}: 28 μM).

From the comparison of these NO production inhibitory activities, the NO production inhibitory activity of biphenyl-type diarylheptanoids (acerogenin E (**248**) (IC_{50}: 24 μM) and acerogenin K (**249**) (IC_{50}: 25 μM)) showed higher NO production inhibitory activity when compared to the

NO production inhibitory activity of diphenyl ether type diarylheptanoids (acerogenin A (**246**) (IC_{50}: 74 μM) and acerogenin B (**247**) (IC_{50}: 88 μM)), and straight (linear) chain-type diarylheptanoid ((-)-centrolobol (**3**) (IC_{50}: 73 μM)). This suggests that the NO production inhibitory activity of biphenyl-type diarylheptanoids is higher than that of diphenyl ether-type diarylheptanoids and straight (linear) chain-type diarylheptanoids [118].

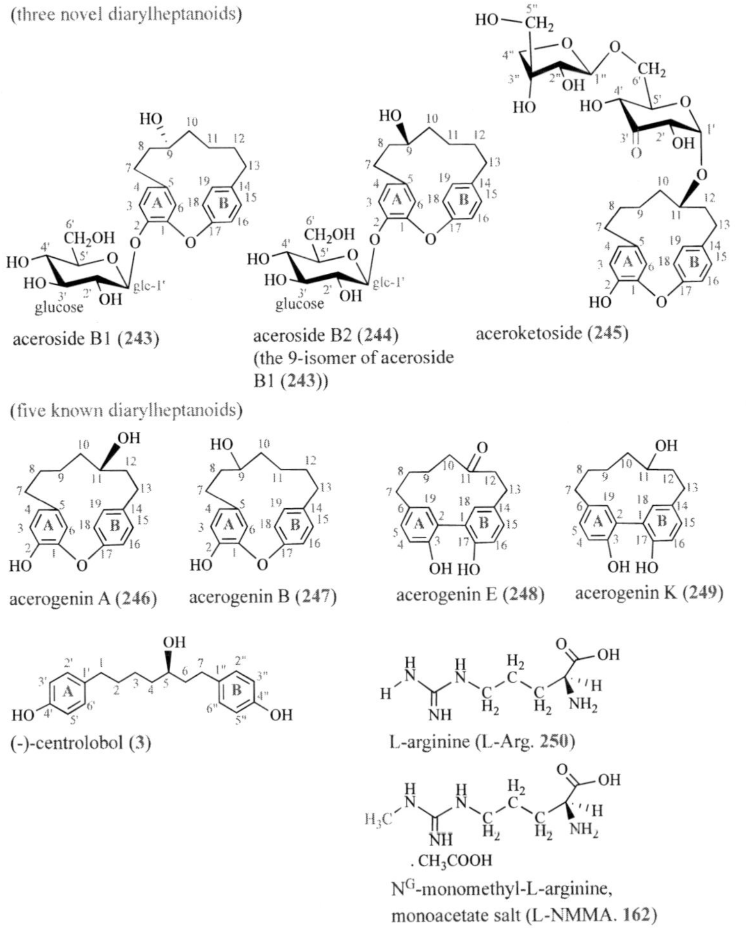

Figure 63. Three novel diarylheptanoids of aceroside B1 (**243**), aceroside B2 (**244**) and aceroketoside (**245**) together with five known diarylheptanoids of acerogenin A (**246**), acerogenin B (**247**), acerogenin E (**248**), acerogenin K (**249**), and (-)-centrolobol (**3**) from the methanolic extract of *Acer nikoense* Maxim. stem bark.

L-Arginine (L-Arg. **250**) and N^G-monomethyl-L-arginine, monoacetate salt (L-NMMA. **162**).

2.9. Order Zingiberales

2.9.1. Zingiberaceae

2.9.1.1. Alpinia

2.9.1.1.1. *Alpinia katsumadai*

In Japan, the seeds of the plant have been used aromatic stomachic. In 1983, Kuroyanagi *et al.* confirmed four novel diarylheptanoids of (5*R*)-*trans*-1,7-diphenyl-5-hydroxy-6-hepten-3-one (**251**), (3*S*,5*S*)-*trans*-1,7-diphenyl-3,5-dihydroxy-1-heptene (**252**), *trans*-1,7-diphenyl-5-hydroxy-1-heptene (**253**) and *trans,trans*-1,7-diphenyl-5-hydroxy-4,6-heptadien-3-one (**254**) (Figure 64) together with two known diarylheptanoids of (3*S*,5*R*)-3,5-dihydroxy-1,7-diphenylheptane (**255**) and *trans,trans*-1,7-diphenyl-4,6-heptadien-3-one (**256**) (Figure 64) from the seeds of *Alpinia katsumadai* Hayata [143].

(Four novel diarylheptanoids)

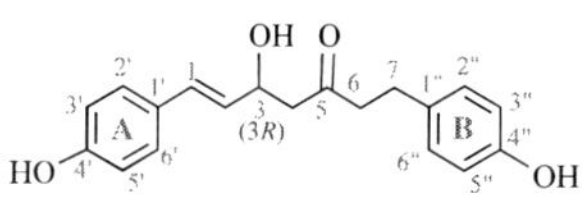

(5*R*)-*trans*-1,7-diphenyl-5-hydroxy-6-hepten-3-one (**251**)

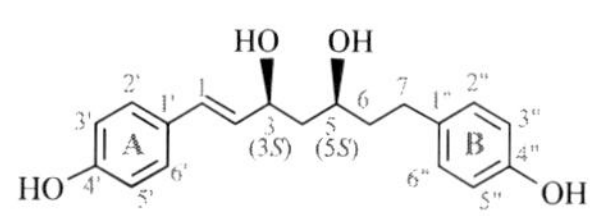

(3*S*,5*S*)-*trans*-1,7-diphenyl-3,5-dihydroxy-1-heptene (**252**)

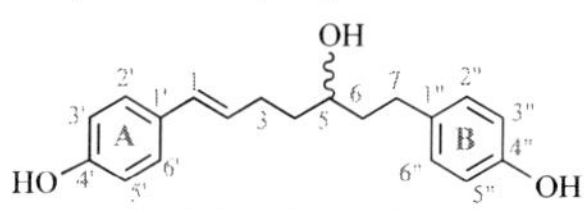

trans-1,7-diphenyl-5-hydroxy-1-heptene (**253**)

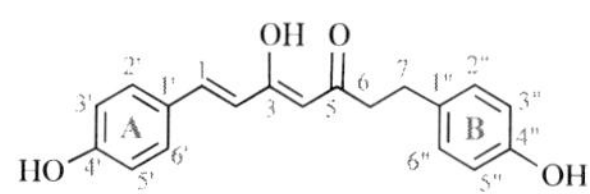

trans,trans-1,7-diphenyl-5-hydroxy-4,6-heptadien-3-one (**254**)

(Two known diarylheptanoids)

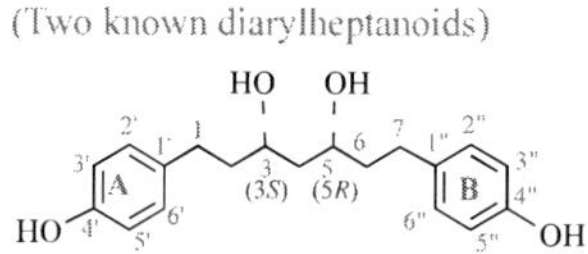

(3*S*,5*R*)-3,5-dihydroxy-1,7-diphenylheptane (**255**)

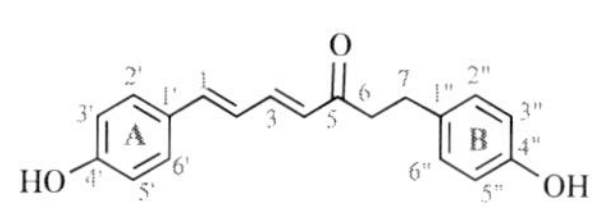

trans,trans-1,7-diphenyl-4,6-heptadien-3-one (**256**)

Figure 64. Four novel diarylheptanoids of (5*R*)-*trans*-1,7-diphenyl-5-hydroxy-6-hepten-3-one (**251**), (3*S*,5*S*)-*trans*-1,7-diphenyl-3,5-dihydroxy-1-heptene (**252**), *trans*-1,7-diphenyl-5-hydroxy-1-heptene (**253**) and *trans,trans*-1,7-diphenyl-5-hydroxy-4,6-heptadien-3-one (**254**) together with two known diarylheptanoids of (3*S*,5*R*)-3,5-dihydroxy-1,7-diphenylheptane (**255**) and *trans,trans*-1,7-diphenyl-4,6-heptadien-3-one (**256**) from the seeds of *Alpinia katsumadai* Hayata.

2.9.1.1.2. *Alpinia officinarum*

2.9.1.1.2.1. *Alpinia officinarum* /2006

In 2006, An N *et al.* identified one novel diarylheptanoid: *trans,trans*-1(3'-methoxy-4'-hydroxyphenyl)-7-phenyl-5-ol-4,6-dien-3-heptanone (**257**) along with five known diarylheptanoids: *trans,trans*-1,7-diphenyl-5-ol-4,6-dien-3-heptanone (**258**) [143], 1,7-diphenyl-5-ol-3-heptanone (**259**) [144], 1,7-diphenyl-4-en-3-heptanone (**260**) [145], 7-(4"-hydroxyphenyl)-1-phenyl-5-ol-3-heptanone (**261**) [146], and 7-(4"-hydroxy-3"-methoxy-phenyl)-1-phenyl-5-ol-3-heptanone (**262**) [144] (Figure 65) from the rhizomes of *Alpinia officinarum* [147].

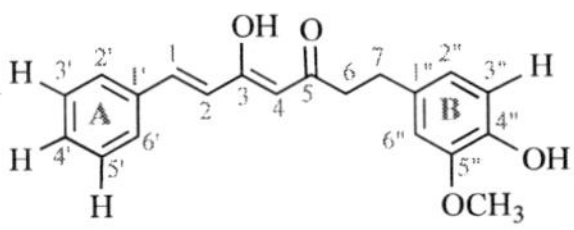

trans,trans-1(3'-methoxy-4'-hydroxyphenyl)-7-phenyl-5-ol-4,6-dien-3-heptanone (**257**)

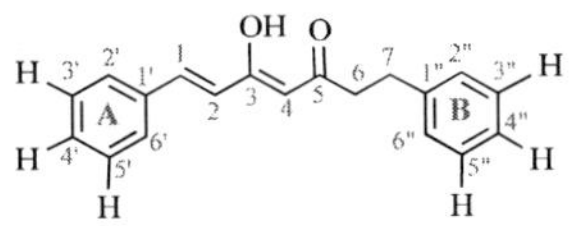

trans,trans-1,7-diphenyl-5-ol-4,6-dien-3-heptanone (**258**)

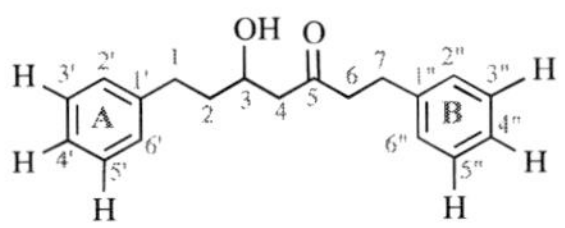

1,7-diphenyl-5-ol-3-heptanone (**259**)

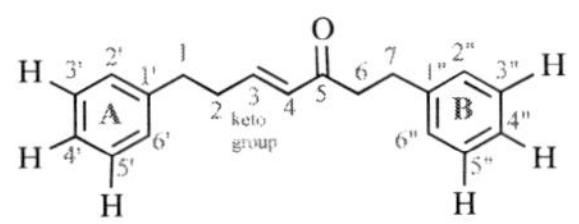

1,7-diphenyl-4-en-3-heptanone (**260**)

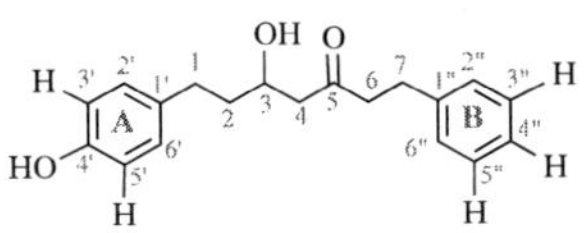

7-(4"-hydroxyphenyl)-1-phenyl-5-ol-3-heptanone (**261**)

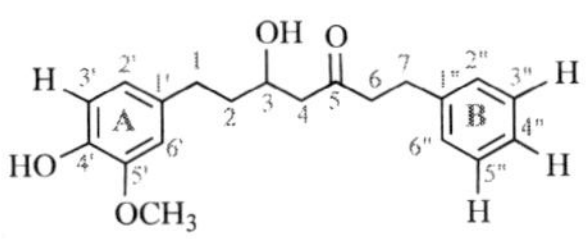

7-(4"-hydroxy-3"-methoxyphenyl)-1-phenyl-5-ol-3-heptanone (**262**)

Figure 65. One novel diarylheptanoid: *trans,trans*-1(3'-methoxy-4'-hydroxyphenyl)-7-phenyl-5-ol-4,6-dien-3-heptanone (**257**), and five known diarylheptanoids: *trans,trans*-1,7-diphenyl-5-ol-4,6-dien-3-heptanone (**258**), 1,7-diphenyl-5-ol-3-heptanone (**259**), 1,7-diphenyl-4-en-heptanone (**260**), 7-(4"-hydroxyphenyl)-1-phenyl-5-ol-3-heptanone (**261**), and 7-(4"-hydroxy-3"-methoxyphenyl)-1-phenyl-5-ol-3-heptanone (**262**) from the rhizomes of *Alp. officinarum*.

2.9.1.1.2.2. *Alpinia officinarum*/2008

In 2008, An N *et al.* identified two novel diarylheptanoids, (5*S*)-5-hydroxy-7-(3,4-hydroxyphenyl)-1-phenyl-3-heptanone (**263**) and (5*R*)-5-

hydroxy-7-(3-methoxy-4,5-dihydroxyphenyl)-1-phenyl-3-heptanone (**264**) Figure 66) along with two known diarylheptanoids, (5*R*)-5-hydroxy-1-(3,4-hydroxyphenyl)-7-(4-hydroxy-3-methoxyphenyl)-3-heptanone (**265**) [148] and 7-(3,4-hydroxyphenyl)-1-(4-hydroxy-3-methoxyphenyl)-4-en-3-heptanone (**266**) [148] (Figure 66) from the rhizomes of *Alpinia officinarum* Hance.

On the cytotoxicity of four diarylheptanoids (**263** - **266**) against three human hepatocarcinoma (HepG2), human breast tumor (MCF-7) and human CNS glioblastoma (SF-268/ATCC) cell lines using the MTT (3-(4,5-dimethylthiazol-2-yl)-2,5-diphenyl tetrazolium bromide) assay, first, *in vitro* cytotoxicity (IC_{50} μg/mL) for human hepatoma (HepG2) was the highest 7-(3,4-hydroxyphenyl)-1-(4-hydroxy-3-methoxyphenyl)-4-en-3-heptanone (**266**) (6), followed by (5*R*)-5-hydroxy-1-(3,4-hydroxyphenyl)-7-(4-hydroxy-3-methoxyphenyl)-3-heptanone (**265**) (21), (5*S*)-5-hydroxy-7-(3,4-hydroxyphenyl)-1-phenyl-3-heptanone (**263**) (25), and (5*R*)-5-hydroxy-7-(3-methoxy-4,5-dihydroxyphenyl)-1-phenyl-3-heptanone (**264**) (60), respectively.

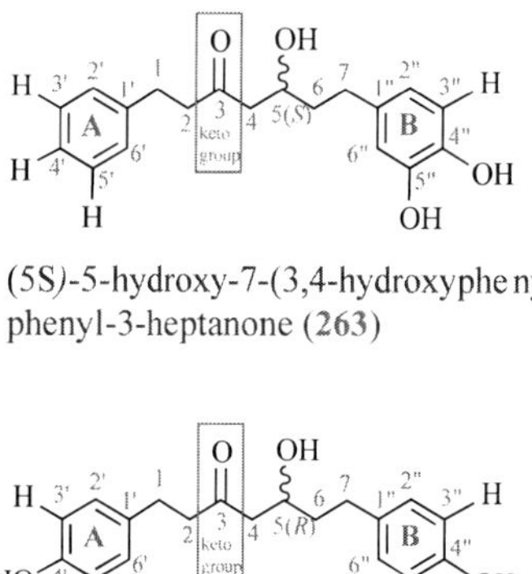

(5S)-5-hydroxy-7-(3,4-hydroxyphenyl)-1-phenyl-3-heptanone (**263**)

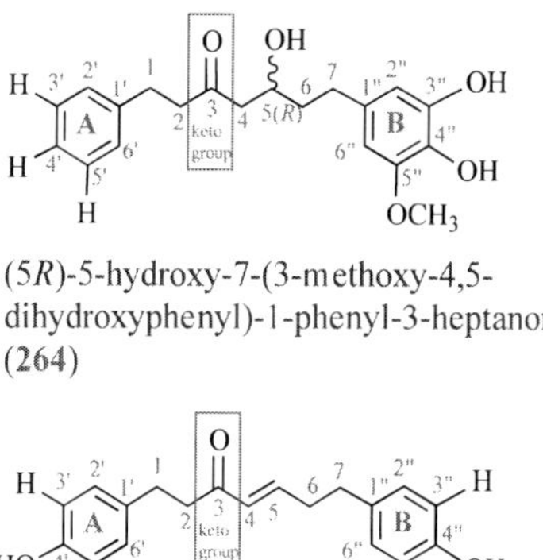

(5*R*)-5-hydroxy-7-(3-methoxy-4,5-dihydroxyphenyl)-1-phenyl-3-heptanone (**264**)

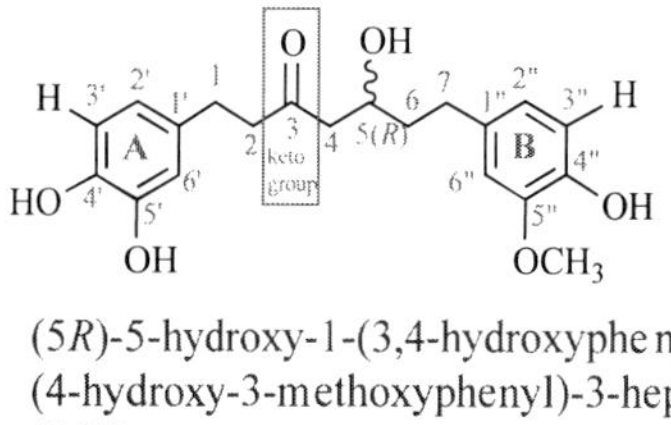

(5*R*)-5-hydroxy-1-(3,4-hydroxyphenyl)-7-(4-hydroxy-3-methoxyphenyl)-3-heptanone (**265**)

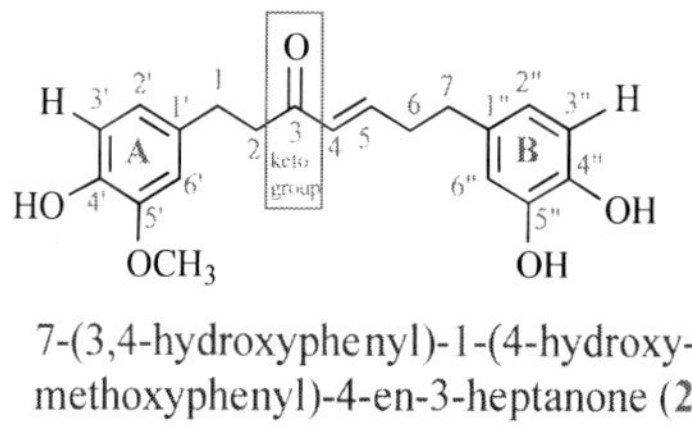

7-(3,4-hydroxyphenyl)-1-(4-hydroxy-3-methoxyphenyl)-4-en-3-heptanone (**266**)

Figure 66. Two novel diarylheptanoids, (5*S*)-5-hydroxy-7-(3,4-hydroxyphenyl)-1-phenyl-3-heptanone (**263**) and (5*R*)-5-hydroxy-7-(3-methoxy-4,5-dihydroxyphenyl)-1-phenyl-heptanone (**264**), and two known diarylheptanoids, (5*R*)-5-hydroxy-1-(3,4-hydroxyphenyl)-7-(4-hydroxy-3-methoxyphenyl)-3-heptanone (**265**) and 7-(3,4-hydroxyphenyl)-1-(4-hydroxy-3-methoxyphenyl)-4-en-3-heptanone (**266**) from the rhizomes of *Alpinia officinarum* Hance.

Second, *in vitro* cytotoxicity (IC_{50} μg/mL) for human breast tumor (MCF-7) was the highest 7-(3,4-hydroxyphenyl)-1-(4-hydroxy-3-methoxyphenyl)-4-en-3-heptanone (**266**) (7), followed by (5*S*)-5-hydroxy-7-(3,4-hydroxyphenyl)-1-phenyl-3-heptanone (**263**) (28), (5*R*)-5-hydroxy-1-(3,4-hydroxyphenyl)-7-(4-hydroxy-3-methoxyphenyl)-3-heptanone (**265**) (35), and (5*R*)-5-hydroxy-7-(3-methoxy-4,5-dihydroxyphenyl)-1-phenyl-3-heptanone (**264**) (47), respectively.

Third, *in vitro* cytotoxicity (IC_{50} μg/mL) for human CNS glioblastoma (SF-268/ATCC) cell lines was the highest 7-(3,4-hydroxyphenyl)-1-(4-hydroxy-3-methoxyphenyl)-4-en-3-heptanone (**266**) (10), followed by (5*S*)-5-hydroxy-7-(3,4-hydroxyphenyl)-1-phenyl-3-heptanone (**263**) (26), (5*R*)-5-hydroxy-1-(3,4-hydroxyphenyl)-7-(4-hydroxy-3-methoxyphenyl)-3-heptanone (**265**) (29), and (5*R*)-5-hydroxy-7-(3-methoxy-4,5-dihydroxyphenyl)-1-phenyl-3-heptanone (**264**) (32), respectively.

From the above results, 7-(3,4-hydroxyphenyl)-1-(4-hydroxy-3-methoxyphenyl)-4-en-3-heptanone (**266**) showed the highest cytotoxicity against three human hepatocarcinoma (HepG2), human breast tumor (MCF-7) and human CNS glioblastoma (SF-268/ATCC) cell lines among four diarylheptanoids (**263** - **266**) [149].

2.9.1.1.2.3. *Alpinia officinarum*/2014/1

In 2014, Dan L *et al.* identified a novel dimeric diarylheptanoid alpinin B (**267**) (Figure 67) along with three known diarylheptanoids, 1,7-diphenyl-3,5-heptanedione (**268**), (*4E*)-1,7-diphenylhept-4-en-3-one (**270**) and (*4E*)-7-(4-hydroxyphenyl)-1-phenylhept-4-en-3-one (**271**) (Figure 67) from the the rhizomes of *Alpinia officinarum* Hance. Two diarylheptanoid units (unit-I and unit-II) of alpinin B (**267**) were 1,7-diphenyl-3,5-heptanedione (unit-I. **268**) [150] and 1,7-diphenyl-heptan-3-one (unit-II. **269**) (Figure 67) [151], respectively.

On the cytotoxicity of four diarylheptanoids (**267**, **268**, **270**, **271**) against two human glioblastoma T98G and the murine melanoma B16F10 cell lines using the methylthiazole tetrazolium (MTT) assay, (*4E*)-1,7-diphenylhept-4-en-3-one (**270**) was cytotoxic to human glioblastoma T98G cell line (50% inhibitory concentration (IC_{50}): 27 μmol/L). However, alpinin B (**267**) was inactive against two human glioblastoma T98G and the murine melanoma B16F10 cell lines. 5-Fluorouracil (5-FU. **272**) (Figure 67) was used as positive control [152].

From these results, it suggests that α,β-unsaturated sites on the linear chain may play an important role on the cytotoxicity of diarylheptanoids (**267**, **268**, **270**, **271**) against two human glioblastoma T98G and the murine melanoma B16F10 cell lines [153].

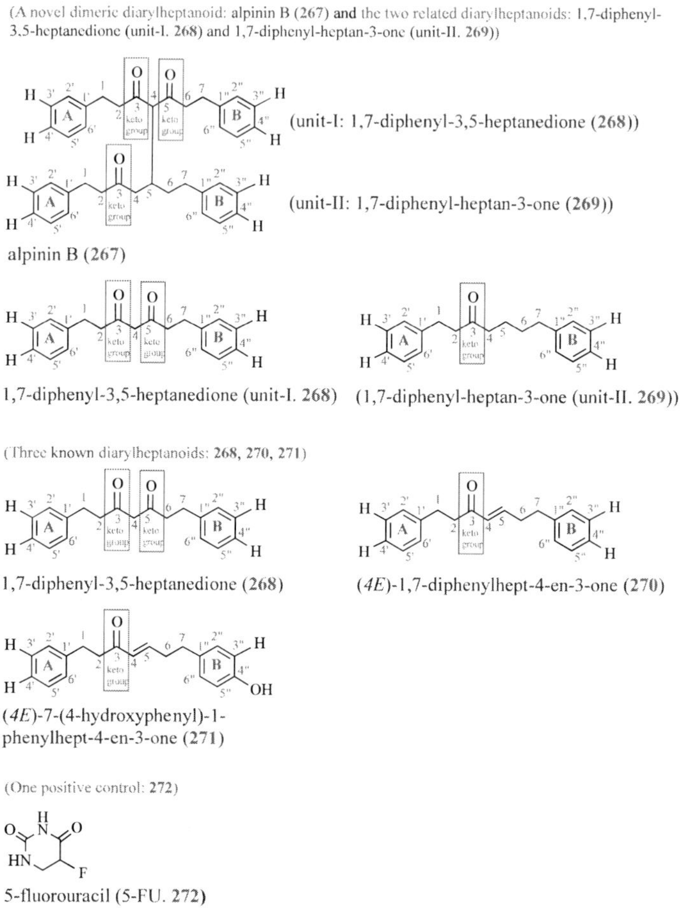

Figure 67. A novel dimeric diarylheptanoid : alpinin B (267) and the two rela diarylheptanoids (1,7-diphenyl-3,5-heptanedione (unit-I. 268) and 1,7-diphenyl-heptan-3-one (unit-II. 269)), and three known diarylheptanoids: 1,7-diphenyl-3,5-heptanedione (268), (*4E*)-1,7-diphenylhept-4-en-3-one (270) and (*4E*)-7-(4-hydroxyphenyl)-1-phenylhept-4-en-3-on (271) from the the rhizomes of *Alpinia officinarum* Hance. A positive control: 5-fluorouracil (5-FU. 272).

2.9.1.1.2.4. *Alpinia officinarum*/2014/2

In 2014, Liu D *et al.* identified two novel dimeric diarylheptanoids: alpinin C (**273**) and alpinin D (**274**), a new natural product of diarylheptanoid 7-(4-hydroxyphenyl)-1-phenyl-3-heptanone (**275**) (Figure 68) [144] along with three known diarylheptanoids: 5*S*-ethoxyl-7-(4-hydroxy-3-methoxyphenyl)-1-phenyl-3-heptanone **276**) [154], 5*R*-hydroxy-7-(4-hydroxy-3-methoxyphenyl)-1-phenyl-3-heptanone (**277**) [155] and (4*E*,6*E*)-5-hydroxy-1-(4-hydroxy-3-methoxyphenyl)-7-phenyl-hepta-4,6-dien-3-one (**278**) [147] (Figure 68) from the rhizomes of *Alpinia officinarum* Hance.

On the *in vitro* cytotoxicity (IC_{50}: µg/mL) of six diarylheptanoids (**273**, **274**, **275**, **276**, **277**, **278**) against five human hepatoma) (HepG2), human breast adenocarcinoma (MCF-7), human Caucasian glioblastoma (T98G) and murine melanoma cells (B16-F10) cancer cell lines, a noncancerous lung (IMR-90), and one positive control 5-fluorouracil (5-FU. **272**) by using the MTT colorimetric method, first, each dose of 100 µg/mL in six diarylheptanoids (**273**, **274**, **275**, **276**, **277**, **278)** did not affect the cytotoxicity of a noncancerous lung (IMR-90).

Second, *in vitro* cytotoxicity (IC_{50}: µg/mL) for human hepatoma) (HepG2) was the highest 5-fluorouracil (5-FU. **272**) (20.31), followed by (4*E*,6*E*)-5-hydroxy-1-(4-hydroxy-3-methoxyphenyl)-7-phenylhepta-4,6-dien-3-one (**278**) (22.68), alpinin C (**273**) (90.05), **275** - **277** (>50), and **274** (>80), respectively.

Third, *in vitro* cytotoxicity (IC_{50}: µg/mL) for human breast adenocarcinoma (MCF-7) was the highest **278** (12.37), followed by 5-fluorouracil (5-FU. **272**) (12.37), **274** (20.747), **273** (38.54), and **275** - **277** (>50), respectively.

Fourth, *in vitro* cytotoxicity (IC_{50} µg/mL) for human Caucasian glioblastoma (T98G) was the highest **278** (8.46), followed by 5-fluorouracil (5-FU. **272**) (30.74), **273** (35.43), and **274**, **275**, **276** and **277** (>80), respectively.

Fifth, *in vitro* cytotoxicity (IC_{50}: µg/mL) for murine melanoma cells (B16-F10) was the highest **278** (4.44), followed by 5-fluorouracil (5-FU.

272) (22.82), **277** (41.650), **273** (66.45), **275** (>50), and **274** and **276** (>80), respectively.

From above results, alpinin C (**273**) showed selective cytotoxicity against human human breast adenocarcinoma (MCF-7) and human Caucasian glioblastoma (T98G). (4*E*,6*E*)-5-Hydroxy-1-(4-hydroxy-3-methoxyphenyl)-7-phenylhepta-4,6-dien-3-one (**278**) showed significant cytotoxicity against all four tumor cell lines (HepG2, MCF-7, T98G, B16-F10) [156].

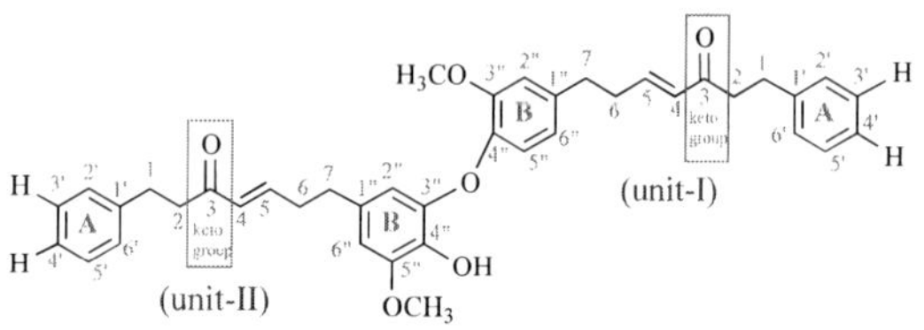

alpinin C (**273**)

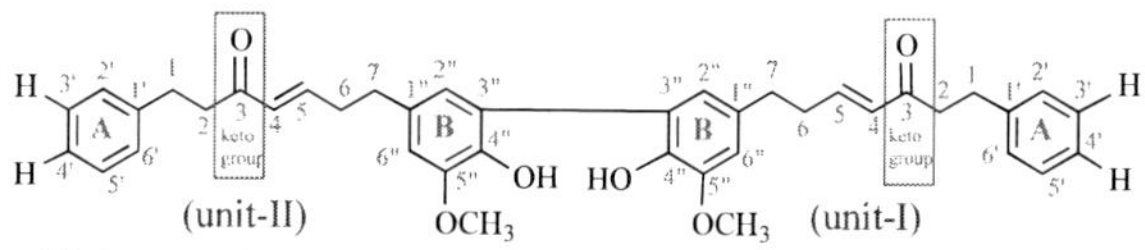

alpinin D (**274**)

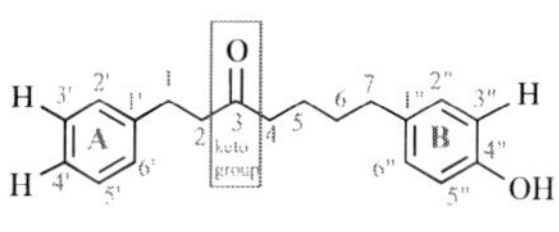

7-(4-hydroxyphenyl)-1-phenyl-3-heptanone (**275**)

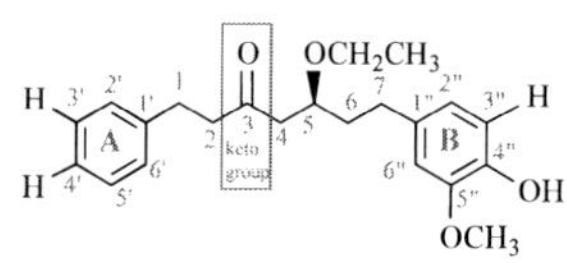

5*S*-ethoxyl-7-(4-hydroxy-3-methoxyphenyl)-1-phenyl-3-heptanone (**276**)

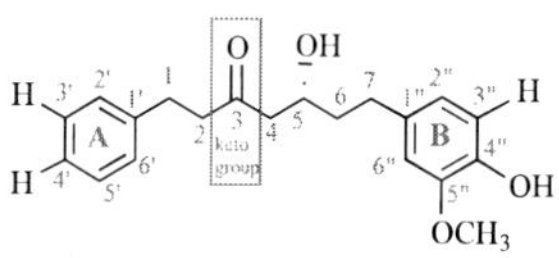

5*R*-hydroxy-7-(4-hydroxy-3-methoxyphenyl)-1-phenyl-3-heptanone (**277**)

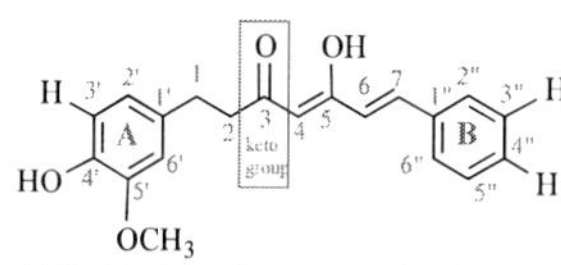

(4*E*,6*E*)-5-hydroxy-1-(4-hydroxy-3-methoxyphenyl)-7-phenylhepta-4,6-dien-3-one (**278**)

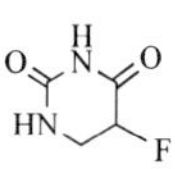

5-fluorouracil (5-FU. **272**)

Figure 68. Two novel dimeric diarylheptanoids: alpinin C (**273**) and alpinin D (**274**), a novel diarylheptanoid: 7-(4-hydroxyphenyl)-1-phenyl-3-heptanone (**275**), and tl diarylheptanoids: 5*S*-ethoxyl-7-(4-hydroxy-3-methoxyphenyl)-1-phenyl-3-heptanone (**276**), 5*R*-hydroxy-7-(4-hydroxy-3-methoxyphenyl)-1-phenyl-3-heptanone (**277**) and (4*E*,6*E*)-5-hydroxy-1-(4-hydroxy-3-methoxyphenyl)-7-phenylhepta-4,6-dien-3-one (**278**) from the the rhizomes of *Alpinia officinarum* Hance. A positive control: 5-fluorouracil (5-FU. **272**).

2.9.1.1.3. *Alpinia pinnanensis*

2.9.1.1.3.1. *Alpinia pinnanensis*

In 2005, Giang PM *et al.* identified three novel acyclic diarylheptanoids: alpinnanin A (**279**), alpinnanin B (**267**), and alpinnanin C (**273**) (Figure 69) along with one known acyclic diarylheptanoid: (3*S*,5*S*)-*trans*-3,5-dihydroxy-1,7-diphenyl-1-heptene ((3*S*,5*S*)-*trans*-1,7-diphenyl-3,5-dihydroxy-1-heptene. **252**) [143] (Figure 69) from the rhizomes of *Alpinia pinnanensis* T. L. WU et SENJEN [157].

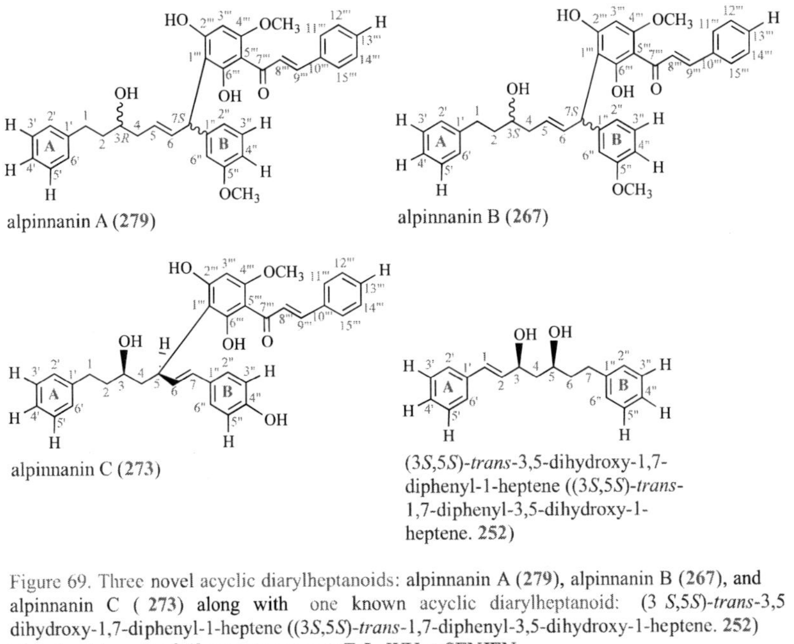

Figure 69. Three novel acyclic diarylheptanoids: alpinnanin A (**279**), alpinnanin B (**267**), and alpinnanin C (**273**) along with one known acyclic diarylheptanoid: (3 *S*,5*S*)-*trans*-3,5 dihydroxy-1,7-diphenyl-1-heptene ((3*S*,5*S*)-*trans*-1,7-diphenyl-3,5-dihydroxy-1-heptene. **252**) from the rhizomes of *Alpinia pinnanensis* T. L. WU et SENJEN.

2.9.1.2. Amomum

2.9.1.2.1. *Amomum muricarpum* ELMER

2.9.1.2.1.1. *Amomum muricarpum* ELMER/2006

In 2006, Giang *et al.* identified two novel linear-diarylheptanoids - muricarpone A ((5*R*)-5-methoxy-1,7-*bis*(3,4-dihydroxyphenyl)-3-heptanone. **280**) and muricarpone B (1,7-*bis*(3,4-dihydroxyphenyl)-3-heptanone. **281**), and three known linear-diarylheptanoids - 1,7-di-(3’,4’-dihydroxyphenyl)-4-hepten-3-one (**282**), 1-(3’,4’-dihydroxyphenyl)-7-(4”-hydroxyphenyl)-4-hepten-3-one (**283**) and 1,7-*bis(p*-hydroxyphenyl)-4-hepten-3-one (1,7-*bis*-(4-hydroxyphenyl)-4-hepten-3-one. **106**) (Figure 70) from the oven-dried rhizomes of *Amomum muricarpum* [158].

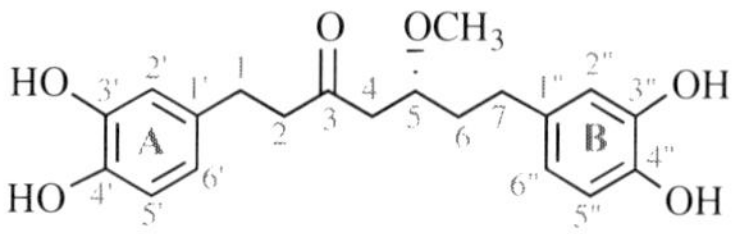

muricarpone A ((5*R*)-5-methoxy-1,7-*bis*(3,4-dihydroxyphenyl)-3-heptanone (**280**)

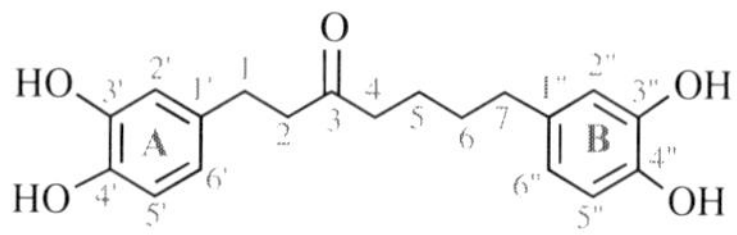

muricarpone B (1,7-*bis*(3,4-dihydroxyphenyl)-3-heptanone (**281**)

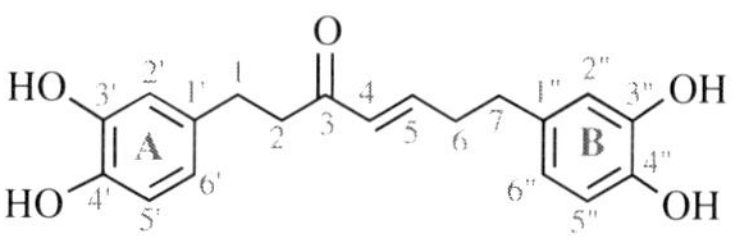

1,7-di-(3’,4’-dihydroxyphenyl)-4-hepten-3-one (**282**)

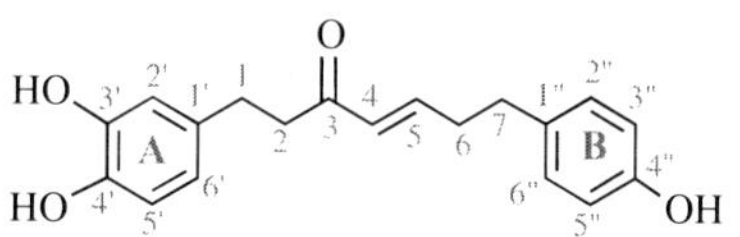

1-(3’,4’-dihydroxyphenyl)-7-(4”-hydroxyphenyl)-4-hepten-3-one (**283**)

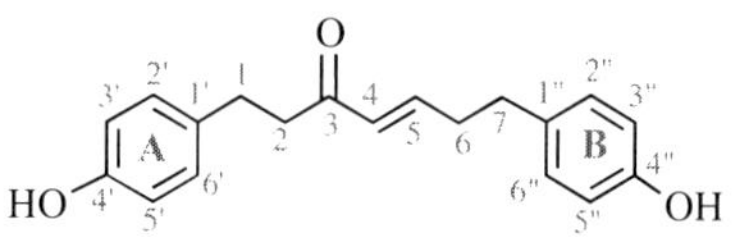

1,7-*bis(p*-hydroxyphenyl)-4-hepten-3-one (1,7-*bis*-(4-hydroxyphenyl)-4-hepten-3-one. **106**)

Figure 70. Two novel linear-diarylheptanoids – muricarpone A ((5*R*)-5-methoxy-1,7-*bis*(3,4-dihydroxyphenyl)-3-heptanone. **280**) and muricarpone B (1,7-*bis*(3,4-dihydroxyphenyl)-3-heptanone. **281**), and three known linear-diarylheptanoids – 1,7-di-(3’,4’-dihydroxyphenyl)-4-hepten-3-one (**282**), 1-(3’,4’-dihydroxyphenyl)-7-(4”-hydroxyphenyl)-4-hepten-3-one (o**283**) and 1,7-*bis(p*-hydroxyphenyl)-4-hepten-3-one (1,7-*bis*-(4-hydroxyphenyl)-4-hepten-3-one. **106**) from the oven-dried rhizomes of *Amomum muricarpum*.

2.9.1.2.1.2. *Amomum muricarpum* ELMER/2012

In 2012, Giang *et al.* identified one novel linear-diarylheptanoid - muricarpin (1-(4’-hydroxyphenyl)-7-(3”,4”-dihydroxyphenyl)-heptan-3-one. **284**), and four known linear-diarylheptanoids - 1,7-*bis*(3,4-dihydroxyphenyl)heptan-3-yl acetate (**285**), 1-(4'-hydroxyphenyl)-7-(3",4"-dihydroxyphenyl)heptan-3-yl acetate (**286**), 1-(3',4'-hydroxyphenyl)-7-(4"-hydroxyphenyl)-heptan-3-one (**287**) and (5*R*)-5-hydroxy-1,7-*bis*(4-hydroxyphenyl)-3-heptanone (**288**) (Figure 71) from the rhizomes of *Amomum muricarpum* Elmer [159].

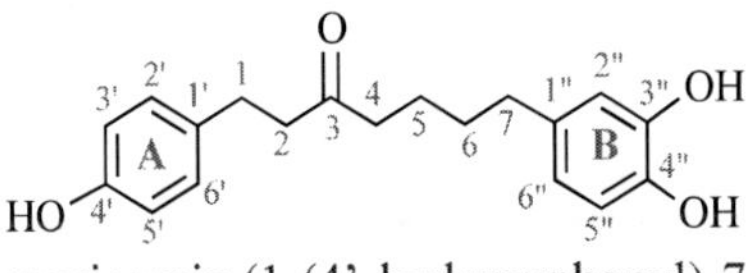

muricarpin (1-(4'-hydroxyphenyl)-7-(3",4"-dihydroxyphenyl)-heptan-3-one (**284**)

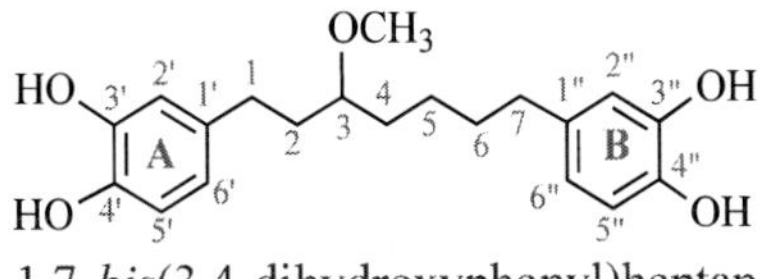

1,7-*bis*(3,4-dihydroxyphenyl)heptan-3-yl acetate (**285**)

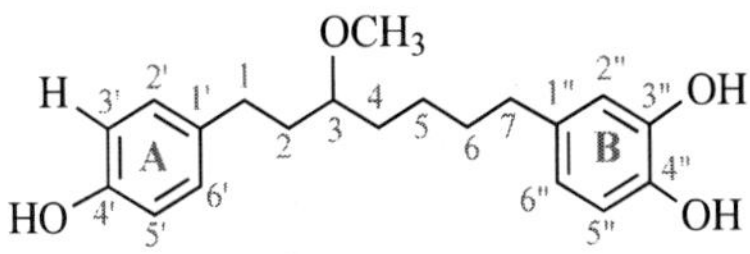

1-(4'-hydroxyphenyl)-7-(3",4"-dihydroxyphenyl)heptan-3-yl acetate (**286**)

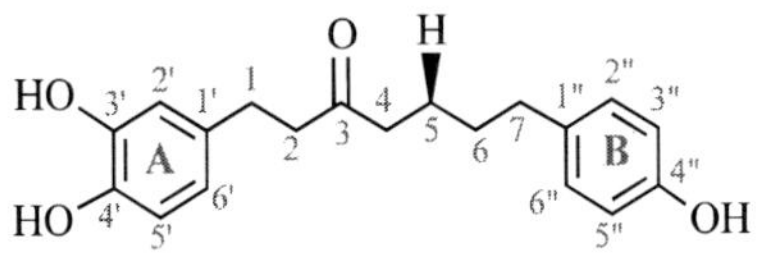

1-(3',4'-hydroxyphenyl)-7-(4"-hydroxyphenyl)-heptan-3-one (**287**)

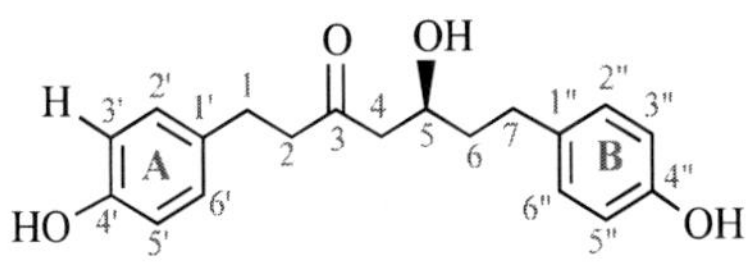

(5*R*)-5-hydroxy-1,7-*bis*(4-hydroxyphenyl)-3-heptanone (**288**)

Figure 71. One novel linear-diarylheptanoid – muricarpin (1-(4'-hydroxyphenyl)-7-(3",4"-dihydroxyphenyl)-heptan-3-one. **284**), and four known linear-diarylheptanoids – 1,7-*bis*(3,4-dihydroxyphenyl)heptan-3-yl acetate (**285**), 1-(4'-hydroxyphenyl)-7-(3",4"-dihydroxyphenyl)heptan-3-yl acetate (**286**), 1-(3',4'-hydroxyphenyl)-7-(4"-hydroxyphenyl)-heptan-3-one (**287**) and (5*R*)-5-hydroxy-1,7-*bis*(4-hydroxyphenyl)-3-heptanone (**288**) from the rhizomes of *Amomum muricarpum* Elmer.

2.9.1.3. Curcuma

The genus Curcuma found in Japan is *Curcuma domestica* Valeton (*Curcuma longa* L.) (Photos 10, 11, and 12).

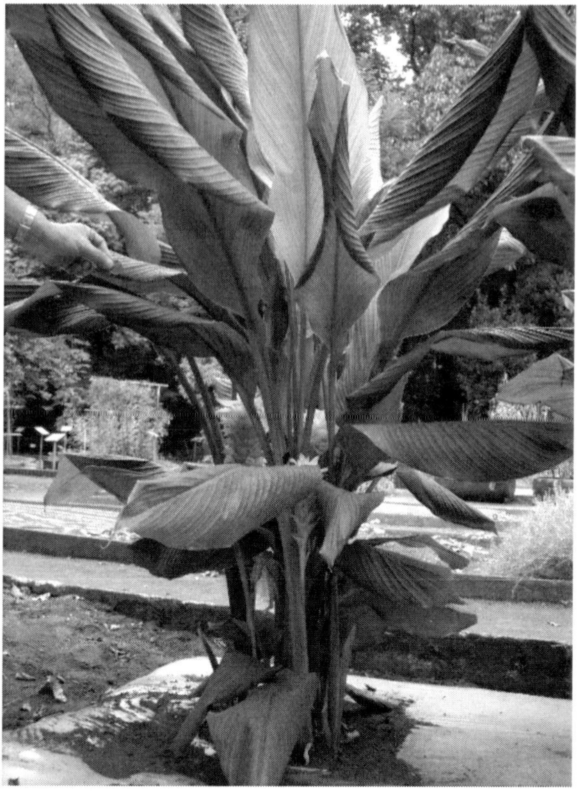

Photo 10. Whole tree of turmeric. Photographed by Noboru Motohashi at Tokyo Metropolitan Medicinal Garden, Tokyo, Japan. 8/28/2007 Tue.

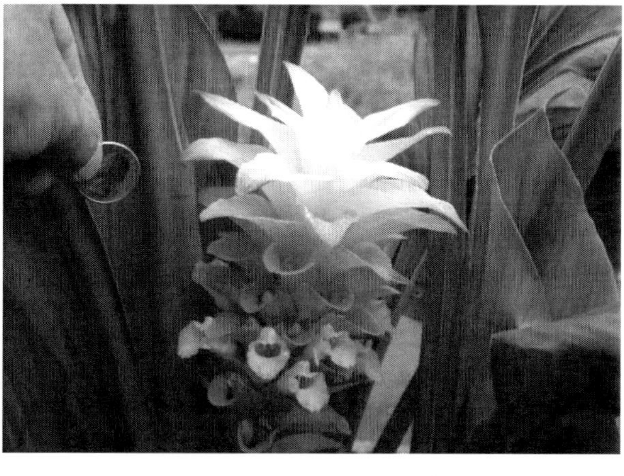

Photo 11. Spikes (new leaves and flowers) of turmeric. Photographed by Noboru Motohashi at Tokyo Metropolitan Medicinal Garden, Tokyo, Japan. 8/28/2007 Tue.

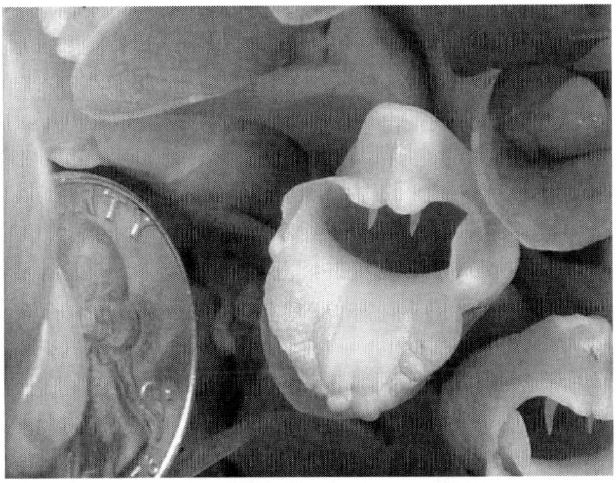

Photo 12. (Macrophoto) Flowers of turmeric. Photographed by Noboru Motohashi at Tokyo Metropolitan Medicinal Garden, Tokyo, Japan. 8/28/2007 Tue.

2.9.1.3.1. *Curcuma kwangsiensis*

In 2011, Li *et al.* confirmed eleven novel diarylheptanoids (**289** - **299**) (Figure 72) of *rel*-(3*R*,5*S*)-3,5-dihydroxy-1-(3,4-dihydroxyphenyl)-7-(4-hydroxyphenyl)-heptane (**289**), *rel*-(3*R*,5*S*)-3,5-dihydroxy-1-(4-hydroxy-3-methoxyphenyl)-7-(4-hydroxyphenyl)-heptane (**290**), *rel*-(3*R*,5*S*)-3,5-dihydroxy-1-(3-methoxy-4,5-dihydroxyphenyl)-7-(4-hydroxyphenyl)-heptane (**291**), (5*S*)-5-hydroxy-1-(4-hydroxyphenyl)-7-phenyl-3-heptanone (**292**), (5*S*)-5-hydroxy-1-(4-hydroxyphenyl)-7-(3,4-dihydroxyphenyl)-3-heptanone (**293**), (5*S*)-5-hydroxy-1-(4-hydroxy-3-methoxyphenyl)-7-(4-hydroxyphenyl)-3-heptanone (**294**), (3*R*,5*R*)-3-acetoxy-5-hydroxy-1,7-*bis*(4-hydroxyphenyl)-heptane (**295**), (3*R*,5*R*)-3-acetoxy-5-hydroxy-1,7-*bis*(3,4-dihydroxyphenyl)-heptane (**296**), (3*R*,5*R*)-3,5-diacetoxy-1-(3,4-dihydroxyphenyl)-7-(4-hydroxyphenyl)-heptane (**297**), (3*S*,5*S*)-3-acetoxy-5-hydroxy-1-(3,4-dihydroxyphenyl)-7-(4-hydroxyphenyl)-heptane (**298**) and (3*R*,5*S*)-3-acetoxy-5-hydroxy-1-(3,4-dihydroxyphenyl)-7-(4-hydroxy-phenyl)-heptane (**299**) (Figure 72) together with seven known diarylheptanoids (**300, 301, 302** - **306**) (Figure 72(continued 1)) of (3*R*,5*R*)-3,5-dihydroxy-1,7-*bis*(4-hydroxyphenyl)-heptane (**300**) [111],

(3*R*,5*R*)-3,5-dihydroxy-1-(3,4-dihydroxyphenyl)-7-(4-hydroxyphenyl)-heptane (**301**) [111], (3*R*,5*R*)-3,5-dihydroxy-1-(4-hydroxy-3-methoxy-phenyl)-7-(3,4-dihydroxyphenyl)-heptane (**302**) [111], (3*R*,5*R*)-3,5-diacetoxy-1,7-*bis*(3,4-dihydroxyhenyl)-heptane (**303**) [148], (3*R*,5*S*)-3,5-dihydroxy-1,7-*bis*(4-hydroxyhenyl)-heptane (**304**) [160], (5*S*)-5-hydroxy-1,7-*bis*(4-hydroxyhenyl)-heptane-3-one (**305**) [161] and (5*S*)-5-hydroxy-1-(4-hydroxy-3-methoxy-henyl)-7-(3,4-dihydroxyphenyl)-heptane-3-one (**306**) [162] (Figure 72(continued 1)) from the rhizomes of *Curcuma kwangsiensis*.

On the scavenging activity of 18 diarylheptanoids against active-oxygen NO species, an indole acetate non-steroidal anti-inflammatory drug indomethacin (**307**) (Figure 72(continued 1)) (IC_{50}: 12.96±1.16 μM), and hydrocortisone (**308**) (Figure 72(continued 1)) (IC_{50}: 40.64 ± 3.22 μM) having weak anti-inflammatory action of glucocorticoid were used as positive controls.

Among 18 diarylheptanoids, quenching effect (IC_{50}±SD: in the range 2.41±0.18 μM to 3.13±0.33 μM) against NO-species by three diarylheptanoids of *rel*-(3*R*,5*S*)-3,5-dihydroxy-1-(3,4-dihydroxyphenyl)-7-(4-hydroxyphenyl)-heptane (**289**), *rel*-(3*R*,5*S*)-3,5-dihydroxy-1-(4-hydroxy-3-methoxyphenyl)-7-(4-hydroxyphenyl)-heptane (**290**) and *rel*-(3*R*,5*S*)-3,5-dihydroxy-1-(3-methoxy-4,5-dihydroxyphenyl)-7-(4-hydroxyphenyl)-heptane (**291**) showed higher quenching effect of NO-species when compared to that (NO-species-quenching effect) of any other 15 diarylheptanoids (IC_{50}±SD: in the range 7.98±0.66 μM to >100 μM).

From the above results, the structural features of the diarylheptanoid skeleton appear to greatly influence the elimination effect on NO-species: In other words, the conformation of C-3 and C-5 on the diarylheptanoid skeleton is highly likely to affect the inhibitory effect on NO formation. In fact, three diarylheptanoids (**289**, **290**, **291**) with *two syn(cis) conformation type of hydroxyl groups in C-3 and C-5* showed significantly inhibitory activity [163].

(eleven novel diarylheptanoids: **289** - **299**)

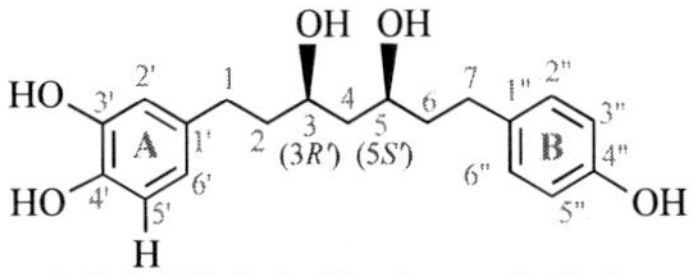

rel-(3*R*,5*S*)-3,5-dihydroxy-1-(3,4-dihydroxyphenyl)-7-(4-hydroxyphenyl)-heptane (**289**)

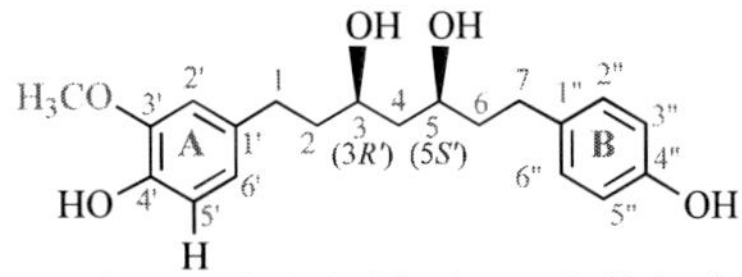

rel-(3*R*,5*S*)-3,5-dihydroxy-1-(4-hydroxy-3-methoxyphenyl)-7-(4-hydroxyphenyl)-heptane (**290**)

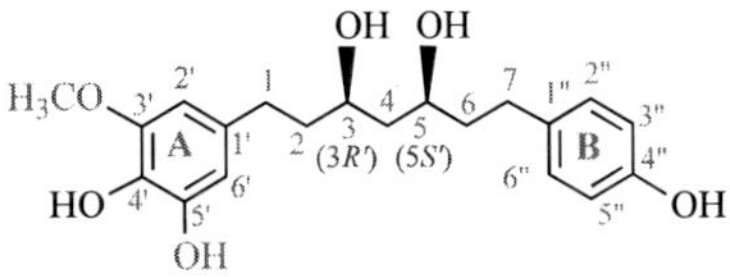

r*el*-(3R,5S*)*-3,5-dihydroxy-1-(3-methoxy-4,5-dihydroxyphenyl)-7-(4-hydroxyphenyl)-heptane (**291**)

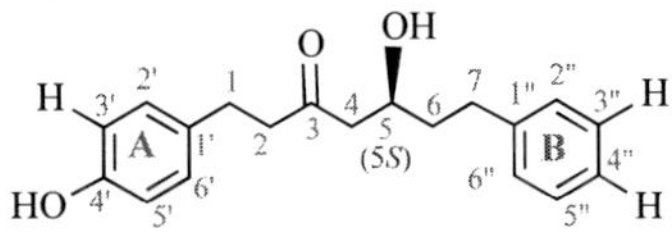

(5*S*)-5-hydroxy-1-(4-hydroxyphenyl)-7-phenyl-3-heptanone (**292**)

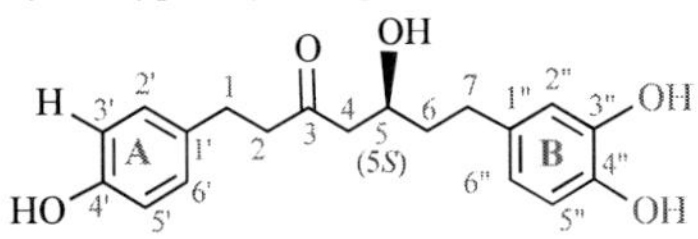

(5*S*)-5-hydroxy-1-(4-hydroxyphenyl)-7-(3,4-dihydroxyphenyl)-3-heptanone (**293**)

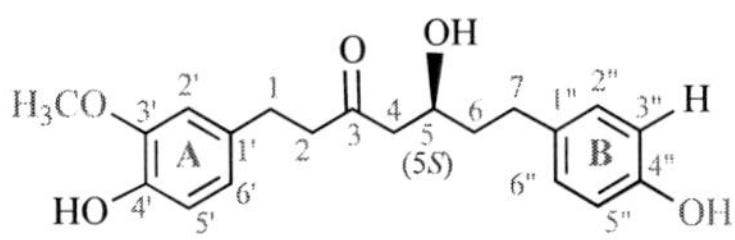

(5*S*)-5-hydroxy-1-(4-hydroxy-3-methoxyphenyl)-7-(4-hydroxyphenyl)-3-heptanone (**294**)

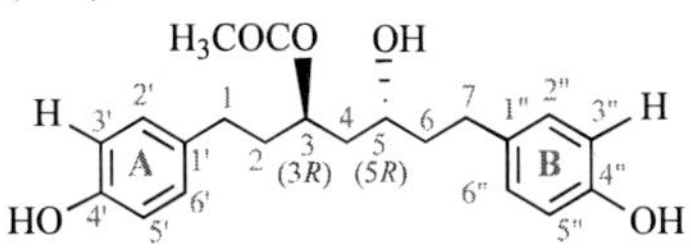

(3*R*,5*R*)-3-acetoxy-5-hydroxy-1,7-*bis*(4-hydroxyphenyl)-heptane (**295**)

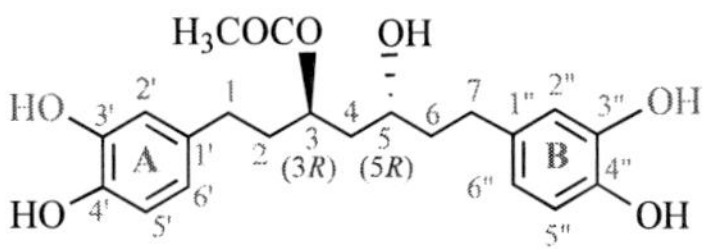

(3R,5R*)*-3-acetoxy-5-hydroxy-1,7-b*is(*3,4-dihydroxyphenyl)-heptane (**296**)

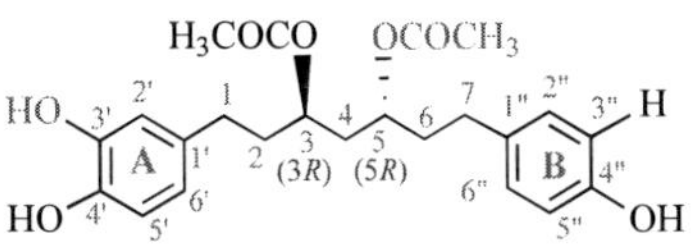

(3R,5R*)*-3,5-diacetoxy-1-(3,4-dihydroxyphenyl)-7-(4-hydroxyphenyl)-heptane (**297**)

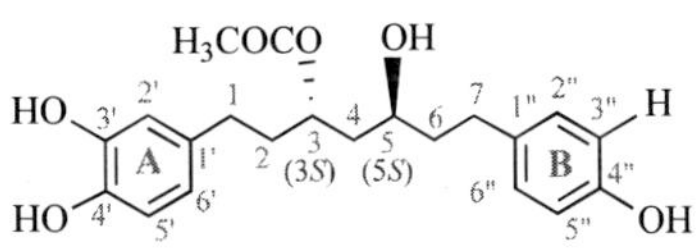

(3S,5S*)*-3-acetoxy-5-hydroxy-1-(3,4-dihydroxyphenyl)-7-(4-hydroxyphenyl)-heptane (**298**)

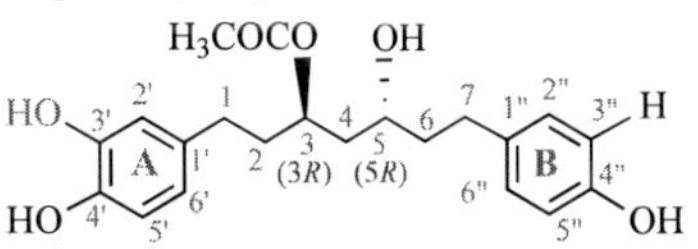

(3*R*,5*S*)-3-acetoxy-5-hydroxy-1-(3,4-dihydroxyphenyl)-7-(4-hydroxyphenyl)-heptane (**299**)

Figure 72. Eleven novel diarylheptanoids (**289** - **299**) from the rhizomes of *Curcuma kwangsiensis*.

(seven known diarylheptanoids)

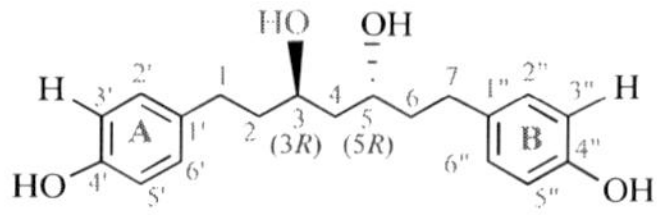

(3*R*,5*R*)-3,5-dihydroxy-1,7-*bis*(4-hydroxyphenyl)-heptane (**300**)

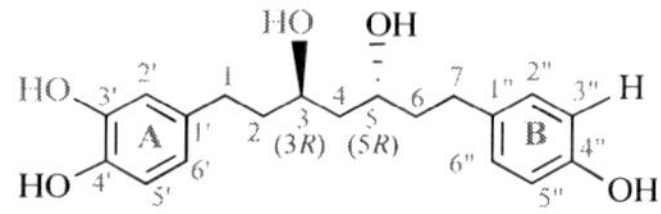

(3R,5R)-3,5-dihydroxy-1-(3,4-dihydroxyphenyl)-7-(4-hydroxyphenyl)-heptane (**301**)

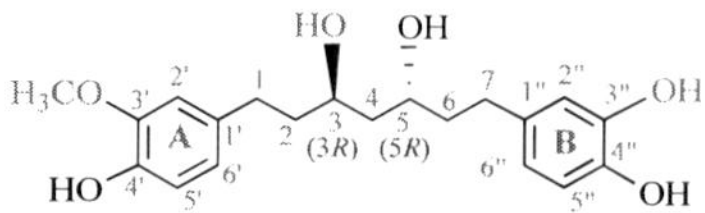

(3*R*,5*R*)-3,5-dihydroxy-1-(4-hydroxy-3-methoxyphenyl)-7-(3,4-dihydroxyphenyl)-heptane (**302**)

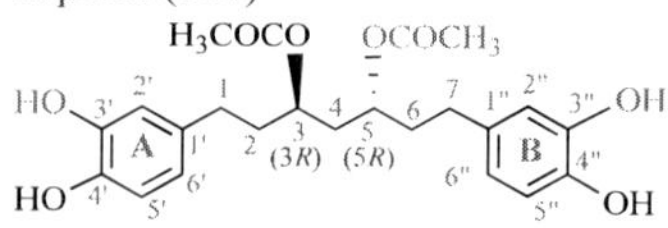

(3*R*,5*R*)-3,5-diacetoxy-1,7-*bis*(3,4-dihydroxyhenyl)-heptane (**303**)

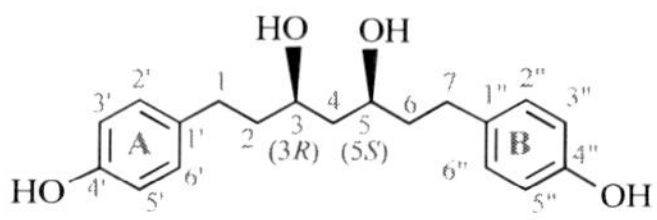

(3*R*,5*S*)-3,5-dihydroxy-1,7-*bis*(4-hydroxyhenyl)-heptane (**304**)

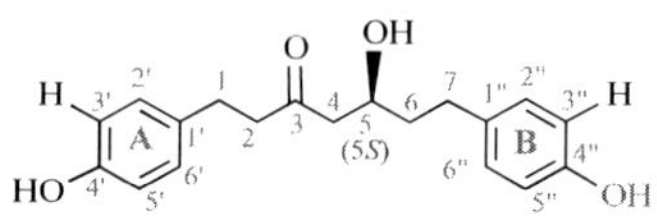

(5*S*)-5-hydroxy-1,7-*bis*(4-hydroxyhenyl)-heptane-3-one (**305**

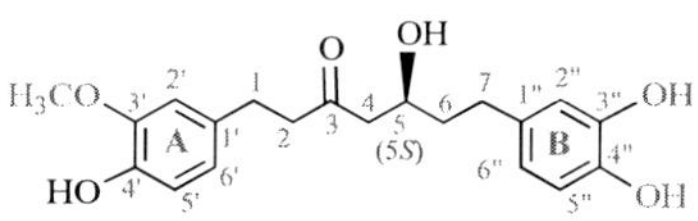

(5S)-5-hydroxy-1-(4-hydroxy-3-methoxy-henyl)-7-(3,4-dihydroxyphenyl)-heptane-3-one (**306**)

(two positive controls (**307**, **308**))

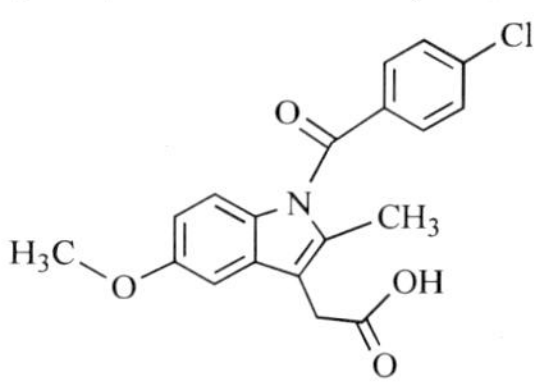

indomethacin (**307**)

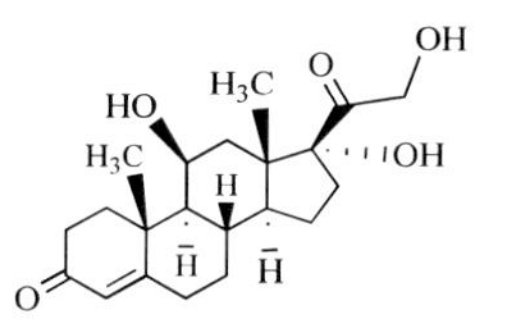

hydrocortisone (**308**)

Figure 72(continued 1). Seven known diarylheptanoids (**300, 301, 302** - **306**) from the rhizomes of *Curcuma kwangsiensis*. Two positive controls (**307**, **308**).

2.9.1.4. *Hedychium*

2.9.1.4.1. *Hedychium coronarium* (Giger Lily)

In 2015, Lin *et al.* confirmed the presence of seven new diarylheptanoids (**309** - **315**) such as three hedycoropyrans (hedycoropyran

A (**309**), hedycoropyran B (**310**), hedycoropyran C (**311**)) (Figure 73) with a tetrahydropyran moiety, and four hedycorofurans (hedycorofuran A (**312**), hedycorofuran B (**313**), hedycorofuran C (**314**), hedycorofuran D (**315**)) (Figure 73) with a tetrahydrofuran moiety from the rhizome of *Hedychium coronarium* [164].

(Three hedycoropyrans)

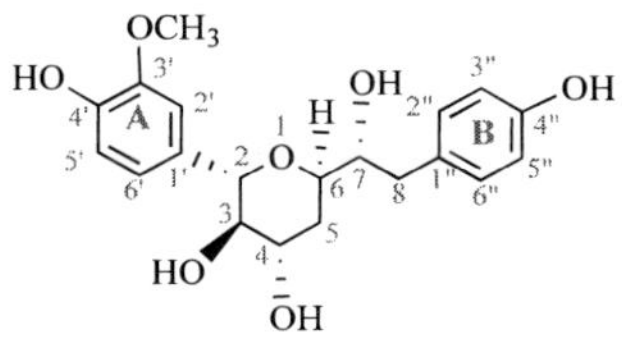

hedycoropyran A (**309**)

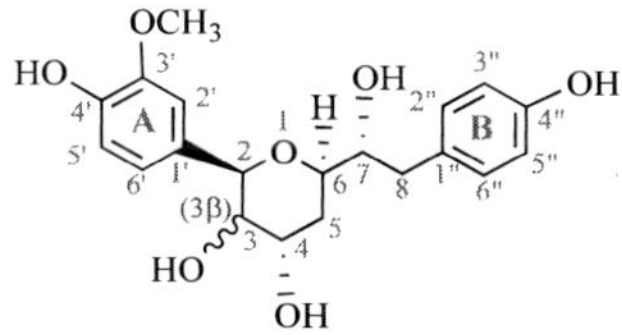

hedycoropyran B (**310**)

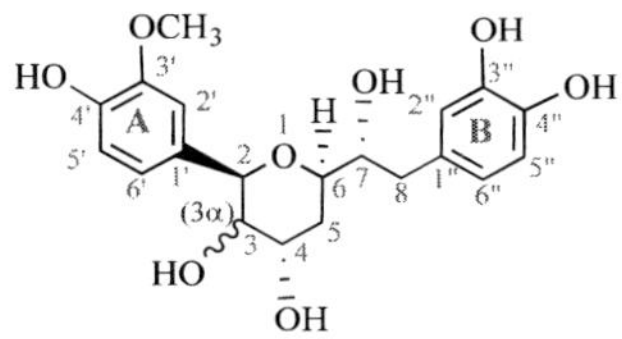

hedycoropyran C (**311**)

(Four hedycorofurans)

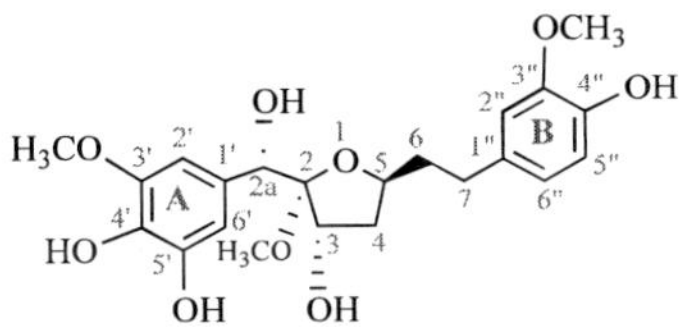

hedycorofuran A (**312**)

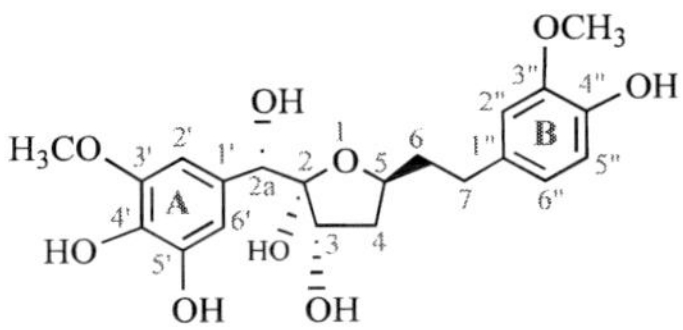

hedycorofuran B (**313**)

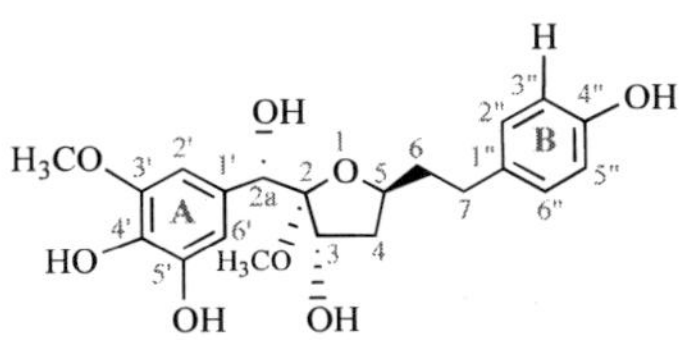

hedycorofuran C (**314**)

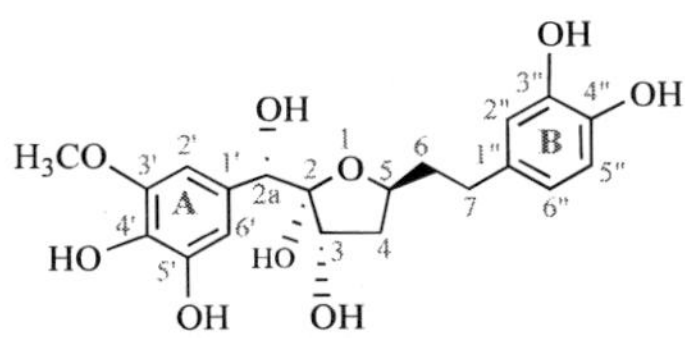

hedycorofuran D (**315**)

Figure 73. Three hedycoropyrans (hedycoropyran A (**309**), hedycoropyran B (**310**), hedycoropyran C (**311**)) with a tetrahydropyran moiety, and four hedycorofurans (hedycorofuran A (**312**), hedycorofuran B (**313**), hedycorofuran C (**314**), hedycorofuran D (**315**)) with a tetrahydrofuran moiety from the rhizome of *Hedychium coronarium*.

2.9.1.5. *Renealmia*

2.9.1.5.1. *Renealmia exaltata*

In 2002, Sekiguchi *et al.* confirmed the presence of two novel diarylheptanoids with a tetrahydrofuran ring of renealtin A (**316**) and renealtin B (**317**) (Figure 74) from the seeds of *Renealmia exaltata* [165].

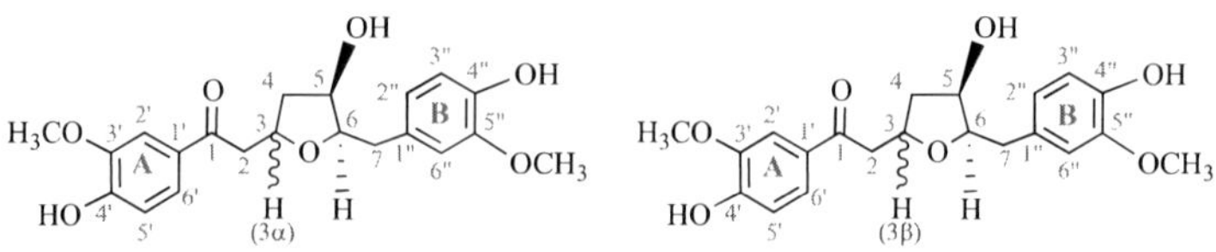

renealtin A (**316**) renealtin B (**317**)

Figure 74. Renealtin A (**316**) and renealtin B (**317**) from the seeds of *Renealmia exaltata*.

2.9.1.5.2. *Renealmia nicolaioides* Loes

In 2019, Gevú *et al.* isolated one novel diarylheptanoid (1*R*,2*S*,5*S*)-2-hydroxy-1,7(*p*-hydroxyphenyl)-centrolobine (**318**)) (Figure 75) with two known diarylheptanoids, 1,7-*bis*(4-hydroxyphenyl)-(1*E*)-1-hepten-3-one (**319**) and 5*R*-1,7-*bis*(4-hydroxyphenyl)-1*E*-hepten-5-ol (**320**) (Figure 75) from the rhizome of *Renealmia nicolaioides* Loes [166].

(one novel diarylheptanoid)

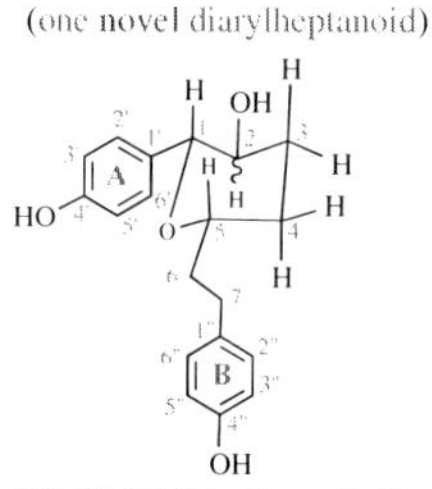

(1*R*,2*S*,5*S*)-2-hydroxy-1,7(*p*-hydroxyphenyl)-centrolobine (**318**)

(two known diarylheptanoids)

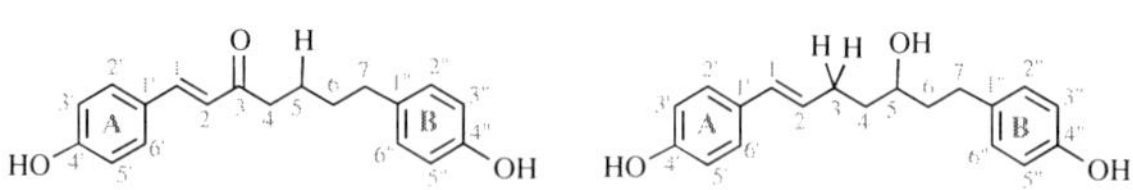

1,7-*bis*(4-hydroxyphenyl)-(1*E*)-1-hepten-3-one (**319**) 5*R*-1,7-*bis*(4-hydroxyphenyl)-1*E*-hepten-5-ol (**320**)

Figure 75. One novel diarylheptanoid (1*R*,2*S*,5*S*)-2-hydroxy-1,7(*p*-hydroxyphenyl)-centrolobine (**318**) with two known diarylheptanoids, 1,7-*bis*(4-hydroxyphenyl)-(1*E*)-1-hepten-3-one (**319**) and 5*R*-1,7-*bis*(4-hydroxyphenyl)-1*E*-hepten-5-ol (**320**).

2.9.1.6. *Zingiber*

2.9.1.6.1. *Zingiber officinale* L

2.9.1.6.1.1. *Zingiber officinale* L. (Ginger)/2012/1

In 2012, Peng F *et al.* identified five known linear diarylheptanoids (**321-325**): 3,5-dioxo-1,7-*bis*(3-methoxy-4-hydroxy)-phenyl-heptane (1,7-*bis*(4-hydroxy-3-methoxyphenyl)heptanes-3,5-dione (**321**) [167], gingerenones A ((*E*)-1,7-*bis*(4-hydroxy-3-methoxyphenyl)hept-4-en-3-one (**322**) [168], 3,5-diacetoxy-1-(3-methoxy-4,5-dihydroxy-phenyl)-7-(4-hydroxy-3-methoxyphenyl)heptane (1-(3,4-dihydroxy-5-methoxyphenyl)-7-(4-hydroxy-3-methoxyphenyl)heptane-3,5-diyl diacetate (**323**) [169], 1,7-*bis(*4-hydroxy-3- methoxyphenyl)heptane-3,5-diol (**324**) [170] and 7-(3,4-dihydroxy-5-methoxyphenyl)-5-hydroxy-1-(4-hydroxy-3-methoxyphenyl)heptan-3-one (**325**) [162] (Figure 76), and three known epoxidic diarylheptanoids (**326-328**): 1,5-epoxy-3-hydroxy-1-(3,4-hydroxy-5-methoxyphenyl)-7-(4-hydroxy-3-methoxyphenyl)heptane. (5-((2*S*,4*S*,6*S*)-4-hydroxy-6-(3-hydroxy-4-methoxyphenethyl)tetrahydro-2*H*-pyran-2-yl)-3-methoxybenzene-1,2-diol (**326**) [171], 1,5-epoxy-3-hydroxy-1-(3,4-hydroxy-5-methoxyphenyl)-7-(4-hydroxy-3-methoxyphenyl)-heptane (5-((2*S*,4*R*,6*S*)-4-hydroxy-6-(3-hydroxy-4-methoxyphenethyl)-tetrahydro-2*H*-pyran-2-yl)-3-methoxybenzene-1,2-diol (**327**) [171] and 5-[4-hydroxy-6-(4-hydroxyphenethyl)tetrahydro-2*H*-pyran-2-yl]-3-methoxy-benzene-1,2-diol (5-((2*S*,4*R*,6*S*)-4-hydroxy-6-(4-hydroxyphe-nethyl)tetra-hydro-2*H*-pyran-2-yl)-3-methoxybenzene-1,2-diol (**328**) [172] (Figure 76(continued 1)) from the root bark of fresh *Zingiber officinale* L.

First, on their 2,2-diphenyl-1-picrylhydrazyl (DPPH) free radical scavenging activity (50% effective concentration (EC_{50})) (μM) among five known linear diarylheptanoids (**321-325**) and three known epoxidic diarylheptanoids (**326-328**), **324** (EC_{50}: around 22), **325** (EC_{50}: around 25), **326** (EC_{50}: around 30), **327** (EC_{50}: around 35) and **328** (EC_{50}: around 25) showed their stronger quenching ability of DPPH radicals when compared to that of positive control curcumin (**58**) (EC_{50}: around 40).

EC_{50} (μM) of other two positive controls were quercetin (**329**) (EC_{50}: around 10) and L-ascorbic acid (vitamin C. **93**) (EC_{50}: around 70) (Figure 76(continued 1)), respectively.

Among eight known diarylheptanoids (**321-328**), EC_{50} (μM) of 1,7-*bis(*4-hydroxy-3- methoxyphenyl)heptane-3,5-diol (**324**) (EC_{50}: around 22) with two 1,3 hydroxy moieties were more effective when compared to those(EC_{50} values) of 3,5-dioxo-1,7-*bis*(3-methoxy-4-hydroxy)-phenyl-heptane (1,7-*bis*(4-hydroxy-3-methoxyphenyl)heptanes-3,5-dione (**321**) (EC_{50}: around 52) with 1,3-dioxo counterparts or 7-(3,4-dihydroxy-5-methoxyphenyl)-5-hydroxy-1-(4-hydroxy-3-methoxyphenyl)heptan-3-one (**325**) (EC_{50}: around 25) with 3-hydroxy-1-one counterparts.

This suggests that diarylheptanoids with some hydroxyl substitutions in ginger phenols play an important role in 2,2-diphenyl-1-picrylhydrazyl (DPPH) free radical scavenging activity (EC_{50} (μM)).

The gingerenones A ((*E*)-1,7-*bis*(4-hydroxy-3-methoxyphenyl)hept-4-en-3-one (**322**) (EC_{50}: around 50) with diarylheptanoid-independent enone moiety showed lower DPPH free radical scavenging activity when compared to a conjugated dienone analog curcumin (**58**) (EC_{50}: around 40) of 3,5-dioxo-1,7-*bis*(3-methoxy-4-hydroxy)-phenyl-heptane (1,7-*bis*(4-hydroxy-3-methoxyphenyl)heptanes-3,5-dione (**321**) (EC_{50}: around 50).

Thus, conjugation appeared to enhance DPPH free radical scavenging activity when comparing 3,5-dioxo-1,7-*bis*(3-methoxy-4-hydroxy)-phenyl-heptane (1,7-*bis*(4-hydroxy-3-methoxyphenyl)heptanes-3,5-dione (**321**) (EC_{50}: around 50) to curcumin (**58**) (EC_{50}: around 40). However, gingerenones A ((*E*)-1,7-*bis*(4-hydroxy-3-methoxyphenyl)hept-4-en-3-one (**322**) (EC_{50}: around 50) with an independent enone moiety did not increase the DPPH free radical scavenging activity of diarylheptanoids. The substituted 1,7-*bis(*4-hydroxy-3-methoxyphenyl)heptane-3,5-diol (**324**) (EC_{50}: around 22) having two aliphatic hydroxyl groups showed the highest DPPH free radical scavenging activity among eight known diarylheptanoids (**321-328**). Additionally, the DPPH free radical scavenging activity (EC_{50}) of ginger diarylheptanoids tends to be higher in dry ginger than in fresh ginger [173]. In general, ginger diarylheptanoids isolates also appear to have higher DPPH free radical scavenging activity in proportion to the number of conjugates and hydroxyl substitutions [174].

Second, on inhibitory effects (inhibition rate: %) of five known linear diarylheptanoids (**321-325**), three known epoxidic diarylheptanoids (**326-328**), and two reference samples curcumin (**58**) and quercetin (**329**) at each 250 μM concentration against rat brain homogenates lipid peroxidation (LPO), curcumin (**58**) was the highest around 85, followed by 5-[4-hydroxy-6-(4-hydroxyphenethyl)tetrahydro-2*H*-pyran-2-yl]-3-methoxy-benzene-1,2-diol (5-((2*S*,4*R*,6*S*)-4-hydroxy-6-(4-hydroxyphenethyl)tetra-hydro-2*H*-pyran-2-yl)-3-methoxybenzene-1,2-diol (**328**) (around 84), 3,5-diacetoxy-1-(3-methoxy-4,5-dihydroxy-phenyl)-7-(4-hydroxy-3-methoxy-phenyl)heptane (1-(3,4-dihydroxy-5-methoxyphenyl)-7-(4-hydroxy-3-methoxyphenyl)heptane-3,5-diyl diacetate (**323**) (around 70), 7-(3,4-dihydroxy-5-methoxyphenyl)-5-hydroxy-1-(4-hydroxy-3-methoxyphenyl)-heptan-3-one (**325**) (around 68), 1,5-epoxy-3-hydroxy-1-(3,4-hydroxy-5-methoxyphenyl)-7-(4-hydroxy-3-methoxyphenyl)heptane. (5-((2*S*,4*S*,6*S*)-4-hydroxy-6-(3-hydroxy-4-methoxyphenethyl)tetrahydro-2*H*-pyran-2-yl)-3-methoxybenzene-1,2-diol (**326**) (around 65), gingerenones A ((*E*)-1,7-*bis*(4-hydroxy-3-methoxyphenyl)hept-4-en-3-one (**322**) (around 60) and quercetin (**329**) (around 60), 3,5-dioxo-1,7-*bis*(3-methoxy-4-hydroxy)-phenyl-heptane (1,7-*bis*(4-hydroxy-3-methoxyphenyl)heptanes-3,5-dione (**321**) (around 55), 1,5-epoxy-3-hydroxy-1-(3,4-hydroxy-5-methoxy-phenyl)-7-(4-hydroxy-3-methoxyphenyl)heptane (5-((2*S*,4*R*,6*S*)-4-hydroxy -6-(3-hydroxy-4-methoxyphenethyl)tetrahydro-2*H*-pyran-2-yl)-3-methoxy-benzene-1,2-diol (**327**) (around 52) and 1,7-*bis(*4-hydroxy-3- methoxy-phenyl)heptane-3,5-diol (**324**) (around 38), respectively.

From the above results, inhibition rates (%) of five diarylheptanoids (**322, 323, 325, 326** and **328**) showed higher decreasing effect of lipid peroxidation (LPO) of rat brain homogenates when compared to that (inhibition rates (%)) of quercetin (**329**) (inhibition rate: 59.4±4.5%) at 250 μM concentration. However, the inhibition rates (%) of five diarylheptanoids (**322, 323, 325, 326** and **328**) showed lower lipid peroxidation (LPO) inhibitory effect than that of curcumin (**58**) (inhibition rate: 83.2±7.4%).

Interestingly, the experimental results for the rat brain homogenate differed from the previously reported mouse liver homogenate results [172]. For example, reduction of LPO by 1,5-epoxy-3-hydroxy-1-(3,4-hydroxy-5-methoxyphenyl)-7-(4-hydroxy-3-methoxyphenyl)heptane. (5-((2*S*,4*S*,6*S*)-4-Hydroxy-6-(3-hydroxy-4-methoxyphenethyl)tetrahydro-2*H*-pyran-2-yl)-3-methoxybenzene-1,2-diol (**326**) and 1,5-epoxy-3-hydroxy-1-(3,4-hydroxy-5-methoxyphenyl)-7-(4-hydroxy-3-methoxyphenyl)heptane (5-((2*S*,4*R*,6*S*)-4-hydroxy-6-(3-hydroxy-4-methoxyphenethyl)tetrahydro-2*H*-pyran-2-yl)-3-methoxybenzene-1,2-diol (**327**) on mouse liver microsomal homogenates showed a higher lipid peroxidation (LPO) decreasing effect when compared to that (reduction of LPO) of rat brain homogenates. Similarly, quercetin (**329**) also inhibited rat brain homogenate lipid peroxidation (LPO) by only approximately 60% at a concentration of 250 μM compared to mouse liver microsomes. These differences in lipid peroxidation (LPO) inhibitory activity can be explained by reports suggesting that homogenate lipid peroxidation is higher than microsomal lipid peroxidation [175]. Therefore, five diarylheptanoids (**322, 323, 325, 326** and **328**) are expected to have a lower homogenate LPO inhibitory activity than microsomal lipid peroxidation (LPO) inhibitory activity. Among five diarylheptanoids (**322, 323, 325, 326** and **328**), diarylheptanoid **328** showed the highest inhibitory activity against rat brain homogenate lipid peroxidation (LPO).

Therefore, from the results of DPPH radical scavenging ability by the above eight diarylheptanoids (**321-328**), it suggest that diarylheptanoids with a *cis*-substituted hydroxyl six-membered ether moiety and a *para*-substituted demethoxylated phenyl group can be the potential lead compounds for anti-lipid peroxidation. In general, there was a clear correlation between the DPPH radical scavenging effect of ginger phenols and their ability to scavenge lipid peroxidation (LPO), except for diarylheptanoid **324**, which showed a relatively weak inhibitory effect on rat brain homogenate lipid peroxidation (LPO) (inhibition rate: 36.9±4.1%).

Third, regarding cytotoxicity (50% inhibitory concentration (IC_{50} values in μM)) of eight diarylheptanoids (**321-328**) against 9 types of tumor cells (human oral epidermal carcinoma KB cell lines (SIBS #TCHu 73), human hepatocellular carcinoma BEL-7404 cell lines (SIBS #TCHu 64), murine macrophage-like lymphoid P388D1 cell line, human chronic granulocytic leukemia K562 cell lines (SIBS #TCHu 29), human promyelocytic leukemia HL-60 cell lines (SIBS #TCHu 23), human lung epithelial adenocarcinoma A549 cell lines (SIBS #TCHu 5), human cervical carcinoma HeLa cell lines (SIBS #TCHu 19), human nasopharyngeal carcinoma CNE cell lines (SIBS #TCHu 13) and human prostatic carcinoma PC3 cell lines (SIBS #TCHu 41)), diarylheptanoid **324** showed low cytotoxicity ($IC_{50} > 300$) against eight other tumor cell lines except for the HeLa cell lines (IC_{50}: 191.0±16.5).

On the other hand, diarylheptanoids: **322** (IC_{50}: in the range 8.8 ± 2.6 (for KB) to 114.3 ± 14.2 (for PC-3)) and **323** (IC_{50}: in the range 62.0 ± 10.7 (for CNE) to 137.0 ± 15.1 (for P388D1)), and curcumin (**58**) (IC_{50}: in the range 14.9 ± 2.6 (for HL-60) to 58.8 ± 9.4 (for A549)) are all cytotoxic to 9 types of tumor cells.

Gingerenones A ((*E*)-1,7-*bis*(4-hydroxy-3-methoxyphenyl)hept-4-en-3-one (**322**) (IC_{50}: 8.8 ± 2.6 (for KB); 9.0 ± 2.3 (for BEL7404); 6.0 ± 3.2 (for HL-60) and 15.4 ± 3.2 (for Hela)) showed the significant cytotoxicity (50% inhibitory concentration (IC50 values in μM)) when compared to that (IC_{50}) of the control sample cisplatin (C-DDP. **229**) (IC_{50}: 13.0 ± 2.4 (for KB); 10.2 ± 2.6 (for BEL7404); 9.4 ± 1.6 (for HL-60) and 9.4 ± 1.6 (for Hela)) (Figure 76(continued 1)).

From within-group comparison of each pair of diarylheptanoids, 1,3 dioxo-diarylheptanoid **321** was always more cytotoxic than its 1,3-dihydroxy counterpart diarylheptanoid **324**. This fact was found to be consistent with the preferential activity of shogaol over gingerol.

Interestingly, gingerenones A ((*E*)-1,7-*bis*(4-hydroxy-3-methoxyphenyl)hept-4-en-3-one (**322**), a diarylheptanoid with an enone group, showed almost the similar cytotoxicity spectrum as their dienone counterpart, curcumin (**58**), except for PC3 cell lines (SIBS #TCHu 41) (IC_{50}: 114.3±14.2). However, two comparable diarylheptanoids with the enone removed: 3,5-dioxo-1,7-*bis*(3-methoxy-4-hydroxy)-phenyl-heptane (1,7-*bis*(4-hydroxy-3-methoxyphenyl)heptanes-3,5-dione (**321**) and 7-(3,4-

dihydroxy-5-methoxyphenyl)-5-hydroxy-1-(4-hydroxy-3-methoxy-phenyl)heptan-3-one (**325**), significantly reduced their cytotoxicity.

Fourth, regarding other biological activities, among eight diarylheptanoids (**321-328**), several diarylheptanoids exhibited their neuro-protection of rat pheochromocytoma (PC12) cells against H_2O_2-induced injury, inhibition of xanthine oxidase (XO) (**323-328**) showed modest inhibition of XO), inhibitory effects on monoamine oxidase-A (MAO-A), protective properties on H_2O_2-induced rat primary liver cell injury (**326**, **328**), a distinct quantitative structure-activity relationships (QSAR) for the cytotoxicity of diarylheptanoids (**323**, **325**, **326**, **328**) against nine cultured tumor cell lines using chemical descriptors of chemical components, and α-glucosidase inhibition of diarylheptanoids.

(Five known linear diarylheptanoids (**321-325**))

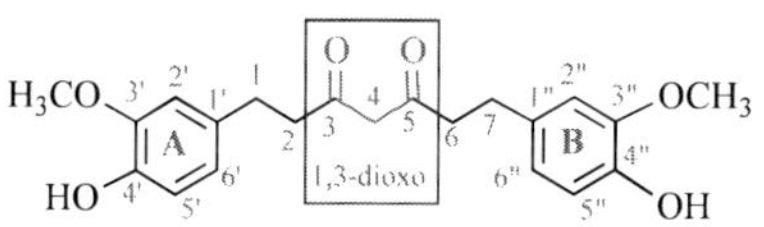

3,5-dioxo-1,7-*bis*(3-methoxy-4-hydroxy)-phenyl-heptane (1,7-*bis*(4-hydroxy-3-methoxyphenyl)heptanes-3,5-dione (**321**)

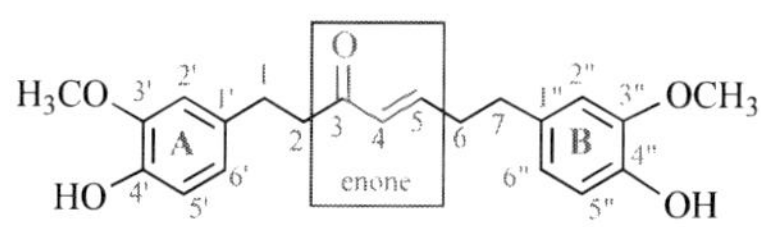

gingerenones A ((*E*)-1,7-*bis*(4-hydroxy-3-methoxyphenyl)hept-4-en-3-one (**322**)

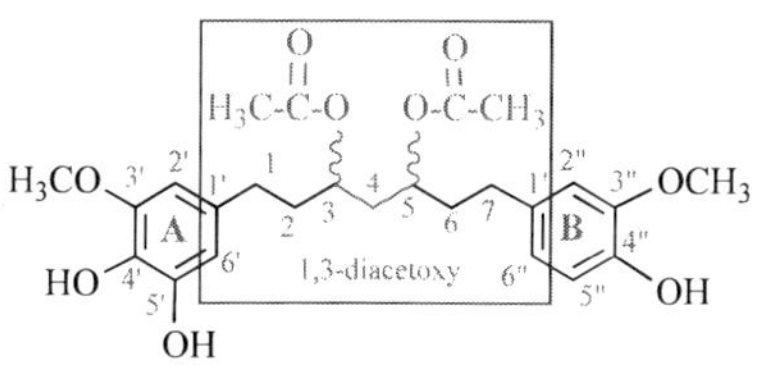

3,5-diacetoxy-1-(3-methoxy-4,5-dihydroxy-phenyl)-7-(4-hydroxy-3-methoxyphenyl)heptane (1-(3,4-dihydroxy-5-methoxyphenyl)-7-(4-hydroxy-3-methoxyphenyl)heptane-3,5-diyl diacetate (**323**)

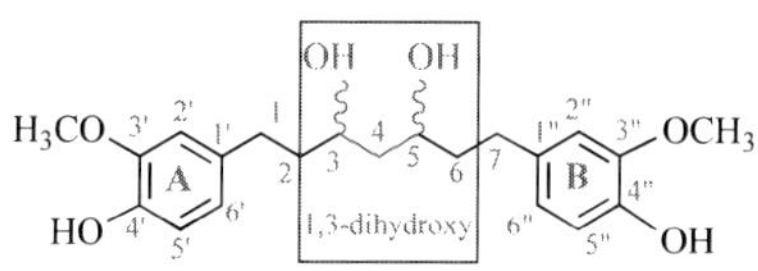

1,7-*bis*(4-hydroxy-3- methoxyphenyl)heptane-3,5-diol (**324**)

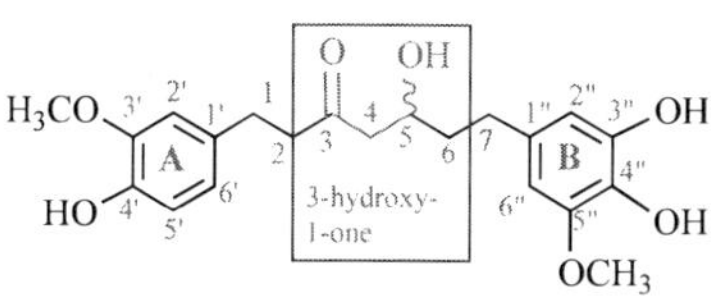

7-(3,4-dihydroxy-5-methoxyphenyl)-5-hydroxy-1-(4-hydroxy-3-methoxyphenyl)heptan-3-one (**325**)

Figure 76. Five known linear diarylheptanoids (**321-325**) from the root bark of fresh *Zingiber officinale* L..

(three known epoxidic diarylheptanoids (**326-328**))

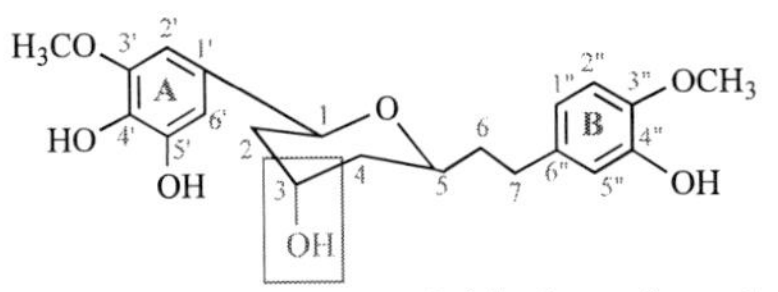

1,5-epoxy-3-hydroxy-1-(3,4-hydroxy-5-m ethoxyphenyl)-7-(4-hydroxy-3-methoxyphenyl)heptane. (5-((2*S*,4*S*,6*S*)-4-hydroxy-6-(3-hydroxy-4-m ethoxyphenethyl)tetrahydro-2*H*-pyran-2-yl)-3-methoxybenzene-1,2-diol (**326**)

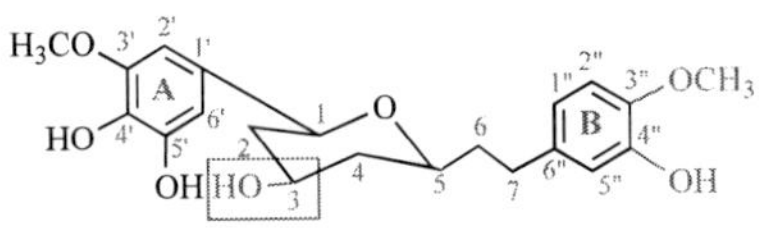

1,5-epoxy-3-hydroxy-1-(3,4-hydroxy-5-m ethoxyphenyl)-7-(4-hydroxy-3-methoxyphenyl)heptane (5-((2*S*,4*R*,6*S*)-4-hydroxy-6-(3-hydroxy-4-m ethoxyphenethyl)tetrahydro-2*H*-pyran-2-yl)-3-methoxybenzene-1,2-diol (**327**)

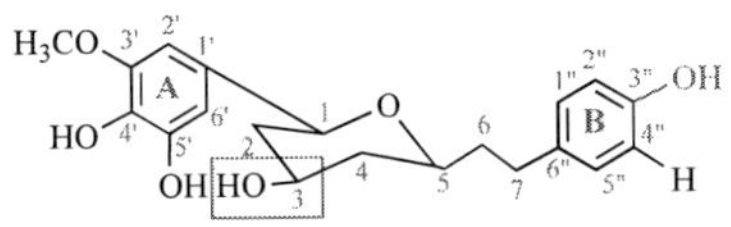

5-[4-hydroxy-6-(4-hydroxyphe nethyl)tetrahydro-2*H*-pyran-2-yl]-3-methoxybenzene-1,2-diol (5-((2*S*,4*R*,6*S*)-4-hydroxy-6-(4-hydroxyphenethyl)tetrahydro-2*H*-pyran-2-yl)-3-methoxybenzene-1,2-diol (**328**)

(four positive controls (**58, 329, 93, 229**))

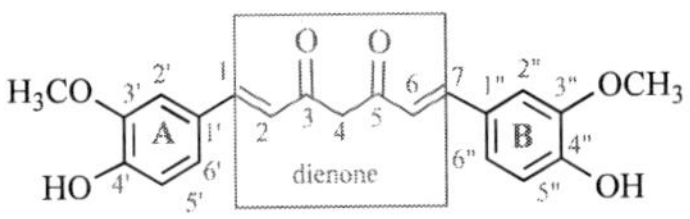

curcumin (**58**)

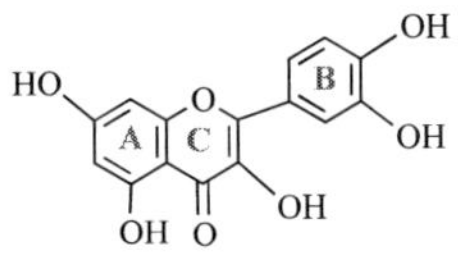

quercetin (**329**)

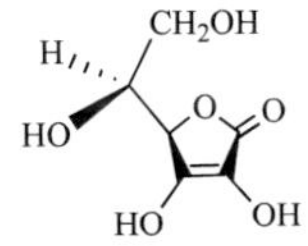

L-ascorbic acid (vitamin C. **93**)

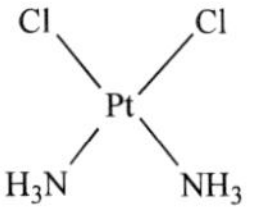

cisplatin (C-DDP. **229**)

Figure 76(continued 1). Three known epoxidic diarylheptanoids (**326-328**) from the root bark of fresh *Zingiber officinale* L.. Four positive controls (**58, 329, 93, 229**): curcumin (**58**), quercetin (**329**), L-ascorbic acid (vitamin C. **93**) and cisplatin (C-DDP. **229**).

From the above results, diarylheptanoids showed potent antioxidant activity, cytotoxicity at low micromolar concentrations, moderate inhibitory activity against xanthine oxidase (XO), monoamine oxidase-A

(MAO-A) and α-glucosidase inhibitions, and PC-12 and protection against H_2O_2-induced rat primary hepatocyte damage. Furthermore, quantitative structure-activity relationship (QSAR) analysis suggested that the cytotoxic potency of diarylheptanoids could be predicted by molecular descriptors related to lipophilicity and reactivity of diarylheptanoids [176].

2.9.1.6.1.2. *Zingiber officinale* L./2012/2

In 2012, Li N *et al.* identified one novel diarylheptanoid: (4*E*,6*E*)-7-(3,4-dihydroxy-5-methoxyphenyl)-1-(4-hydroxy-3-methoxyphenyl)-hepta-4,6-dien-3-one (**330**) along with ten known diarylheptanoids: tetrahydrocurcumin (**331**) [177, 178], curcumin (**58**) [178, 179], 5-hydroxy-1,7-*bis*(4-hydroxy-3-methoxyphenyl)heptan-3-one (**332**) [180], gingerenone A (**322**) [177, 180], 7-(3,4-dihydroxyphenyl)-5-hydroxy-1-(4-hydroxy-3-methoxyphenyl)heptan-3-one (**333**) [180], (*E*)-1,7-*bis*(4-hydroxy-3-methoxyphenyl)hept-1-ene-3,5-dione (**334**) [181], (*E*)-7-(4-hydroxy-3-methoxyphenyl)-1-(4-hydroxyphenyl)-hept-1-ene-3,5-dione (**335**) [181], shogasulfonic acid A (**336**) [182], 1,5-epoxy-3-hydroxy-1-(3,4-dihydroxy-5-methoxyphenyl)-7-(4-hydroxy-3-methoxyphenyl)-heptane (**337**) [171] and (3*S*,5*S*)-3,5-diacetoxy-1,7-*bis*(3,4-dihydroxy-phenyl)heptane (**338**) [148] (Figure 77) from the rhizomes of *Zingiber officinale*.

First, on the antioxidant activities (IC_{50}/(μmol/L)) of 11 kinds of diarylheptanoids by DPPH radical scavenging assay using L-ascorbic acid (vitamin C. **93**) (Figure 77) as control sample, 7-(3,4-dihydroxyphenyl)-5-hydroxy-1-(4-hydroxy-3-methoxyphenyl)heptan-3-one (**333**) was the highest 11.2, followed by gingerenone A (**322**) (12.6), tetrahydrocurcumin (**331**) (14.5), 5-hydroxy-1,7-*bis*(4-hydroxy-3-methoxyphenyl)heptan-3-one (**322**) (15.3), (*E*)-1,7-*bis*(4-hydroxy-3-methoxyphenyl)hept-1-ene-3,5-dione (**334**) (16.4), (3*S*,5*S*)-3,5-diacetoxy-1,7-*bis*(3,4-dihydroxyphenyl)-heptane (**338**) (20.2), (4*E*,6*E*)-7-(3,4-dihydroxy-5-methoxyphenyl)-1-(4-hydroxy-3-methoxyphenyl)-hepta-4,6-dien-3-one (**330**) (24.3), methoxyphenyl)heptane (**337**) (24.4), curcumin (**58**) (25.7), (*E*)-7-(4-hydroxy-3-methoxyphenyl)-1-(4-hydroxyphenyl)-hept-1-ene-3,5-dione

(**335**) (29.8), and shogasulfonic acid A (**336**) (41.8), respectively. A control L-ascorbic acid (vitamin C. **93**) was 26.7.

From the above results, among 11 kinds of diarylheptanoids (**330**, **331**, **58**, **332**, **322**, **333** - **338**), 9 kinds of diarylheptanoids (**330**, **331**, **58**, **332**, **322**, **333**, **334**, **337**, **338**) exhibited their marked DPPH radical scavenging activities (IC_{50}/(μmol/L)) with respective IC_{50} values of 24.3, 14.5, 25.7, 15.3, 12.6, 11.2, 16.4, 24.4 and 20.2 when compared to that (IC_{50}/(μmol/L)) of the positive control ascorbic acid (IC_{50}: 26.7). DPPH radical scavenging activity (IC_{50}/(μmol/L)) of ((*E*)-7-(4-hydroxy-3-methoxyphenyl)-1-(4-hydroxyphenyl)-hept-1-ene-3,5-dione (**335**) (29.8) showed an IC_{50} value (26.7) which is almost equivalent to control L-ascorbic acid (vitamin C. **93**). Shogasulfonic acid A (**336**) showed moderate DPPH radical scavenging activity (IC_{50}/(μmol/L): 41.8).

11 kinds of diarylheptanoids (**330**, **331**, **58**, **332**, **322**, **333** - **338**) are analogs of diarylheptanoids and have the same Ph-C7-Ph skeleton. Comparing the IC_{50} values of these 11 kinds of diarylheptanoids (**330**, **331**, **58**, **332**, **322**, **333** - **338**), it is clear that the DPPH radical scavenging activity of these diarylheptanoids depends heavily on the introduction of electron-donating groups (hydroxyl and methoxy) to the *ortho* position of the 4-hydroxyl group. And, phenoxyl groups in diarylheptanoids can make a greater contribution to DPPH radical scavenging activity when compared to methoxyphenoxyl groups. For example, 7-(3,4-dihydroxyphenyl)-5-hydroxy-1-(4-hydroxy-3-methoxyphenyl)heptan-3-one (**333**) with four electron donating groups (three phenoxyl and one methoxyphenoxyl) 3-one) showed the highest DPPH radical scavenging activity (IC_{50}: 11.2). (*E*)-7-(4-hydroxy-3-methoxyphenyl)-1-(4-hydroxyphenyl)-hept-1-ene-3,5-dione (**335**) (IC_{50}/(μmol/L): 29.8) having three electron donating groups (two phenoxyl groups and one methoxyphenoxyl group) showed relatively weaker DPPH radical scavenging activity when compared to diarylheptanoids with four or five electron donating groups, with the exception of shogasulfonic acid A (**336**). Thus, the relatively low IC_{50} value of shogasulfonic acid A (**336**) (IC_{50}/(μmol/L): 41.8) when compared to other diarylheptanoids indicates apparently that the introduction of

sulfonic acid group is responsible for the decrease in DPPH radical scavenging activity.

It suggests that the structure-activity relationship (SAR) of diarylheptanoids for DPPH radical scavenging activity is effective for predicting the biological activity of *Zingiber officinale* and for further promoting the rational use of *Zingiber officinale* for the prevention and treatment of oxidative damage.

Second, on their cytotoxic activity (IC_{50}/(μmol/L)) towards HeLa cell line of 11 kinds of diarylheptanoids, gingerenone A (**322**) was the highest 6.4, followed by curcumin (**58**) (16.5), (*E*)-1,7-*bis*(4-hydroxy-3-methoxyphenyl)hept-1-ene-3,5-dione (**334**) (22.4), (*E*)-7-(4-hydroxy-3-methoxyphenyl)-1-(4-hydroxyphenyl)-hept-1-ene-3,5-dione (**335**) (23.5), 7-(3,4-dihydroxyphenyl)-5-hydroxy-1-(4-hydroxy-3-methoxyphenyl)-heptan-3-one (**333**) (41.5), respectively. And six other diarylheptanoids: (4*E*,6*E*)-7-(3,4-dihydroxy-5-methoxyphenyl)-1-(4-hydroxy-3-methoxy-phenyl)-hepta-4,6-dien-3-one (**330**), tetrahydro-curcumin (**331**), 5-hydroxy-1,7-*bis*(4-hydroxy-3-methoxyphenyl)heptan-3-one (original **#4**), shogasulfonic acid A (**336**), 1,5-epoxy-3-hydroxy-1-(3,4-dihydroxy-5-methoxyphenyl)-7-(4-hydroxy-3-methoxyphenyl)heptane (**337**) and (3*S*,5*S*)-3,5-diacetoxy-1,7-*bis*(3,4-dihydroxyphenyl)heptane (**338**) were all IC_{50}: >100 μmol/L.

Third, on their cytotoxic activity (IC_{50}/(μmol/L)) towards MNK-45 cell line of 11 kinds of diarylheptanoids, gingerenone A (**322**) was the highest 7.8, followed by (*E*)-1,7-*bis*(4-hydroxy-3-methoxyphenyl)hept-1-ene-3,5-dione (**334**) (15.7), (*E*)-7-(4-hydroxy-3-methoxyphenyl)-1-(4-hydroxyphenyl)-hept-1-ene-3,5-dione (**335**) (25.5) and curcumin (**58**) (36.8), respectively. And six other diarylheptanoids: (4*E*,6*E*)-7-(3,4-dihydroxy-5-methoxyphenyl)-1-(4-hydroxy-3-methoxyphenyl)-hepta-4,6-dien-3-one (**330**), tetrahydrocurcumin (**331**), 5-hydroxy-1,7-*bis*(4-hydroxy-3-methoxyphenyl)heptan-3-one (**332**), 7-(3,4-dihydroxyphenyl)-5-hydroxy -1-(4-hydroxy-3-methoxyphenyl)heptan-3-one (**333**), shogasulfonic acid A (**336**), 1,5-epoxy-3-hydroxy-1-(3,4-dihydroxy-5-methoxyphenyl)-7-(4-hydroxy-3-methoxyphenyl)heptane (**337**) and (3*S*,5*S*)-3,5-diacetoxy-1,7-*bis*(3,4-dihydroxyphenyl)heptane (**338**) were all IC_{50}: >100 μmol/L.

(one novel diarylheptanoid)

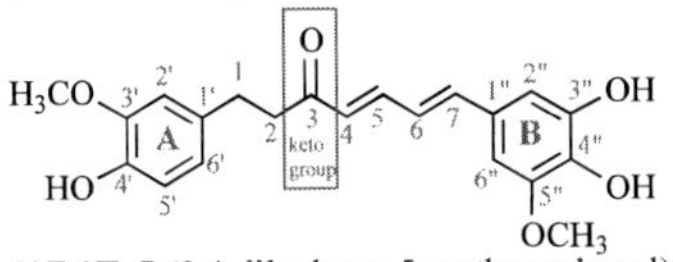

(4*E*,6*E*)-7-(3,4-dihydroxy-5-methoxyphenyl)-1-(4-hydroxy-3-methoxyphenyl)-hepta-4,6-dien-3-one (**330**)

(ten known diarylheptanoids)

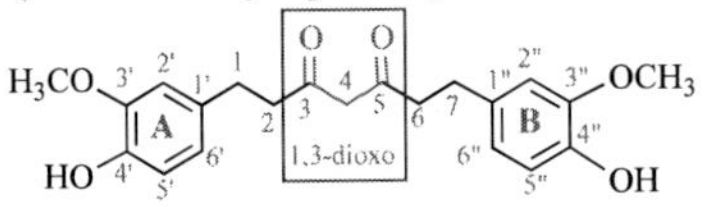

tetrahydrocurcumin (**331**)

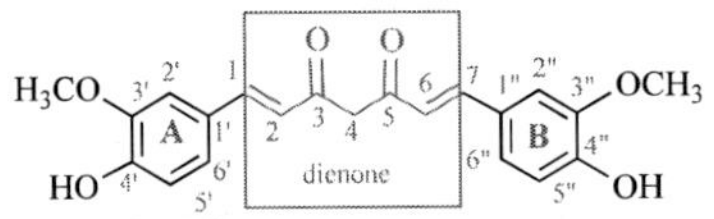

curcumin (**58**)

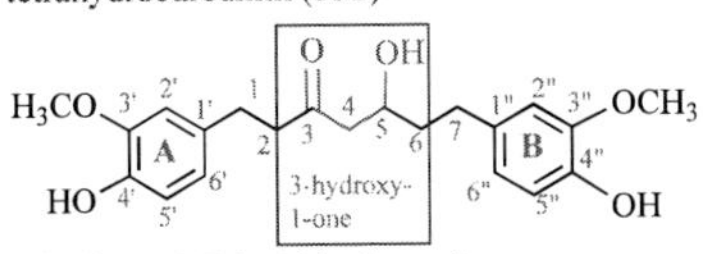

5-hydroxy-1,7-*bis*(4-hydroxy-3-methoxyphenyl)heptan-3-one (**332**)

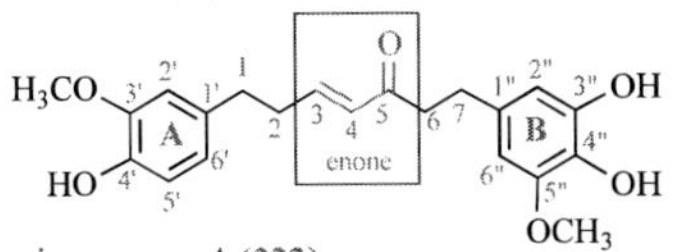

gingerenone A (**322**)

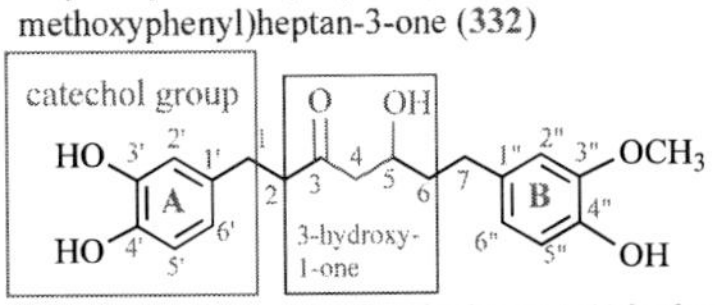

7-(3,4-dihydroxyphenyl)-5-hydroxy-1-(4-hydroxy-3-methoxyphenyl)heptan-3-one (**333**)

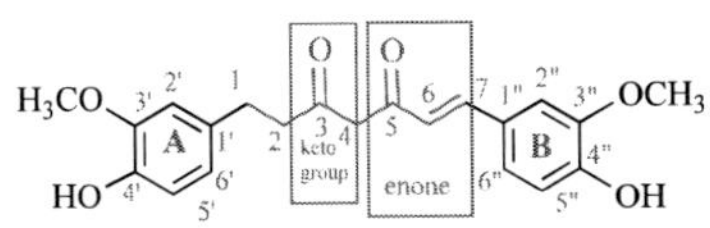

(*E*)-1,7-*bis*(4-hydroxy-3-methoxyphenyl)hept-1-ene-3,5-dione (**334**)

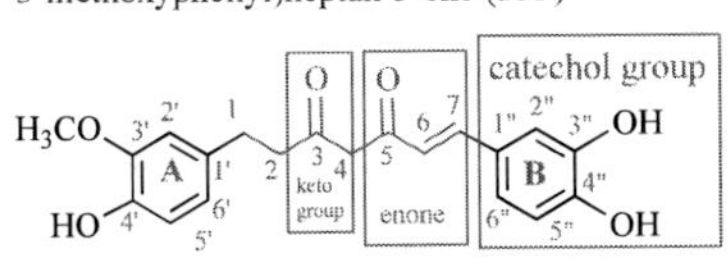

(*E*)-7-(4-hydroxy-3-methoxyphenyl)-1-(4-hydroxyphenyl)-hept-1-ene- 3,5-dione (**335**)

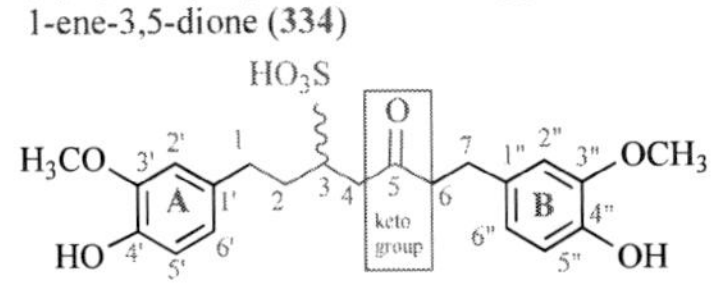

shogasulfonic acid A (**336**)

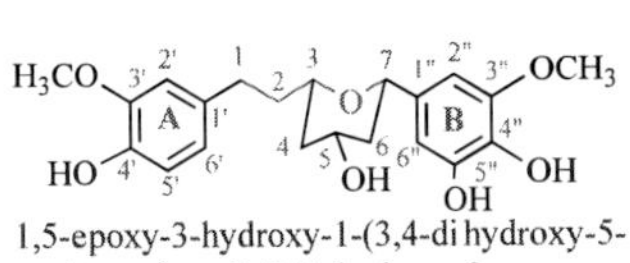

1,5-epoxy-3-hydroxy-1-(3,4-di hydroxy-5-methoxyphenyl)-7-(4-hydroxy-3-methoxyphenyl)heptane (**337**)

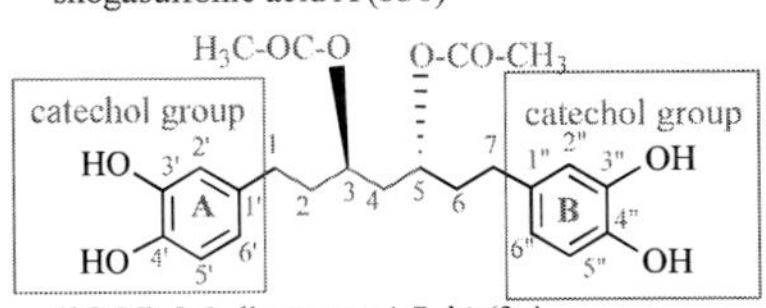

(3*S*,5*S*)-3,5-diacetoxy-1,7-*bis*(3,4-dihydroxyphenyl)heptane (**338**)

Figure 77. One novel diarylheptanoid: (4*E*,6*E*)-7-(3,4-dihydroxy-5-methoxyphenyl)-1-(4-hydroxy-3-methoxyphenyl)-hepta-4,6-dien-3-one (**330**) along with ten known diarylheptanoids: tetrahydrocurcumin (**331**), curcumin (**58**), 5-hydroxy-1,7-*bis*(4-hydroxy-3-methoxyphenyl)heptan-3-one (**332**), gingerenone A (**322**), 7-(3,4-dihydroxyphenyl)-5-hydroxy-1-(4-hydroxy-3-methoxyphenyl)heptan-3-one (**333**), (*E*)-1,7-*bis*(4-hydroxy-3-methoxyphenyl)hept-1-ene-3,5-dione (**334**), (*E*)-7-(4-hydroxy-3-methoxyphenyl)-1-(4-hydroxyphenyl)-hept-1-ene- 3,5-dione (**335**), shogasulfonic acid A (**336**), 1,5-epoxy-3-hydroxy-1-(3,4-dihydroxy-5-methoxyphenyl)-7-(4-hydroxy-3- methoxyphenyl)heptane (**337**) and (3*S*,5*S*)-3,5-diacetoxy-1,7-*bis*(3,4-dihydroxyphenyl)heptane (**338**) from the rhizomes of *Zingiber officinale*.

From the above results among 11 kinds of diarylheptanoids (**330**, **331**, **58**, **332**, **322**, **333** - **338**) using HeLa cell lines and MNK-45 cell lines by methylthiazole tetrazolium (MTT) assay, five diarylheptanoids (**58**, **322** and **333** - **335**) showed anticancer activity against HeLa cell lines. Four diarylheptanoids (**58**, **322**, **334** and **335**) displayed growth inhibition against MNK-45 cell lines. Interestingly, a diarylheptanoid gingerenone A (**322**) showed the highest cytotoxic activity against both HeLa cell lines (IC_{50}/(μmol/L): 6.4) and MNK-45 cell lines (IC_{50}/(μmol/L): 7.8).

Among 11 kinds of diarylheptanoids (**330**, **331**, **58**, **332**, **322**, **333** - **338**), some diarylheptanoids exhibited their high specific tumor cytotoxicity, suggesting that they may be lead compounds for new cancer chemotherapeutic agents [183].

2.9.1.6.2. *Zingiber mioga*/2015

In 2015, Han JS *et al.* identified diarylheptanoid pungent components: tetrahydrocurcumin (**331**), galanganol C (**339**) and gingerenone A (**322**) (Figure 78) from the whole plants including above-ground parts and root parts of *Zingiber mioga* (Photos 13, 14, 15, and 16).

The difference between ginger and mioga of Zingiber at the same time was that the rhizome of ginger showed the higher tetrahydrocurcumin (**331**) and diarylhetapnoid content when compared to the rhizome of mioga. However, these pungent diarylheptanoids did not show a consistent relative pattern.

For more accurate discrimination, because ginger and mioga contain five types of pungent diarylheptanoids: 7-(3,4-dihydroxy-5-methoxyphenyl)-5-hydroxy-1-(4-hydroxy-3-methoxyphenyl)-3-heptanone (**340**), 1-(3,4-dihydroxy-5-methoxyphenyl)-5-hydroxy-7-(4-hydroxy-3-methoxyphenyl)-3-heptanone (**341**) (Figure 78), tetrahydrocurcumin (**331**), gingerenone A ((*E*)-1,7-*bis*(4-hydroxy-3-methoxyphenyl)hept-4-en-3-one. **322**) and galanganol C (**339**), respectively, in addition to each rhizome, it was also identified by differences in diarylheptanoid content from different parts such as stems and leaves on the ground.

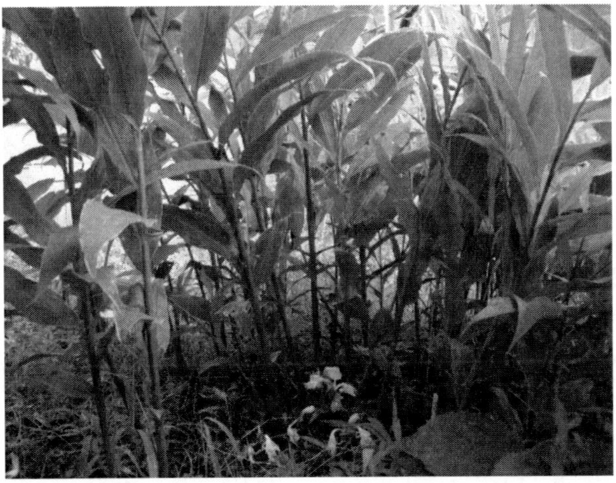

Photo 13. Whole plants of mioga at home garden of author Noboru Motohashi in Tokyo, Japan. Photographed by Noboru Motohashi. 7/21/2007 Sat.

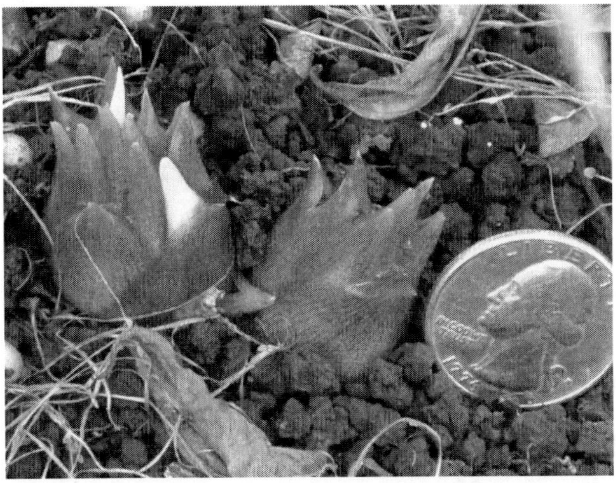

Photo 14. Miyoga sprouts at home garden of author Noboru Motohashi in Tokyo, Japan. Photographed by Noboru Motohashi. 7/21/2007 Sat.

Then, from the discrimination method using the structure-activity relationship *between* the diarylheptanoids contained in each ginger and mioga, *and* their antioxidant activity, it found that there were Pearson's positive coefficient correlation values ($0 < \gamma$ (gamma) < 1) correlations *between* five diarylheptanoids: 7-(3,4-dihydroxy-5-methoxyphenyl)-5-

hydroxy-1-(4-hydroxy-3-methoxyphenyl)-3-heptanone (**340**) or 1-(3,4-dihydroxy-5-methoxyphenyl)-5-hydroxy-7-(4-hydroxy-3-methoxyphenyl)-3-heptanone (**341**), tetrahydrocurcumin (**331**), gingerenone A (**322**) and galanganol C (**339**) in ginger and mioga *with* antioxidant activity and total phenol content (TPC) assay.

It was shown that the identification of rhizomes and aboveground parts of *Zingiber mioga* and *Zingiber officinale* could be distinguished and identified based on their biological activities determined by the different contents of metabolites such as diarylheptanoids contained in both, and non-targeting and unbiased metabolomics suitable for comprehensive analysis of intracellular metabolism. The different relative content of metabolites in the two species and plant parts resulted in their different antioxidant activities. These profiled metabolites, such as diarylheptanoids, provide their own characteristic relative content for different species and sites, then it might be a more accurate biomarker to distinguish between *Zingiber mioga* and *Zingiber officinale*. This approach is not limited to Zingiber species, but suggests that it is expected to be more accurate, faster and widely applicable to many other medicinal and edible plants [184].

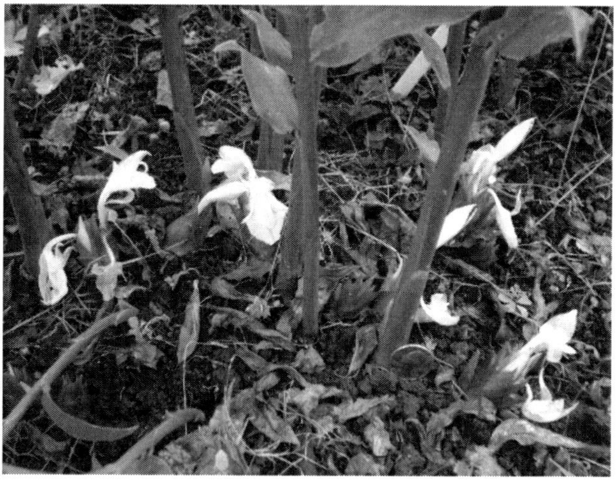

Photo 15. Flowers of mioga at home garden of author Noboru Motohashi in Tokyo, Japan. Photographed by Noboru Motohashi. 7/21/2007 Sat.

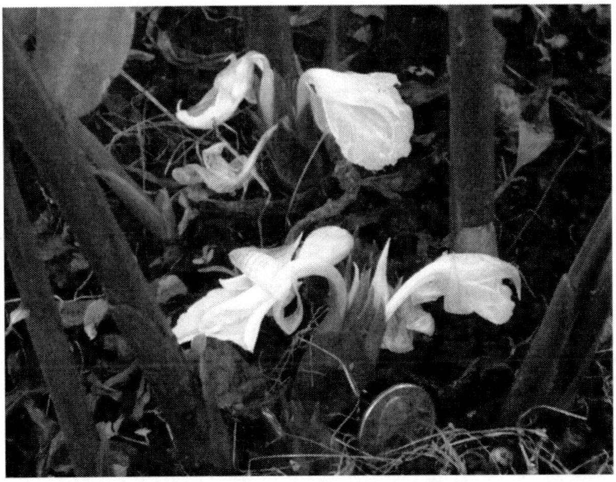

Photo 16. (Macrophoto) Flowers of mioga at home garden of author Noboru Motohashi in Tokyo, Japan. Photographed by Noboru Motohashi. 7/21/2007 Sat.

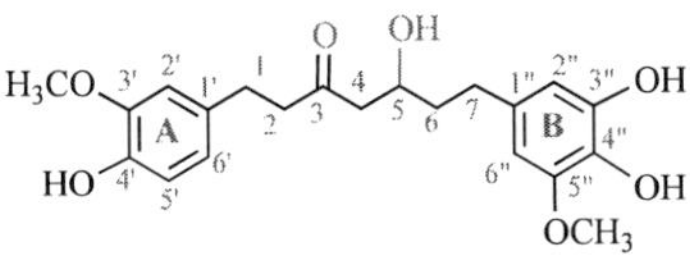

7-(3,4-dihydroxy-5-methoxyphenyl)-5-hydroxy-1-(4-hydroxy-3-methoxyphenyl)-3-heptanone (**340**)

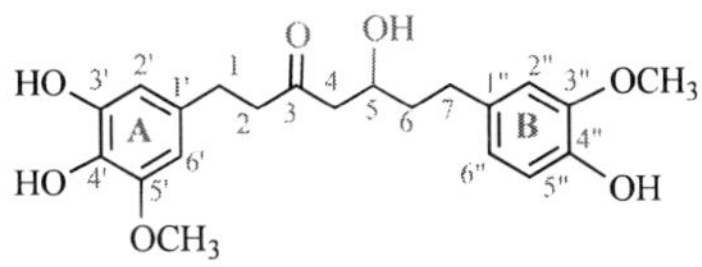

1-(3,4-dihydroxy-5-methoxyphenyl)-5-hydroxy-7-(4-hydroxy-3-methoxyphenyl)-3-heptanone (**341**)

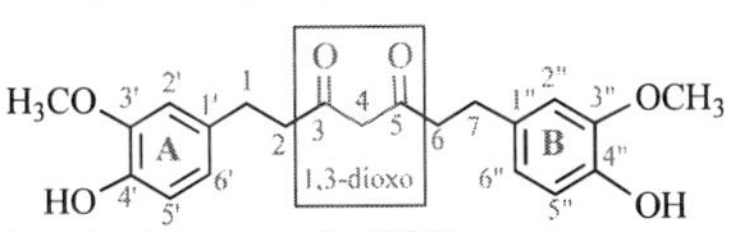

tetrahydrocurcumin (**331**)

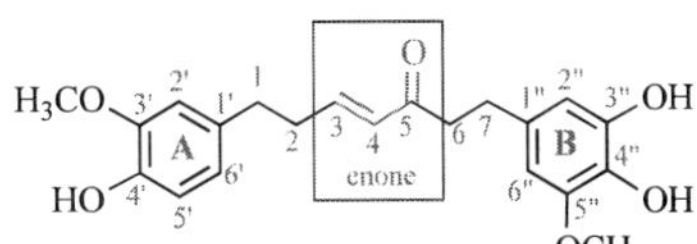

gingerenone A ((*E*)-1,7-*bis*(4-hydroxy-3-methoxyphenyl)hept-4-en-3-one. **322**)

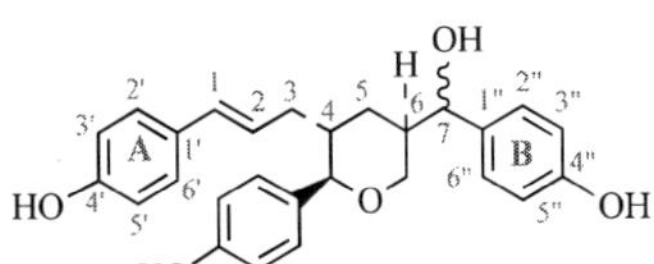

galanganol C (**339**)

Figure 78. Five types of diarylheptanoids commonly contained in the whole plants including above-ground parts and root parts of *Zingiber mioga* and *Zingiber officinale*: 7-(3,4-dihydroxy-5-methoxyphenyl)-5-hydroxy-1-(4-hydroxy-3-methoxyphenyl)-3-heptanone (**340**), 1-(3,4-dihydroxy-5-methoxyphenyl)-5-hydroxy-7-(4-hydroxy-3-methoxyphenyl)-3-heptanone (**341**), tetrahydrocurcumin (**331**), gingerenone A ((*E*)-1,7-*bis*(4-hydroxy-3-methoxyphenyl)hept-4-en-3-one. **322**) and galanganol C (**339**).

Conclusion

Since ancient time, a typical diarylheptanoid curcumin, a yellow edible pigment in turmeric, has been widely used as a flavor and dye in India and its surrounding countries since ancient times. In particular, among curcumonoids (diarylheptanoids), curcumin I, curcumin II, and curcumin III have been elucidated by many researchers not only in the food area but also in human health effects.

Curcumonoids are roughly classified into linear-diarylheptanoids and cyclic-diarylheptanoids. In addition, because there are more glycosides of these two diarylheptanoids, diarylheptanoids form an enormous derivative.

In Chapter 1, plants containing diarylheptanoids were alphabetically started from the order, followed by family, genus, and plant name. Next, this Chapter introduced as much as possible the biological activities of each plant shown in papers.

In particular, their specific contents on diarylheptanoids (curcuminoids) in plants were introduced according to the following description:

At least 9 orders, 12 families and 27 genera are known to contain plant diarylheptanoids as follows: **order Fagales** contain the most versatile 3 families 8 genera including family Betulaceae 5 genera (Alnus, Betula, Carpinus, Corylus and Ostrya), family Myricaceae 2 genera (Morella and Myrica), and family Casuarinaceae 1 genus (Casuarina). This is followed by **order Zingiberales**: 1 family 6 genera (Alpinia, Amomum, Curcuma, Hedychium, Renealmia, and Zingiber) of family Zingiberaceae; **order Sapindales**: 2 families 3 genera of family Burseraceae 2 genera (Boswellia and Garuga), and family Sapindaceae 1 genus (Acer); **order Juglandales**: 2 families 4 genera of Juglandaceae 3 genera (Juglans, Platycarya, and Pterocarya) and Rhoipteleaceae 1 genus (Rhoiptelea); **order Fabales**: 1 family Leguminosae 1 genus (Centrolobium); **order Dioscoreales**: 1 family Dioscoreaceae 2 genera (Dioscorea and Tacca); **order Ericale**: 1 family Actinidiaceae 1 genus (Clematoclethra); **order Gentiales**: 1 family Rubiaceae 1 genus (Pyrostria); and **order Santalales**: 1 family Santalaceae 1 genus (Viscum), respectively.

Regarding the structure-activity relationship of diarylheptanoids, the presence of catechol group, keto group, gallate group, vanillyl (vanilloyl) group, 1,3-dioxo group, enone site, 1,3-dihydroxy site and 3-hydroxy-1-one, dienone site in the diarylheptanoid skeleton enhances active oxygen scavenging, antitumor and anti-inflammatory properties. On the contrary, 1,3-diacetoxy group *etc.* have a function to reduce these biological activities.

New modified products such as diarylheptanoids as lead compounds can be expected to contribute to drug development, such as the emergence of new chemotherapeutic agents.

REFERENCES

[1] Craveiro AA, Prado ADC, Gottlieb OR, Albuquerque PCWD. Diarylheptanoids of *Centrolobium species*. *Phytochemistry* 9(8), 1869-1875, 1970.

[2] Alegrio LV, Braz-filho R, Gottlieb OR. Diarylheptanoids and isoflavonoids from *Centrolobium species*. *Phytochemistry* 28(9), 2359-2362, 1989.

[3] Guo JX, Kimura T, But PPH, Sung CK. *International collation of traditional and folk medicine: Northeast Asia (International Collation of Traditional & Folk Medicine Vol.)* Vol. 4. 2001. World Scientific Pub Co Inc (1600), Singapore.

[4] Benson DR, Silvester WB. Biology of Frankia strains, actinomycete symbionts of actinorhizal plants. *Microbiol Rev* 57(2), 293-319, 1993.

[5] Shayanmehr F, Jalall GF, Hosseinzadeh CA, Youseffzadeh H, Zare H. Pollen morphology of the genus *Alnus Mill.* in hyrcanian forests, north of Iran. *Applied Ecology and Enviromental Reserach* 13(3), 833-847, 2015.

[6] Asakawa Y, Genjida F, Hayashi S, Matsuura T. A new ketck from *Alunus firma* Sieb. et Zucc. (Betulaceae). *Tetrahedron Letters* 38, 3235-3237, 1969.

[7] Asakawa Y. Chemical constituents of *Alnus firma* (Butulaceae). I. Phenyl propane derivatives isolated from *Alnus firma*. *Chem Parm Bull* 43(7), 2223-2229, 1970.

[8] Yang XW, Wang JS, Ma YL, Xiao HT, Zuo YQ, Lin H, He HP, Li L, Hao XJ. Bioactive phenols from the leaves of *Baccaurea ramiflora*. *Planta Med* 73(13), 1415-1417, 2007.

[9] Kuroyanagi M, Shimomae M, Nagashima Y, Muto N, Okuda T, Kawahara N, Nakane T, Sano T. New diarylheptanoids from *Alnus japonica* and their antioxidative activity. *Chem Pharm Bull (Tokyo)* 53(12), 1519-1523, 2005.

[10] Sunnerheim-Sjöberg K, Knutsson P. Platyphylloside: metabolism and digestibility reduction *in vitro*. *J Chem Ecol* 21(9), 1339–1347, 1995.

[11] Sunnerheim K, Palo RT, Theander O, Knutsson PG. Chemical defense in birch. Platyphylloside: a phenol from *Betula pendula* inhibiting digestibility. *J Chem Ecol* 14, 549-560, 1988.

[12] Šmite E, Lundgren LN, Andersson R. Arylbutanoid and diarylheptanoid glycosides from inner bark of *Betula pendula*. *Phytochemistry* 32(2), 365-369, 1993.

[13] Giang PM, Son PT, Matsunami K, Otsuka H. New diarylheptanoids from *Amomum muricarpum* Elmer. *Chem Pharm Bull* 54(1), 139-140, 2006.

[14] Wada H, Tachibana H, Fuchino H, Tanaka N. Three new diarylheptanoid glycosides from *Alnus japonica*. *Chem Pharm Bull* 46(6), 1054-1055, 1998.

[15] Gonzalez-laredo RF, Chen J, Karchesy YM, Karchesy JJ. Four new diarylheptanoid glycosides from *Alnus rubra* bark. *Nat Prod Lett* 13(2), 75-80, 1999.

[16] Lee MA, Lee HK, Kim SH, Kim YC, Sung SH. Chemical constituents of *Alnus firma* and their inhibitory activity on lipopolysaccharide-induced nitric oxide production in BV2 microglia. *Planta Med* 76(10), 1007-1010, 2010.

[17] Roze L, Bikovens O, Telysheva G. Determination and separation of diarylheptanoids from alder growing in Latvia. *Environment.*

Technology. Resources Proceedings of the 8th International Scientific and Practical Conference. Volume 1, 329-332, 2011.

[18] Fenech M. The cytokinesis-block micronucleus technique: a detailed description of the method and its application to genotoxicity studies in human populations. *Mutat Res* 285(1), 35-44, 1993.

[19] Heim KE, Tagliaferro AR, Bobilya DJ. Flavonoid antioxidants: chemistry, metabolism and structure-activity relationships. *J Nutr Biochem* 13(10), 572-584, 2002.

[20] Stanković M, Tesević V, Vajs V, Todorović N, Milosavljević S, Godevac D. Antioxidant properties of grape seed extract on human lymphocyte oxidative defence. *Planta Med* 74(7), 730-735, 2008.

[21] Vucković I, Vajs V, Stanković M, Tesević V, Milosavljević S. A new prenylated flavanonol from *Seseli annuum* roots showing protective effect on human lymphocytes DNA. *Chem Biodivers* 7(3), 698-704, 2010.

[22] Novaković M, Stanković M, Vučković I, Todorović N, Trifunović S, Tešević V, Vajs V, Milosavljević S. Diarylheptanoids from *Alnus glutinosa* bark and their chemoprotective effect on human lymphocytes DNA. *Planta Med* 79(6), 499-505, 2013.

[23] Chen J, Gonzalez-Laredo RF, Karchesy JJ. Minor diarylheptanoid glycosides of *Alnus rubra* bark. *Phytochemistry* 53(8), 971-973, 2000.

[24] Gonzalez-Laredo RF, Helm RF, Chen J, Karchesy JJ. Two acylated diarylheptanoid glycosides from red alder bark. *Nat Prod Lett* 61(10), 1292-1294, 1998.

[25] Ohta S, Aoki T, Hirata T, Suga T. The structures of four diarylheptanoid glycosides from the female flowers of *Alnus serrulatoides*. *J Chem Soc Perkin Trans 1*, 1635-1642, 1984.

[26] Lee SS, Chen SC, Chin CKO, Chen CH, Kuo CM. Chemical constituents from *Alnus formosana* Burke. II. Polar constituents from the leaves. *Nat Prod Commun* 1(6), 461-464, 2006.

[27] Lee KK, Bahler BD, Hofmann GA, Mattern MR, Johnson RK, Kingston DGI. Isolation and structure elucidation of new PKCa inhibitors from *Pinus flexilis*. *J Nat Prod* 61(11), 1407-1409, 1998.

[28] Mshvildadze V, Legault J, Lavoie S, Gauthier C, Pichette A. Anticancer diarylheptanoid glycosides from the inner bark of *Betula papyrifera*. *Phytochemistry* 68(20), 2531-2536, 2007.

[29] Choi SE, Kim KH, Kwon JH, Kim SB, Kim HW, Lee MW. Cytotoxic activities of diarylheptanoids from *Alnus japonica*. *Arch Pharm Res* 31(10), 1287-1289, 2008.

[30] Andjelkovic T, Pesic M, Bankovic J, Tanic N, Markovic ID, Ruzdijic S. Synergistic effects of the purine analog sulfinosine and curcumin on the multidrug resistant human non-small cell lung carcinoma cell line (NCI-H460/R). *Cancer Biol Ther* 7(7), 1024-1032, 2008.

[31] Pesic M, Markovic JZ, Jankovic D, Kanazir S, Markovic ID, Rakic L, Ruzdijic S. Induced resistance in the human non small cell lung carcinoma (NCI-H460) cell line *in vitro* by anticancer drugs. *J Chemother* 18(1), 66-73, 2006.

[32] Ahmed S, Othman NH. Honey as apotential natural anticancer agent: A review of its mechanisms. *Evidence-Based Complementary and Alternative Medicine* Volume 2013, Article ID 829070, 7 pages. <http://dx.doi.org/10.1155/2013/829070>.

[33] Novaković M, Pešić M, Trifunović S, Vučković I, Todorović N, Podolski-Renić A, Dinić J, Stojković S, Tešević V, Vajs V, Milosavljević S. Diarylheptanoids from the bark of black alder inhibit the growth of sensitive and multi-drug resistant non-small cell lung carcinoma cells. *Phytochemistry* 97, 46-54, 2014.

[34] Terazawa, M, M. Miyake M, Okuyama H. Phenolic compounds in living tissue of woods. V. Reddish orange staining in keyamahannoki (*Alnus hirsuta*) and hannoki (*A. japonica*) [Betulaceae] caused by the interaction of hirsutoside and catechol oxidase after cutting the woods. *Mokuzai Gakkaishi* 30(7), 601-607, 1984.

[35] Sati SC, Sati N, Sati OP. Bioactive constituents and medicinal importance of genus Alnus. *Pharmacognosy Rev* 5(10), 174-183, 2011.

[36] Terazawa M, Okuyama H, Miyake M, Sasaki M. Phenolic compounds in living tissue of woods IV. Hirsutoside from the green bark of keyamahannoki (*Alnus hirsuta*) [Betulaceae] and its seasonal variations in the living tissues of hannoki (*A. japonica*). *Mokuzai Gakkaishi* 30(7), 587-600, 1984.

[37] Jin W, Cai XF, Na M, Lee JJ, Bae K. Triterpenoids and diarylheptanoids from *Alnus hirsuta* inhibit HIF-1 in AGS cells. *Arch Pharm Res* 30(4), 412-418, 2007.

[38] Nomura M, Tokoroyama T, Kubota T. Biarylheptanoids and other constituents from wood of *Alnus japonica*. *Phytochemistry* 20(5), 1097–1104, 1981.

[39] Aoki T, Ohta S, Suga T. Triterpenoids, diarylheptanoids and their glycosides in the flowers of *Alnus speies*. *Phytochemistry* 29(11), 3611-3614, 1990.

[40] Oyanagui Y. Reevaluation of assay methods and establishment of kit for superoxide dismutase activity. *Anal Biochem* 142(2), 290-296, 1984.

[41] Ahnfelt-Rønne I, Nielsen OH. The antiinflammatory moiety of sulfasalazine, 5-aminosalicylic acid, is a radical scavenger. *Agents Actions* 21(1-2), 191-194, 1987.

[42] Ibrahim SR, Fouad MA, Abdel-Lateff A, Okino T, Mohamed GA. Alnuheptanoid A: a new diarylheptanoid derivative from *Alnus japonica*. *Nat Prod Res* 28(20), 1765-1771, 2014.

[43] Dugas AJ Jr, Castañeda-Acosta J, Bonin GC, Price KL, Fischer NH, Winston GW. Evaluation of the total peroxyl radical-scavenging capacity of flavonoids: structure-activity relationships. *J Nat Prod* 63(3), 327-331, 2000.

[44] Mohamed GA, Ibrahim SRM, Elkhayat ES, Ross SA, Sayed HM, El-Moghazy SAM, El-Shanawany MA. Blepharisides A and B, new flavonol glycosides from *Blepharis ciliaris* growing in Saudi Arabia. *Phytochem Lett* 11, 177-182, 2015.

[45] Ibrahim SRM, Mohamed GA, Al-Musayeib NM. New constituents from the rhizomes of Egyptian *Iris germanica* L. *Molecules* 17(3), 2587-2598, 2012.

[46] Alcaraz MJ, Jimenez MJ. Flavonoids as antiinflammatory agents. *Fitoterapia* 59, 25-38, 1988.

[47] Bellik Y, Boukraâ L, Alzahrani HA, Bakhotmah BA, Abdellah F, Hammoudi SM and Iguer-Ouada M. Molecular mechanism underlying anti-inflammatory and anti-allergic activities of phytochemicals: an update. *Molecules* 18(1), 322-353, 2012.

[48] Tatli II, Akdemir ZS, Yesilada E and Küpeli E. Antiinflammatory and antinociceptive potential of major phenolics from *Verbascum salviifolium* Boiss. *Z Naturforsch C J Biosci* 63(3-4), 196-202, 2008.

[49] Ibrahim SRM, Mohamed GA, Khedr AIM, Aljaeid BM. Anti-oxidant and anti-Inflammatory cyclic diarylheptanoids from *Alnus japonica* stem bark. *Iran J Pharm Res* 16(Suppl), 83-91, 2017.

[50] Sakakibara K, Mori K, Matsui M. Synthesis of 1,7-diphenyl-1,3-heptadien-5-one, one of the components in the fresh catkin of *Alnus pendula* Masayuki. *Agricultural and Biological Chemistry* 36(10), 1825-1827, 1972.

[51] Suga T, Iwata N, Asakawa Y. Chemical constituents of the male flower of *Alnus pendula* (Betulaceae). *Bulletin of the Chemical Society of Japan* 45(7), 2058-2060, 1972.

[52] Chen J, Gonzalez-Laredo RF, Karchesy JJ. Minor diarylheptanoid glycosides of *Alnus rubra* bark. *Phytochemistry* 53(8), 971-973, 2000.

[53] Lee SJ. *Korea folk medicin*e. Pub. Center of Seoul National University. Seoul, Korea, 1966.

[54] Kim MH, Park KH, Kim SR, Park KJ, Oh MH, Heo JH, Yoon KH, Jun Yin, Yoon KH. Lee MW. Two new phenolic compounds from the leaves of *Alnus sibirica* Fisch. ex Turcz. *Nat Prod Res* 30(2), 206-213, 2016.

[55] Hashimoto T, Tori M, Asakawa Y. Five new diarylheptanoids from the male flowers of *Alnus sieboldiana*. *Chem Pharm Bull* 34(4), 1846-1849, 1986.

[56] Suga T, Ohta S, Aoki T, Hirata T. An X-ray crystallographic study on the absolute configuration of dihydroyashabushiketol and the

solvent-dependence of its optical rotation. *Bull Chem Sot Jpn* 56(11), 3353-3357, 1983.

[57] Asakawa Y. Chemical constituents of *Alnus sieboldiana* (BETULACEAE). III. The synthesis and stereochemistry of yashabushiketols. *Bull Chem Sot Jpn* 45(6), 1794-1797, 1972.

[58] Nomura M, Tokoroyama T, Kubota T. Three new cyclized C9–C1–C9 compounds from *Alnus japonica* steud. *J Chem Soc Chem Commun* 65-66, 1974.

[59] Sasaya T, Izumiyama K. Phenolic compounds from the wood of Keyamahannoki *Alnus hirsuta* TURCZ (Betulaceae). *Res Bull Coll Exp For Hokkaido Univ* 31(1), 23-50, 1974.

[60] Sasaya T. Diarylheptanoids of *Alnus hirsuta* TURCZ (Betulaceae). *Res Bull Coll Exp For Hokkaido Univ* 42(1), 191-205, 1985.

[61] Sawa Y, Sasaya T, Ozawa S. Extractives of the genus Carpinus I. Diarylheptanoids of sawashiba *Carpinus cordata* Blume wood (1). *Mokuzai Gakkaishi* 34(2), 162-168, 1988.

[62] Watanabe N, Sasaya T, Ozawa S. Extractives of the genus Corylus III. Novel diarylheptanoids from the wood of *Corylus sieboldiana* Blume (2). *Mokuzai Gakkaishi* 40(11), 1219–1225, 1994.

[63] Wang J, Dong S, Wang Y, Lu Q, Zhong H, Du G, Zhang L, Cheng Y. Cyclic diarylheptanoids from *Myrica nana* inhibiting nitric oxide release. *Bioorg Med Chem* 16(18), 8510-8515, 2008.

[64] Chiba K, Ichizawa H, Kawai S, Nishida T. α-Glucosidase inhibition activity by cyclic siarylheptanoids from *Alnus sieboldiana*. *Journal of Wood Chemistry and Technology*, 33, 44–51, 2013.

[65] Terazawa M, Koga T, Okuyama H, Miyake M. Phenolic compounds in living tissue of woods III. Platyphylloside, a new diarylheptanoid glucoside from the green back of shirakamba (*Betula platyphylla* Sukatchev *var.* japonica Hara) [Betulaceae]. *Mokuzai Gakkaishi* 30(5), 391-403, 1984.

[66] Fuchino H, Konishi S, Satoh T, Yagi A, Saitsu K, Matsumi T, Tanaka N. Chemical evaluation of *Betula species* in Japan .II. Constituents of *Betula platyphylla* var. japonica. *Chem Pharm Bull* 44(5), 1033–1038, 1996.

[67] Fuchino H, Satoh T, Tanaka N. Chemical evaluation of *Betula species* in Japan. III. Constituents of *Betula maximowicziana* Regel. *Chem Pharm Bull* 44(9), 1748-1753, 1996.

[68] Sasaya T, Sawa Y, Shuji Ozawa S. Extractives of the Genus Carpinus II. Diarylheptanoids of Sawashiba, *Carpinus corldata* Blume, Wood (2). *Mokuzai Gakkaishi* 35(1), 36-41, 1989.

[69] Watanabe N, Sasaya T. Extractives of the Genus Corylus II. Novel diarylheptanoids from the wood of *Corylus sieboldiana* Blume (1). *Mokuzai Gakkaishi* 40(2), 199-203, 1994.

[70] Lee JS, Kim HJ, Park H, Lee YS. New diarylheptanoids from the stems of *Carpinus cordata*. *J Nat Prod* 65(9), 1367-1370, 2002.

[71] Esposito T, Sansone F, Franceschelli S, Del Gaudio P, Picerno P, Aquino RP, Mencherini T. Hazelnut (*Corylus avellana* L.) shells extract: phenolic composition, antioxidant effect and cytotoxic activity on human cancer cell lines. *Int J Mol Sci* 2017 Feb 13;18(2). pii: E392. doi: 10.3390/ijms18020392.

[72] Singldinger B, Dunkel A, Hofmann T. The cyclic diarylheptanoid asadanin as the main contributor to the bitter off-taste in hazelnuts (*Corylus avellana* L.). *J Agric Food Chem* 65(8), 1677-1683, 2017.

[73] Singldinger B, Dunkel A, Bahmann D, Bahmann C, Kadow D, Bisping B, Hofmann T. New taste-active 3-(*O*-β-d-glucosyl)-2-oxoindole-3-acetic acids and diarylheptanoids in Cimiciato-infected hazelnuts. *J Agric Food Chem* 66(18), 4660-4673, 2018.

[74] Yasue M, Miyazaki M, Takahashi T, Imamura H, Honda O. The chemistry of wood extractives. VIII. Constituents of *Ostrya japonica* SARG. *Mokuzai Gakkaishi* 11(3), 111-113, 1965.

[75] Yasue M. The chemistry of wood extractives. IX. The structure of asadanin. (1). *Mokuzai Gakkaishi* 11(4), 146-152 (1965).

[76] [Yasue M. The chemistry of wood extractives. X. The structure of asadanin. (2). *Mokuzai Gakkaishi* 11(4), 153-157, 1965.

[77] Yasue M. The chemistry of wood extractives. XI. The structure of asadanin. (3). *Mokuzai Gakkaishi* 11(5), 202-205, 1965.

[78] YasueY, Imamura H. 材の抽出成分(第 12 報). Asadanin と Epiasadanol の相対配置 (Extracted components of wood (Part 12).

Relative configuration of asadanin and epiasadanol). *木材学会誌 (Journal of the Japan Wood Research Society)* 12, 226-231, 1966.

[79] Yasue M, Imamura H. The chemistry of wood extractives. XIII. The structure of isoasadanol. *Mokuzai Gakkaishi* 12(5), 231-236, 1966.

[80] Yasue M. Studies on the wood extractives of *Ostrya japonica*. On the chemical structures of asadanin and its related compounds (アサダ材の抽出成分に関する研究. 主として Asadanin およびその同族体 の化学構造について). *Ringyo Shikenzyo Kenkyu Houkoku (林業試験場研究報告)* 209, 77-168, 1968.

[81] Kaneda N, Kinghorn AD, Farnsworth NR, Tuchinda P, Udchachon J, Santisuk T, Reutrakul V. Two diarylheptanoids and a lignan from *Casuarina junghuhniana*. *Phytochemistry* 29(10), 3366-3368, 1990.

[82] Herbert J. *Systematic and Biogeography of Myricaceae*; University of St Andrews: St Andrews, UK, 2005.

[83] Hedberg I, Hedberg O, Madati PJ, Mshigeni KE, Mshiu EN, Samuelsson G. Inventory of plants used in traditional medicine in Tanzania. II. Plants of the families Dilleniaceae–Opiliaceae. *J Ethnopharmacol* 9(1), 106-112, 1983.

[84] Schlage C, Mabula C, Mahunnah RLA, Heinrich M. Medicinal plants of the Washambaa (Tanzania): Documentation and ethnopharmacological evaluation. *Plant Biol* 2(1), 83-92, 2000.

[85] Kisangau DP, Lyaruu HV, Hosea KM, Joseph CC. Use of traditional medicines in the management of HIV/AIDS opportunistic infections in Tanzania: a case in the Bukoba rural district. *J Ethnobiol Ethnomed* 2007 Jul 10;3:29.

[86] Getahun A. *Some Common Medicinal and Poisonous Plants Used in Ethiopian Folk Medicine*; Registrated in the Data Bank Prelude; Amare Getahun: Addis Ababa, Ethiopia, 1976.

[87] Teklay A, Abera B, Giday M. An ethnobotanical study of medicinal plants used in Kilte Awulaelo District, Tigray Region of Ethiopia. *J Ethnobiol Ethnomed* 9(1), 1-23, 2013.

[88] Kefalew A, Asfaw Z, Kelbessa E. Ethnobotany of medicinal plants in Ada'a District, East Shewa Zone of Oromia Regional State,

Ethiopia. *J Ethnobiol Ethnomed* 2015 Apr 2;11:25. doi: 10.1186/s13002-015-0014-6.

[89] Kamatenesi-Mugisha M, Oryem-Origa H. Traditional herbal remedies used in the management of sexual impotence and erectile dysfunction in western Uganda. *Afr Health Sci* 5(1), 40-49, 2005.

[90] Kim HH, Oh MH, Park KJ, Heo JH, Lee MW. Anti-inflammatory activity of sulfate-containing phenolic compounds isolated from the leaves of *Myrica rubra*. *Fitoterapia* 92, 188-193, 2014.

[91] Yoshimura M, Yamakami S, Amakura Y, Yoshida T. Diarylheptanoid sulfates and related compounds from *Myrica rubra* bark. *J Nat Prod* 75(10), 1798-1802, 2012.

[92] Sun D, Zhao Z, Wong H, Foo LY. Tannins and other phenolics from *Myrica esculenta* bark. *Phytochemistry* 27(2), 579-583, 1988.

[93] Jones JR, Lebar MD, Jinwal UK, Abisambra JF, Koren J 3rd, Blair L, O'Leary JC, Davey Z, Trotter J, Johnson AG, Weeber E, Eckman CB, Baker BJ, Dickey CA. The diarylheptanoid (+)-a*R*,11*S*-myricanol and two flavones from bayberry (*Myrica cerifera*) destabilize the microtubule-associated protein tau. *J Nat Prod* 74(1), 38-44, 2011.

[94] Joshi BS, Pelletier SW, Newton MG, Lee D, McGaughey GB, Puar MS. Extensive 1D, 2D NMR spectra of some [7.0] metacyclophanes and X-ray analysis of (±)-myricanol. *J Nat Prod* 59(8), 759-764, 1996.

[95] Begley MJ, Campbel RVM, Crombie L, Tuck B, Whiting DA. Constitution and absolute configuration of meta-meta-bridged, strained biphenyls from Myrica nagi; X-ray analysis of 16-bromomyricanol. *J Chem Soc* 3634-3642, 1971.

[96] Matsuda H, Morikawa T, Tao J, Ueda K, Yoshikawa M. Bioactive constituents of Chinese natural medicines. VII. Inhibitors of degranulation in RBL-2H3 cells and absolute stereostructures of three new diarylheptanoid glycosides from the bark of *Myrica rubra*. *Chem Pharm Bull* 50(2), 208-215, 2002.

[97] Tene M, Wabo HK, Kamnaing P, Tsopmo A, Tane P, Ayafor JF, Sterner O. Diarylheptanoids from *Myrica arborea*. *Phytochemistry* 54(8), 975-978, 2000.

[98] Tao J, Morikawa T, Toguchida I, Ando S, Matsuda H, Yoshikawa M. Inhibitors of nitric oxide production from the bark of *Myrica rubra*: Structures of new biphenyl type diarylheptanoid glycosides and taraxerane type triterpene. *Bioorg Med Chem* 10(12), 4005-4012, 2002.

[99] Yaguchi Y, Sakurai N, Nagai M, Inoue T. Constituents of *Myrica rubra*. III.1: Structures of two glycosides of myricanol. *Chem Pharm Bull* 36(4), 1419-1424, 1988.

[100] Sakurai N, Yaguchi Y, Hirakawa T, Nagai M, Inoue T. Two myricanol glycosides from *Myrica rubra* and revision of the structure of isomyricanone. *Phytochemistry* 30(9), 3077-3079, 1991.

[101] Makule E, Schmidt TJ, Heilmann J, Kraus B. Diarylheptanoid glycosides of *Morella salicifolia* bark. *Molecules* 2017 Dec 19;22(12). pii. E2266. doi.

[102] Anthonsen T, Lorentzen GB. Malterud KE, Porson, a new [7,0]-metacyclophane from *Myrica gale* L.. *Acta Chem Scand* B29(4), 529-530, 1976.

[103] Malterud KE, Anthonsen T, Hjortas J. 14-Oxa-[7.1]-metapara-cyclophanes from *Myrica gale* L., a new class of natural products. *Tetrahedron Letters* 35, 3069-3072, 1976.

[104] Nagai M, Dohi J, Morihara M, Sakurai N. Diarylheptanoids from *Myrica gale* var. tomentosa and revised structure of porson. *Chem Pharm Bull* 43(10), 1674-1677, 1995.pdf.

[105] Morihara M, Sakurai N, Iniue T, Kawai K, Nagai M. Two novel diarylheptanoid glucosides from *Myrica gale* var.tomentosa and absolute structure of plane-chiral galeon. *Chem Pharm Bull* 45(5), 820-823, 1997.

[106] Inoue T, Arai Y, Nagai M. Diarylheptanoids in the bark of *Myrica rubra* SIEB. et ZUCC. *Yakugaku Zasshi* 104(1), 37-41, 1984.

[107] Takeda Y, Fujita T, Shingu T, Ogimi C. Studies on the bacterial gall of *Myrica rubra*: Isolation of a new [7, 0]-metacyclophan from the

gall and DL-β-phenyllactic acid from the culture of gall-forming bacteria. *Chem Pharm Bull* 35(6), 2569-2573, 1987.
[108] Zhang Y, Ruan J, Li J, Chao L, Shi W, Yu H, Gao X, Wang T. Bioactive diarylheptanoids and stilbenes from the rhizomes of *Dioscorea septemloba* Thunb. *Fitoterapia* 117, 28-33, 2017.
[109] Ali MS, Tezuka Y, Awale S, Banskota AH, Kadota S. Six new diarylheptanoids from the seeds of *Alpinia blepharocalyx*. *J Nat Prod* 64(3), 289-293, 2001.
[110] Li W, Wang S, Feng J, Xiao Y, Xue X, Zhang H, Wang Y, Liang X. Structure elucidation and NMR assignments for curcuminoids from the rhizomes of *Curcuma longa*. *Magn Reson Chem* 47(10), 902-908, 2009.
[111] Yokosuka A, Mimaki Y, Sakagami H, Sashida Y. New diarylheptanoids and diarylheptanoid glucosides from the rhizomes of *Tacca chantrieri* and their cytotoxic activity. *J Nat Prod* 65(3), 283-289, 2002.
[112] Dong SH, Nikolić D, Simmler C, Qiu F, van Breemen RB, Soejarto DD, Pauli GF, Chen SN. Diarylheptanoids from *Dioscorea villosa* (Wild Yam). *J Nat Prod* 75(12), 2168-2177, 2012.
[113] Guo H, Li BG, Wu ZJ, Zhang GL. Lupane triterpenoids and a diarylheptanoid from *Clematoclethra actinidioides*. *Planta Med* 72(2), 180-183, 2006.
[114] Beniddir MA, Grellier P, Rasoanaivo P, Loiseau PM, Bories C, Dumontet V, Guéritte F, Litaudon M, Diarylheptanoid glucosides from *Pyrostria major* and their antiprotozoal activities. *Eur J Org Chem* 2012(5), 1039-1046, 2012.
[115] Liu J, Meng M, Li C, Huang X, Di D. Simultaneous determination of three diarylheptanoids and an α-tetralone derivative in the green walnut husks (*Juglans regia* L.) by high-performance liquid chromatography with photodiode array detector. *J Chromatgraphy A* 1190(1-2), 80-85, 2008.
[116] Tanaka T, Jiang ZH, Kouno I. Distribution of ellagic acid derivatives and a diarylheptanoid in wood of *Platycarya strobilacea*. *Phytochemistry* 47(5), 851-854, 1998.

[117] Ishida J, Kozuka M, Wang H, Konoshima T, Tokuda H, Okuda M, Yang Mou X, Nishino H, Sakurai N, Lee KH, Nagai M. Antitumor-promoting effects of cyclic diarylheptanoids on Epstein-Barr virus activation and two-stage mouse skin carcinogenesis. *Cancer Lett* 159(2), 135-140, 2000.

[118] Morikawa T, Tao J, Toguchida I, Matsuda H, Yoshikawa M. Structures of new cyclic diarylheptanoids and inhibitors of nitric oxide production from Japanese folk medicine *Acer nikoense*. *J Nat Prod* 66(1), 86-91, 2003.

[119] Liu HB, Cui CB, Cai B, Gu QQ, Zhang DY, Zhao QC, Guan HS. Pterocarine, a new diarylheptanoid from *Pterocarya tonkinesis*, its cell cycle inhibition at G0/G1 phase and induction of apoptosis in HCT-15 and K562 cells. *Chin Chem Lett* 16(2), 215-218, 2005.

[120] Jiang ZH, Tanaka T, Hirata H, Fukuoka R, Kouno I. Three diarylheptanoids from *Rhoiptelea chiliantha*. *Phytochemistry* 43(5), 1049-1054, 1996.

[121] Chun KS, Sohn Y, Kim HS, Kim OH, Park KK, Lee JM, Moon A, Lee SS, Surh YJ. Anti-tumor promoting potential of naturally occurring diarylheptanoids structurally related to curcumin. *Mutat Res* 428(1-2), 49-57, 1999.

[122] Elattar TM, Virji AS. The inhibitory effect of curcumin, genistein, quercetin and cisplatin on the growth of oral cancer cells *in vitro*. *Anticancer Res* 20(3A), 1733-1738, 2000.

[123] Hadi SM, Asad SF, Singh S, Ahmad A. Putative mechanism for anticancer and apoptosis-inducing properties of plant-derived polyphenolic compounds. *IUBMB Life* 50(3), 167-171, 2000.

[124] Ramsewak RS, DeWitt DL, Nair MG. Cytotoxicity, antioxidant and anti-inflammatory activities of curcumins I-III from *Curcuma longa*. *Phytomedicine* 7(4), 303-308, 2000.

[125] Surh Y. Molecular mechanisms of chemopreventive effects of selected dietary and medicinal phenolic substances. *Mutat Res* 428(1-2), 305-327, 1999.

[126] Keserü GM, Nógrádi M. Chemistry of natural diarylheptanoids. In: Atta-ur-Rahman X (ed.), *Studies in natural products chemistry Vol 17*. Elsevier Science, Amsterdam, p. 357, 1995.

[127] Martín-Cordero C, López-Lázaro M, Agudo MA, Navarro E, Trujillo J, Ayuso MJ. A cytotoxic diarylheptanoid from *Viscum cruciatum*. *Phytochemistry* 58(4), 567-569, 2001.

[128] Zhao YL, Wang XY, Sun LX, Fan RH, Bi KS, Yu ZG. Cytotoxic constituents of *Viscum coloratum*. *Z Naturforsch C* 67(3-4), 129-134, 2012.

[129] Lakshmi Niranjan Reddy V, Ravinder K, Srinivasulu M, Venkateshwar Goud T, Malla Reddy S, Srujankumar D, Prabhakar Rao T, Suryanarayana Murty U, Venkateswarlu Y. Two new macrocyclic diaryl ether heptanoids from *Boswellia ovalifoliolata*. *Chem Pharm Bull* 51(9), 1081-1084, 2003.

[130] Kalchhauser H, Krishnamurty HG, Talukdar AC, Schmid W. Isolation and structure determination of two new macrocyclic biaryl ethers from *Garuga gamblei*. *Monatshefte für Chemie* 119(8-9), 1047-1050, 1988.

[131] Kalchhauser H, Krishnamurty. NMR spectral assignment and conformation of macrocyclic biaryl ethers from *Garuga gamblei*. *Mag Reson Chem* 27(7), 635-639, 1989.

[132] Meena M. Haribal, Anil K. Mishra, B.K. Sabata. Isolation and structure of a new macrocyclic, 15-membered biphenyl ether-garuganin-I from *garuga pinnata*. *Tetrahedron* 41(21), 4949-4951, 1985.

[133] Mishra AK, Haribal MM, Sabata BK. Garuganin III, a macrocyclic biphenyl ether from *Garuga pinnata*. *Phytochemistry* 24(10), 2463-2465, 1985.

[134] Ara K, Rahman AH, Hasan CM, Iskander MN, Asakawa Y, Quang DN, Rashid MA. Macrocyclic diarylheptanoids from *Garuga pinnata*. *Phytochemistry* 67(24), 2659-2662, 2006.

[135] Ara K, Haque MR, Kaisar MA, Rahman AHMM, Hasan CM, Rashid MA. A new diarylheptanoid from *Garuga pinnata* Roxb. *Dhaka Univ J Pharm Sci* 11(2), 165-167, 2012.

[136] Nagai M, Kubo W, Fujita M, Inoue T, Matsuo M. Acerogenin A, a novel cyclic diarylheptanoid. *J Chem Soc Chem Commun* 338-339, 1976.

[137] Nagai M, Kubo M, Fujita M, Inoue T, Matsuo M. Studies on the constituents of Aceraceae plants. II. Structure of aceroside I, a glucoside of a novel cyclic diarylheptanoid from *Acer nikoense* Maxim. *Chem Pharm Bull* 26(9), 2805-2810, 1978.

[138] Nagai M, Kenmochi N, Fujita M, Furukawa N, Inoue T. Studies on the constituents of Aceraceae plants. VI. Revised stereochemistry of (-)-centrolobol, and new glycosides from *Acer nikoense. Chem Pharm Bull* 34(3), 1056-1060, 1986.

[139] Kubo M, Inoue T, Nagai M. Studies on the constituents of Aceraceae plants. III. Strucure of acerogenin B from *Acer nikoense* MAXIM. *Chem Pharm Bull* 28(4), 1300-1303, 1980.

[140] Nagumo S, Kaji N, Inoue T. Nagai, M. Studies on the constituents of Aceraceae plants. XI. Two types of cyclic diarylheptanoid from *Acer nikoense. Chem Pharm Bull* 41(7), 1255-1257, 1993.

[141] Nagumo S, Kaji N, Inoue T. Nagai, M. Studies on the constituents of Aceraceae plants. XIII. Diarylheptanoids and other phenolics from *Acer nikoense. Chem Pharm Bull* 44(5), 1086-1089, 1996.

[142] Salerno L, Sorrenti V, Di Giacomo C, Romeo G, Siracusa MA. Progress in the development of selective nitric oxide synthase (NOS) inhibitors. *Curr Pharm Des* 8(3), 177-200, 2002.

[143] Kuroyanagi M, Noro T, Fukushima S, Aiyama R, Ikuta A, Itokawa H, Morita M. Studies on the constituents of the seeds of *Alpinia katsumadai* Hayata. *Chem Pharm Bull* 31(5), 1544-1550, 1983.

[144] Itokawa H, Morita M, Midorikawa I, Aiyama R, Motita M. Diarylheptanoids from the rhizome of *Alpinia officinarum. Chem Pharm Bull* 33(11), 4889-4893, 1985.

[145] Itokawa H, Morita M, Mihashi S. Two new diarylheptanoids from *Alpinia officinarum* HANCE *Chem Pharm Bull* 29(8), 2383-2385, 1981.

[146] Kiuchi F, Shibuya M, Sankawa U. Inhibitors of prostaglandin biosynthesis from *Alpinia officinarum. Chem Pharm Bull* 30(6), 2279-2282, 1982.

[147] An N, Xu LZ, Zou ZM, Yang SL. Diarylheptanoids from *Alpinia officinarum. J Asian Nat Prod Res* 8(7), 637-641, 2006.

[148] Kikuzaki H, Kobayashi M, Nakatani N. Diarylheptanoids from rhizomes of *Zingiber officinale. Phytochemistry* 30(11), 3647-3651, 1991.

[149] An N, Zou ZM, Tian Z, Luo XZ, Yang SL, Xu LZ. Diarylheptanoids from the rhizomes of Alpinia officinarum and their anticancer activity. *Fitoterapia* 79(1), 27-31, 2008.

[150] Athamaprasangsa S, Buntrarongroj U, Dampawan P, Ongkavoranan N, Rukachaisirikul V, Sethijinda S, Sornnarintra M, Sriwub P, Taylor WC. A 1,7-diarylheptanoid from *Alpinia conchigera. Phytochemistry* 37(3), 871-873, 1994.

[151] Itokawa H, Aiyama R, Ikuta A. Synthesis of diarylheptanoids and assessment of their pungency. *Chem Pharm Bull* 31(7), 2491-2496, 1983.

[152] Mosmann T. Rapid colorimetric assay for cellular growth and survival: application to proliferation and cytotoxicity assays. *J Immunol Methods* 65(1-2), 55-63, 1983.

[153] Dan L, Wei Q, Ling Z, Fu-Qin G, Jing-Yu L. A new dimeric diarylheptanoid from the rhizomes of *Alpinia officinarum. Chin J Nat Med* 12(2), 139-141, 2014.

[154] Zhao L, Qu W, Fu J-Q, Liang J-Y. A new diarylheptanoid from the rhizomes of *Alpinia officinarum. Chin J Nat Med* 8(4), 241-243, 2010.

[155] Sun Y, Tabata K, Matsubara H, Kitanaka S, Suzuki T, Yasukawa K. New cytotoxic diarylheptanoids from the Rhizomes of *Alpinia officinarum. Planta Med* 74(40, 427-431, 2008.

[156] Liu D, Liu YW, Guan FQ, Liang JY. New cytotoxic diarylheptanoids from the rhizomes of *Alpinia officinarum* Hance. *Fitoterapia* 76-80, 2014. doi:10.1016/j.fitote.2014.04.008.

[157] Giang PM, Son PT, Matsunami K, Otsuka H. New diarylheptanoids from *Alpinia pinnanensis*. *Chem Pharm Bull* 53(10), 1335-1337, 2005.

[158] Giang PM, Son PT, Matsunami K, Otsuka H. New diarylheptanoids from *Amomum muricarpum* ELMER. *Chem Pharm Bull* 54(1), 139-140, 2006.

[159] Giang PM, Son PT, Matsunami K, Otsuka H. One new and several minor diarylheptanoids from *Amomum muricarpum*. *Nat Prod Res* 26(13), 1195-1200, 2012.

[160] Martin TS, Kikuzaki H, Hisamoto M, Nakatani N. Constituents of amomum tsao-ko and their radical scavenging and antioxidant activities. *Journal of the American Oil Chemists' Society* 77(6), 667, 2000.

[161] Ohta S, Koyama M, Aoki T, Suga T. Absolute configuration of platyphylloside and (−)-centrolobol. *Bull Chem Soc Jpn* 58(8), 2423-2424, 1985.

[162] Ma J, Jin X, Yang L, Li ZL. Diarylheptanoids from the rhizomes of *Zingiber officinale*. *Phytochemistry* 65(8), 1137-1143, 2004.

[163] Li J, Liao CR, Wei JQ, Chen LX, Zhao F, Qiu F. Diarylheptanoids from *Curcuma kwangsiensis* and their inhibitory activity on nitric oxide production in lipopolysaccharide-activated macrophages. *Bioorg Med Chem Lett* 21(18), 5363-5369, 2011.

[164] Lin YS, Lin JH, Chang CC, Lee SS. Tetrahydropyran- and tetrahydrofuran-containing diarylheptanoids from *Hedychium coronarium* rhizomes. *J Nat Prod* 78(2), 181-187, 2015.

[165] Sekiguchi M, Shigemori H, Ohsaki A, Kobayashi J. Renealtins A and B, new diarylheptanoids with a tetrahydrofuran ring from the seeds of *Renealmia exaltata*. *J Nat Prod* 65(3), 375-376, 2002.

[166] Gevú KV, Carvaalho MGD, Silva IGD, Lima HRP, Castro R, Cunha MD. Phenolic compounds from the rhizome of *Renealmia nicolaioides* Loes.: a new diarylheptanoid. *Anais da Academia Brasileira de Ciências* (*Annals of the Brazilian Academy of Sciences*) 91(1), e20180312, 2019.

[167] Sui Z, Salto R, Li J, Craik C, Ortiz de Montellano PR. Inhibition of the HIV-1 and HIV-2 proteases by curcumin and curcumin boron complexes. *Bioorg Med Chem* 1(6), 415-422, 1993.

[168] Endo K, Kanno E, Oshima Y. Structures of antifungal diarylheptenones, gingerenones A, B, C and isogingerenone B, isolated from the rhizomes of *Zingiber officinale*. *Phytochemistry* 29(3), 797-799, 1990.

[169] Zhou CX, Zhang XY, Dong XW, Tao QF, Dou H, Zhang RP, Ke Huang KX, Li XK, Chen CX, Zeng S, Zhao Y. Three new diarylheptanoids and their antioxidant property. *Chin Chem Lett* 18(10), 1243-1246, 2007.

[170] Kikuzaki H, UsuguchiI J, Nakatani N. Constituents of zingiberaceae. I: diarylheptanoids from the rhizomes of ginger (*Zingiber officinale* ROSCOE). *Chem Pharm Bull* 39(1), 120-122, 1991.

[171] Kikuzaki H, Nakatani N. Cyclic diarylheptanoids from rhizomes of *Zingiber officinale*. *Phytochemistry* 43(1), 273-277, 1996.

[172] Tao QF, Xu Y, Lam RY, Schneider B, Dou H, Leung PS, Shi SY, Zhou CX, Yang LX, Zhang RP, Xiao YC, Wu X, Stöckigt J, Zeng S, Cheng CH, Zhao Y. Diarylheptanoids and a monoterpenoid from the rhizomes of *Zingiber officinale*: antioxidant and cytoprotective properties. *J Nat Prod* 71(1), 12–17, 2008.

[173] Dugasani S, Pichika MR, Nadarajah VD, Balijepalli MK, Tandra S, Korlakunta JN. Comparative antioxidant and anti-inflammatory effects of [6]-gingerol, [8]-gingerol, [10]-gingerol and [6]-shogaol. *J Ethnopharmacol* 127(2), 515-520, 2010.

[174] Simić A, Manojlović D, Segan D, Todorović M. Electrochemical behavior and antioxidant and prooxidant activity of natural phenolics. *Molecules* 12(10), 2327-2340, 2007.

[175] Fraga CG, Leibovitz BE, Tappel AL. Lipid peroxidation measured as thiobarbituric acid-reactive substances in tissue slices: characterization and comparison with homogenates and microsomes. *Free Radic Biol Med* 4(3), 155-161, 1988.

[176] Peng F, Tao Q, Wu X, Dou H, Spencer S, Mang C, Xu L, Sun L, Zhao Y, Li H, Zeng S, Liu G, Hao X. Cytotoxic, cytoprotective and

antioxidant effects of isolated phenolic compounds from fresh ginger. *Fitoterapia* 83(3), 568-585, 2012.

[177] Peng WX, Zhang YD, Yang K, Xiao YC. title (unknown). *Acta Botanica Yunnanica* 9, 125, 2007.

[178] Ley JP, Paetz S, Blings M, Hoffmann-Lücke P, Bertram HJ, Krammer GE. Structural analogues of homoeriodictyol as flavor modifiers. Part III: short chain gingerdione derivatives. *J Agric Food Chem* 56(15), 6656-6664, 2008.

[179] Nakayama R, Tamura Y, Yamanaka H, Kikuzaki H, Nakatani N. Two curcuminoid pigments from *Curcuma domestica*. *Phytochemistry* 33(2), 501-502, 1993.

[180] Jianping Ma, Xiaoling Jin, Li Yang, Zhong-Li Liu. Diarylheptanoids from the rhizomes of *Zingiber officinale*. *Phytochemistry* 65(8), 1137-1143, 2004.

[181] Kamnaing P, Tsopmo A, Tanifum EA, Tchuendem MH, Tane P, Ayafor JF, Sterner O, Rattendi D, Iwu MM, Schuster B, Bacchi C. Trypanocidal diarylheptanoids from *Aframomum letestuianum*. *J Nat Prod* 66(3), 364-367, 2003.

[182] Hori Y, Miura T, Hirai Y, Fukumura M, Nemoto Y, Toriizuka K, Ida Y. Pharmacognostic studies on ginger and related drugs - part 1: five sulfonated compounds from *Zingiberis rhizome* (Shokyo). *Phytochemistry* 62(4), 613-617, 2003.

[183] Li N, Wang L, Zu L, Wang K, Di L, Wang Z. Antioxidant and cytotoxic diarylheptanoids isolated from *Zingiber officinale* rhizomes. *Zhongguo Zhong Yao Za Zhi (Chin J Chem)* 30, 1351-1355, 2012.

[184] Han JS, Lee S, Kim HY, Lee CH. MS-based metabolite profiling of aboveground and root components of *Zingiber mioga* and *officinale*. *Molecules* 20(9), 16170-16185, 2015.

In: *Curcuma longa* and Its Health Effects ISBN: 978-1-53618-083-1
Editor: Noboru Motohashi

Chapter 2

SEAWEEDS CONTAINING CURCUMINOIDS (DIARYLHEPTANOIDS)

***Noboru Motohashi*[1,*]*, Anuradha Vanam*[2,†]*, Jyothirmayi Vadapalli*[3,‡] *and Rao Gollapudi* [4,§]**

[1]Meiji Pharmaceutical University, Tokyo, Japan
[2]Sri Venkateswara University, Tirupathi, AP, India
[3]Acharya Nagarjuna University, Nagarjunanagar, AP, India
[4]University of Kansas, Lawrence, Kansas, USA

ABSTRACT

Seaweed-derived diarylheptanoids are diarylheptanids contained in two orders 3 families from order Alismatales and order Poecilosclerida.

To date, seaweed-derived diarylheptanoids are a very limited order and species. However, characteristic diarylheptanoids from seaweed have been identified. Chapter 2 will be discussed according to the following classification: First, seaweeds containing diarylheptanoids were alphabetically started from the order, followed by family, genus, and

* Corresponding Author's Email: noborumotohashi@jcom.home.ne.jp.
† Corresponding Author's Email: agollapdr@gmail.com.
‡ Corresponding Author's Email: jyothi.galactica@gmail.com.
§ Corresponding Author's Email: gollapudirao@ku.edu.

plant name. In the future, these diarylheptanoids may also be identified from plants. In this sense, it is expected that more kinds of diarylheptanids will be identified from seaweeds in the future.

Keywords: diarylheptanoids, order alismatales, cymodoceaceae, *Cymodocea nodosa*, zosteraceae, zostera, *Zostera marina* (eelgrass), order poecilosclerida, tedaniidae, tedania, *Tedania ignis*

Chemical Constituents in Seaweeds Containing Curcuminoids (Diarylheptanoids)

cymodienol	(**1**)
cymodiene	(**2**)
deoxycymodienol	(**3**)
isocymodiene	(**4**)
methicillin	(**5**)
tetracycline	(**6**)
isotedarene A	(**7**)
Compound 1a	(**8**)
Compound 1b	(**9**)
tedarene A	(**10**)
tedarene B	(**11**)

Abbreviations in Seaweeds Containing Curcuminoids (Diarylheptanoids)

EMRSA	epidemic meticillin-resistant *Staphylococcus aureus*
LPS	lipopolysaccharide
MDR	multidrug resistance
MIC	minimum inhibitory concentration
MRSA	methicillin resistant strains *Staphylococcus aureus*
NSCLC	non-small cell lung cancer
NO	nitric oxide

1. Introduction

Diarylheptanids from seaweed are extremely low compared to diarylheptanids derived from plants. In fact, diarylheptanids from seaweed are known to be found in all three families from two types of order Alismatales and order Poecilosclerida. However, future studies will find seaweed-derived diarylheptanids from many other orders.

2. Seaweeds Containing Curcuminoids (Diarylheptanoids)

2.1. Order Alismatales

2.1.1. Cymodoceaceae

2.1.1.1. Cymodocea

2.1.1.1.1. *Cymodocea nodosa*

In 2005, Kontiza *et al.*, identified two novel diarylheptanoids, cymodienol (**1**) and cymodiene (**2**) (Figure 1) from the specimens of the sea grass *Cymodocea nodosa*.

The cytotoxicity against two types of cancer cells - non-small cell lung cancer (NSCLC)-N6 cells and A549 lung cancer cell lines - was cymodienol (**1**): NSCL-N6 cells (IC_{50} = 84.0 μM) and A549 cells (IC_{50} = 114.6 μM) [1, 2], respectively, showing their strong cytotoxicity. However, cymodiene (**2**) showed only moderate cytotoxicity against both cancer cell lines.

The growth kinetics analysis has shown that the growth inhibition effect of cymodienol (**1**) is irreversible. Because, cessation of cymodienol (**1**) administration after 72 hr treatment did not induce normal growth of the treated cells, so it suggests that the growth inhibitory effect of cymodienol (**1**) is due to progressive cell cycle blockade.

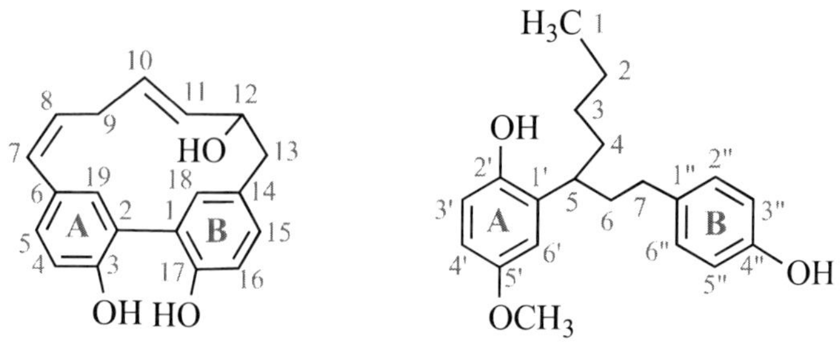

Figure 1. Two novel diarylheptanoids, cymodienol (**1**) and cymodiene (**2**) from the specimens of the sea grass *Cymodocea nodosa*.

Trihydroxy metabolites of dihydroxyheptanoid class are known to exhibit moderate levels of antioxidant activity from biological activity assessment [3, 4].

2.1.1.1.2. Biological Activity of *Cymodocea nodosa*

In 2008, Kontiza *et al.*, isolated two novel diarylheptanoids - deoxycymodienol (**3**) and isocymodiene (**4**), and one known diarylheptanoid cymodienol (**1**) [4] (Figure 2) - from the organic extract of the seagrass marine angiosperm *Cymodocea nodosa*.

The antibacterial properties of these three diarylheptanoids - deoxycymodienol (**3**) and isocymodiene (**4**), and cymodienol (**1**) - were examined.

First, with regard to the minimum inhibitory concentration (MIC) for three types of diarylheptanoids against multi-drug resistant (MDR) *Staphylococcus aureus* and methicillin resistant strains *Staphylococcus aureus* (MRSA), total 6 types of *Staphylococcus aureus* such as resistant bacteria *Staphylococcus aureus* SA1199B (NorA), methicillin (**5**) (Figure 2) - resistant *Staphylococcus aureus* RN4220 (MRSA), an excretion strain *Staphylococcus aureus* XU212 (*TetK*, *mecA*) equipped with *TetK* and *mecK* excretion pumps of *TetK* gene-derived tetracycline resistance gene and *mecA* gene-derived tetracycline (**6**) (Figure 2) resistance gene), the standard (control) *Staphylococcus aureus* ATCC 25923 (negative *Staphylococcus aureus* ATCC 25923. methicillin sensitive

Staphylococcus aureus. MSSA), epidemic meticillin-resistant *Staphylococcus aureus* (EMRSA-15), and an excretion strain *Staphylococcus aureus* CD-1281 (*TetK*) equipped with *TetK* excretion pumps of *TetK* gene-derived tetracycline resistance gene were used.

Among three diarylheptanoids, deoxycymodienol (**3**) showed their activity for three types of resistant bacteria such as SA1199B (NorA) (MIC: 32 μg/mL), RN4220 (MRSA) (MIC: 32 μg/mL), and XU212 (*TetK*, *mecA*) (MIC: 32 μg/mL) as well as the standard (control) *Staphylococcus aureus* ATCC 25923 (MIC: 32 μg/mL). However, antibacterial activity against two types of resistant bacteria, EMRSA-15 と CD-1281 (*TetK*), was not detected.

The antibacterial activity of isocymodiene (**4**) against three types of resistant bacteria is ATCC 25923 (MIC: 64 μg/mL), SA1199B (NorA) (MIC: 32 μg/mL), RN4220 (MRSA) (MIC: 64 μg/mL), and XU212 (*TetK*, *mecA*) (MIC: 64 μg/mL). However, the antibacterial activity of two types of resistant bacteria, EMRSA-15 and CD-1281 (*TetK*), was not detected.

The antibacterial activity of cymodienol (**1**) is 6 types of resistant bacteria (ATCC 25923, SA1199B (NorA), RN4220 (MRSA), XU212 (*TetK*, *mecA*), EMRSA-15, and CD-1281 (*TetK*)) showed each MIC: 64 μg/mL.

From the above results, among three diarylheptanoids, in antibacterial activity against four types of resistant bacteria (ATCC 25923, SA1199B (NorA), RN4220 (MRSA), and XU212 (*TetK*, *mecA*)), deoxycymodienol (**3**) has higher antibacterial activity against three resistant strains (ATCC 25923, RN4220 (MRSA), and XU212 (*TetK*, *mecA*)) than other two diarylheptanoids (**4** and **1**). On the other hand, cymodienol (**1**) showed antibacterial activity against two resistant bacteria, EMRSA-15 and CD-1281 (*TetK*).

Second, regarding mycobacterial activity of three diarylheptanoids (**3**, **4** and **1**) against their fast-growing species of three types of Mycobacterium (mycobacteria) - a mycobacteria in smegma *Mycobacterium smegmatis*, an atypical mycobacteria *M. fortuitum*, and a high temperature desulfurization bacterium *M. phlei*, only cymodienol (**1**) showed MIC: 128 μg/mL against *Mycobacterium smegmatis*.

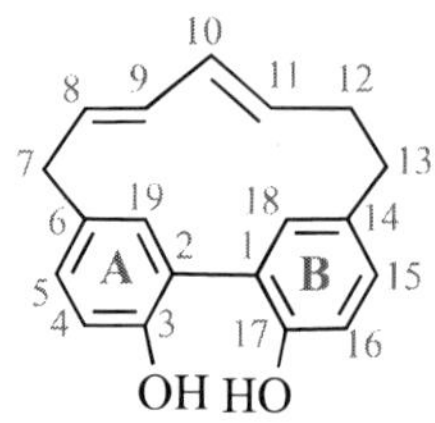

deoxycymodienol (**3**)

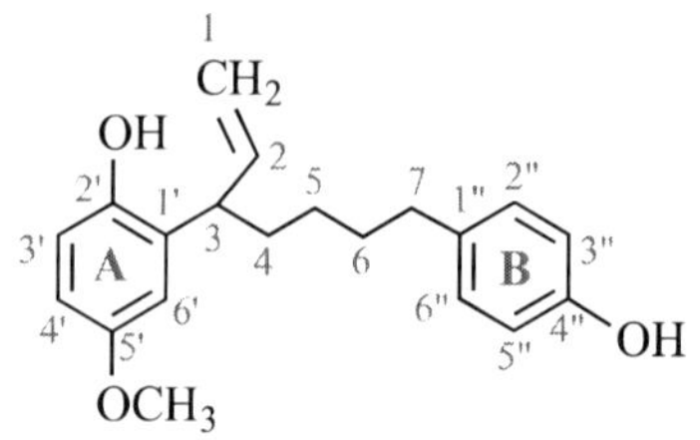

isocymodiene (**4**)

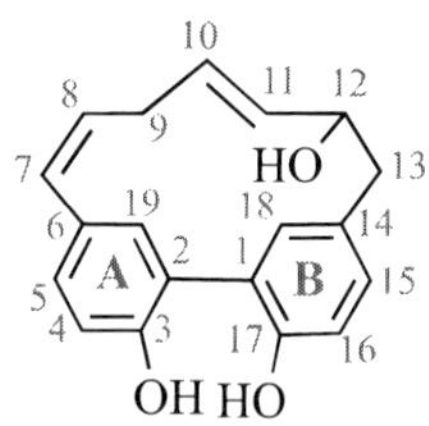

cymodienol (**1**)

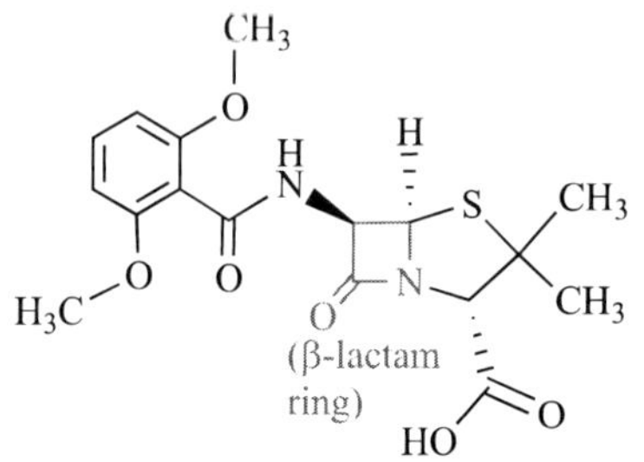

methicillin (**5**)

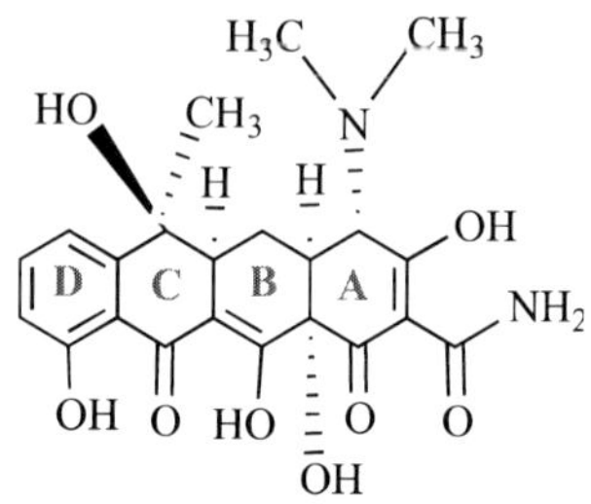

tetracycline (**6**)

Figure 2. Two novel diarylheptanoids (deoxycymodienol (**3**) and isocymodiene (**4**)), and one known diarylheptanoid cymodienol (**1**) from the organic extract of the seagrass marine angiosperm *Cymodocea nodosa*. A narrow spectrum β-lactam antibiotic of the penicillin class methicillin (**5**) and a group of broad-spectrum antibiotics tetracycline antibiotics tetracycline (**6**).

Mycobacterial activity against *M. fortuitum* is highest in isocymodiene (**4**) (MIC: 32 μg/mL), followed by deoxycymodienol (**3**) (MIC: 64 μg/mL), and cymodienol (**1**) (MIC > 128 μg/mL).

Mycobacterial activity against *M. phlei* is highest in cymodienol (**1**) (MIC: 16 μg/mL), followed by isocymodiene (**4**) (MIC: 32 μg/mL), and deoxycymodienol (**3**) (MIC: 64 μg/mL).

From the above results, among three diarylheptanoids, cymodienol (**1**) showed higher mycobacterial activity against *Mycobacterium smegmatis* and *M. phlei*. On the other hand, mycobacterial activity of deoxycymodienol (**3**) and isocymodiene (**4**) against *M. fortuitum* was higher than that of cymodienol (**1**) [5].

2.1.2. Zosteraceae

2.1.2.1. Zostera

2.1.2.1.1. *Zostera marina* (Eelgrass)

2.1.2.1.1.1. *Zostera marina* (Eelgrass)/2019

In 2019, Li Y. *et al.*, identified and confirmed two cyclic diarylheptanoids cymodienol (**1**) (Figure 3) [5], and isotedarene A (**7**) (Figure 3) [6] contained in sponges inhabiting the neotropical region of the South American continent and Central America, including the Caribbean islands and the southern Florida peninsula from *Zostera marina* (eelgrass) [7].

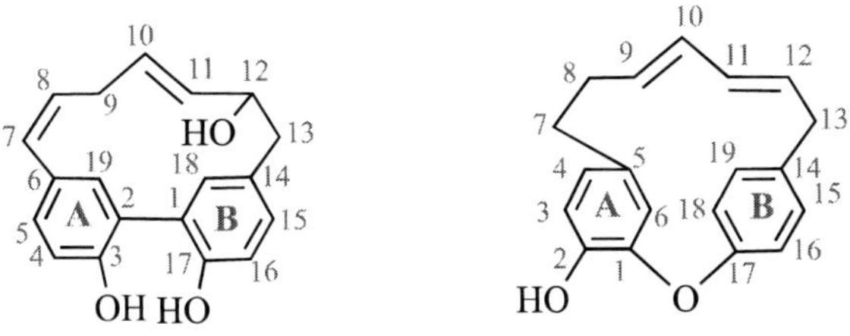

cymodienol (**1**) isotedarene A (**7**)

Figure 3. Two known diarylheptanoids cymodienol (**1**) and isotedarene A (**7**) from *Zostera marina* (eelgrass).

2.1.2.1.1.2. *Zostera marina* (Eelgrass)/2020

In 2020, Grauso L. *et al.*, identified two novel diastereomeric tetracyclic diarylheptanoids: Compound 1a (**8**) and Compound 1b (**9**) (Figure 4) from seagrass *Zostera marina* (eelgrass) [8].

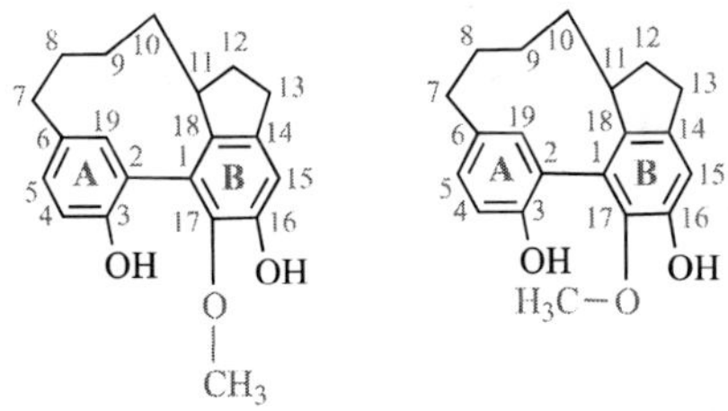

Compound 1a (**8**) Compound 1b (**9**)

Figure 4. Two novel diastereomeric tetracyclic diarylheptanoids: Compound 1a (**8**) and Compound 1b (**9**) from *Zostera marina* (eelgrass).

2.2. Order Poecilosclerida

2.2.1. Tedaniidae

2.2.1.1. Tedania

2.2.1.1.1. *Tedania ignis*

In 2012, Costantino V. *et al.*, identified two novel strained cyclic diarylheptanoids tedarene A (**10**) and tedarene B (**11**) (Figure 5) from a marine sponge *Tedania ignis* (sponge).

Tedarene A (**10**) and tedarene B (**11**) exist as equilibrium mixtures of atropisomers, which are optical isomers with different planar chiralities, *i.e.*, caused by steric hindrance of the bond axis.

Regarding the inhibitory effect of tedarene A (**10**) and tedarene B (**11**) on nitric oxide (NO) production by murine monocyte/macrophages J774 cells stimulated with lipopolysaccharide (LPS) （1 μg/mL）, LPS (1 μg/mL)-induced J774 cells and tedarene A (**10**) or tedarene B (**12**) at three different concentrations (3 μM, 10 μM, 30 μM) were incubated.

As a result, concentrations (10 μM, 30 μM) of tedarene A (**10**) showed a significant inhibitory effect on NO production when compared to LPS-induced control, whereas tedarene B (**11**) did not show the inhibitory effect [9].

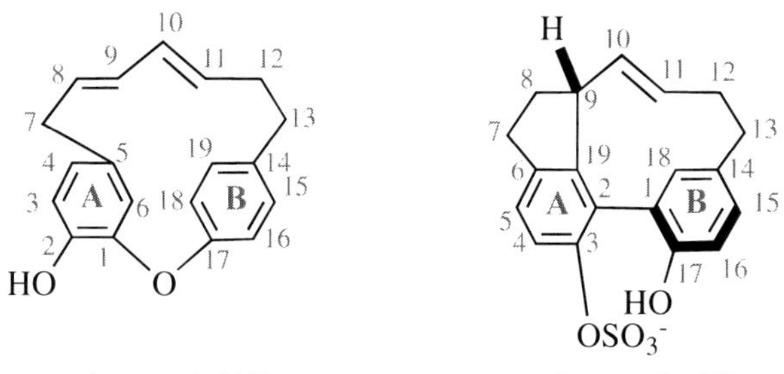

tedarene A (**10**) tedarene B (**11**)

Figure 5. Two novel strained cyclic diarylheptanoids tedarene A (**10**) and tedarene B (**11**) from a marine sponge *Tadania ignis*.

Conclusion

It is known that not only plants but also seaweeds (marine plants) contains diarylheptanoids.

In Chapter 2, seaweeds containing diarylheptanoids were alphabetically started from the order, followed by family, genus, and plant name. At least 2 orders, 3 families and 3 genera are known to contain seaweed diarylheptanoids as follows: **order Alismatales**: 2 families 2 genera of family Cymodoceaceae 1 genus (Cymodoceaceae) and family Zosteraceae 1 genus (Zostera); and **order Poecilosclerida**: 1 family Tedaniidae 1 genus (Tedania), respectively.

For example, diarylheptanoids from *Cymodocea nodosa* exhibited antibacterial properties and mycobacterial activity. Similarly, strained cyclic diarylheptanoids from *Tedania ignis* showed an inhibitory effect on NO production.

Although there are only a few species of seaweed-derived diarylheptanoids known so far, it is highly probable that many new diarylheptanoids will be identified in the future.

New diarylheptanoids are expected to be useful in the prevention and treatment of lifestyle-related diseases such as cancer, myocardial infarction, dementia, hypertension, and diabetes.

References

[1] Roussakis C., Gratas C., Audouin A. F., Le Boterff J., Dabouis C., Andre M. J., Moyon E., Vo N. H., Pradal G., Verbist J. F. Study of *in vitro* drug sensitivity on a newly established cell line from a primary bronchial epidermoid carcinoma of human origin (NSCLCN6). *Anticancer Res* 11(6), 2239-2244, 1991.

[2] Giard D. J., Aaronson S. A., Todaro G. J., Arnstein P., Kersey J. H., Dosik H., Parks W. P. *In vitro* cultivation of human tumors: establishment of cell lines derived from a series of solid tumors. *J Natl Cancer Inst* 51(5), 1417-1423, 1973.

[3] Lee J. S., Kim H. J., Park H., Lee Y. S. New diarylheptanoids from the stems of *Carpinus cordata*. *J Nat Prod* 65(9), 1367-1370, 2002.

[4] Kontiza I., Vagias C., Jakupovic J., Moreau D., Roussakis C., Roussis V. Cymodienol and cymodiene: new cytotoxic diarylheptanoids from the sea grass *Cymodocea nodosa*. *Tetrahedron Lett* 46(16), 2845-2847, 2005.

[5] Kontiza I., Stavri M., Zloh M., Vagias C., Gibbons S., Roussis V. New metabolites with antibacterial activity from the marine angiosperm *Cymodocea nodosa*. *Tetrahedron* 64, 1696-1702, 2008.

[6] *Zostera marina/Tedania ignis* (sponge). *Tedania ignis* (Duchassaing & Michelotti, 1864) (Tedaniidae): http://www.marinespecies.org/porifera/porifera.php?p=taxdetails&id=169565.

[7] Li Y., Mangoni A., Shulha O., Çiçek S. S., Zidorn C. Cyclic diarylheptanoids deoxycymodienol and isotedarene A from *Zostera marina* (Zosteraceae). *Tetrahedron Letters* 60(32), 150930, 2019.

[8] Grauso L., Li Y., Scarpato S., Shulha O., Rárová L., Strnad M., Teta R., Mangoni A., Zidorn C. Structure and conformation of zosteraphenols, tetracyclic diarylheptanoids from the seagrass *Zostera marina*: An NMR and DFT study. *Org Lett* 22(1), 78-82, 2020.

[9] Costantino V., Fattorusso E., Mangoni A., Perinu C., Teta R., Panza E., Ianaro A. Tedarenes A and B: Structural and stereochemical analysis of two new strained cyclic diarylheptanoids from the marine sponge *Tedania ignis*. *J Org Chem* 77(15), 6377-6383, 2012.

In: *Curcuma longa* and Its Health Effects ISBN: 978-1-53618-083-1
Editor: Noboru Motohashi

Chapter 3

BIOLOGICAL ACTIVITY OF CURCUMINOIDS (DIARYLHEPTANOIDS)

Noboru Motohashi[1,*], Anuradha Vanam[2], Jyothirmayi Vadapalli[3] and Rao Gollapudi[4]
[1]Meiji Pharmaceutical University, Tokyo, Japan
[2]Sri Venkateswara University, Tirupathi, AP, India
[3]Acharya Nagarjuna University, Nagarjunanagar, AP, India
[4]University of Kansas, Lawrence, Kansas, USA

ABSTRACT

Naturally occurring diarylheptanoids include both plant-derived and seaweed-derived diarylheptanoids. Diarylheptanoids are known for many biological activities. Therefore, Chapter 3 introduces typical biological activities of diarylheptanoids such as leishmanicidal and antiprotozoal activities, antitumor activities (antitumor promoting effects), anti-inflammatory effects, and inhibitory on nitric oxide production.

* Corresponding Author's Email: noborumotohashi@jcom.home.ne.jp.
† Corresponding Author's Email: agollapdr@gmail.com.
‡ Corresponding Author's Email: jyothi.galactica@gmail.com.
§ Corresponding Author's Email: gollapudirao@ku.edu.

For example, regarding the structure and antitumor properties of diarylheptanoids, α-diketo moiety on cyclic diarylheptanoid showed to be important for antitumor promoting activity.

Keywords: antitumor activity of diarylheptanoids (curcuminoids), leishmanicidal activity, antiprotozoal activity, antitumor activity, antitumor promoting effects, anti-inflammatory effects, inhibitory of nitric oxide production

Chemical Constituents in Biological Activities of Curcuminoids (Diarylheptanoids)

1,7-*bis*[4-hydroxyphenyl]-3-hepten-5-one (**1**)
16-hydroxy-17-*O*-methylacerogenin E (**2**)
acerogenin E (**3**)
15-methoxy-17-*O*-methyl-7-oxoacerogenin E (**4**)
17-*O*-methyl-7-oxoacerogenin E (**5**)
alnusdiol (**6**)
3,5'-dihydroxy-4'-methoxy-3',4"-oxo-1,7-diphenyl-1-heptene (**7**)
myricanone (**8**)
myricanol (**9**)
acerogenin A (**10**)
13-oxomyricanol (**11**)
synthetic Compound (**12**)
synthetic Compound (**13**)
syntheticCompound (**14**)
synthetic Compound (**15**)
synthetic Compound (**16**)
synthetic Compound (**17**)
synthetic myricalactam (**18**)
curcumin (**19**)
TPA (12-*O*-tetradecanoylphorbol-13-acetate. **20**)
7,12-dimethylbenz[*a*]anthracene (DMBA. **21**)
(-)-centrolobol (**22**)

(-)-di-*O*-methylcentrolobol (**23**)
12-dehydroporson (**24**)
porson (**25**)
myricanone oxime (**26**)
myricamine (**27**)
acerogenin K (**28**)
isomyricanone (**29**)
acerogenin C (**30**)
acerogenin C oxime (**31**)
galeon (**32**)
monomethylmyricanone (**33**)
compound 15 (**34**)
compound 16 (**35**)
compound 17 (**36**)
compound 18 (**37**)
acerogenin M (**38**)
aceroside I (**39**)
aceroside III (**40**)
(*R*)-acerogenin B (**41**)
aceroside B_1 (**42**)
acerogenin D (**43**)
aceroside IV (**44**)
quercetin (**45**)
indomethacin (**46**)
myricanol 11-*O*-β-D-glucopyranoside (**47**)
myricanone 5-*O*-β-D-glucopyranoside (**48**)
neomyricanone 5-*O*-β-D-glucopyranoside (**49**)
(+)-*S*-myricanol 5-*O*-β-D-glucopyranoside (**50**)
(+)-*S*-myricanol (**51**)
myricanol glucoside (**52**)
myricanene A 5-*O*-α-L-arabinofuranosyl-(1→6)-β-D-glucopyranoside (**53**)
myricanene A (**54**)

myricanene B 5-*O*-α–L-arabinofuranosyl-(1→6)-β-D-glucopyranoside (**55**)
myricanene B (**56**)
myricanane (**57**)
L-arginine (**58**)
(-)-epigallocatechin (**59**)
(-)-epigallocatechin 3-*O*-gallate (EGCG. **60**)
N^G-monomethyl-L-arginine (L-NMMA. **61**)
myricananin A (**62**)
myricananin B (**63**)
myricananin C (**64**)
myricananin D (65)
myricananin E (**66**)
acetonide of myricananin A (**67**)
acetonide of myricananin B (**68**)
12-hydroxymyricanone (**69**)
alnusonol (**70**)
myricatomentogenin ((+)-3’,4”-epoxy-1-(4’-hydroxylphenyl)-7-(3”-hydroxyphenyl) heptane-3-one. **71**)
actinidione (**72**)

Abbreviations in Biological Activities of Curcuminoids (Diarylheptanoids)

BET	Brauner-Emmet-Teller
EBA-EA	Epstein Barr virus early antigen
iNOS	inducible nitric oxide synthase
IC_{50}	50% inhibitory concentration
ID_{50}	50% inhibitory dose
IL-1β	interleukin-1β
LPS	lipopolysaccharide

NO	nitric oxide
NOS	nitric oxide synthase
TNF–α	tumor necrosis factor–α

1. Introduction

Diarylheptanoids have many kinds of health effects including antioxidant effects. Diarylheptanoids include Leishmanicidal and antiprotozoal activities, especially cyclic diarylheptanoids are known to have antitumor promoting effects (antitumor promoting effects), anti-inflammatory effects, and inhibitory on nitric oxide production. In Chapter 3, new biological activities of diarylheptanoids were introduced in addition to the biological activities of Chapter 1 and Chapter 2.

2. Biological Activity of Diarylheptanoids

2.1. Leishmanicidal and Antiprotozoal Activities for the Genus Leishmania, a Genus of Flagellates

Leishmaniasis is a parasitic disease that occurs when a type of parasitic protozoa, Leishmania, infects vertebrates through the transmission of very small sand flies, and infects these cells.

In 2004, Takahashi *et al.*, examined the Leishmanicidal and antiprotozoal activities by seven diarylheptanoids 1,7-*bis*[4-hydroxy-phenyl]-3-hepten-5-one (**1**) from *Betula platyphylla* var. japonica [1], 16-hydroxy-17-*O*-methylacerogenin E (**2**) from *Betula maximowicziana* Regel [2], acerogenin E (**3**) from *Betula platyphylla* var. japonica [1], 15-methoxy-17-*O*-methyl-7-oxoacerogenin E (**4**) from inner bark of *Betula davurica* Pall [3], 17-*O*-methyl-7-oxoacerogenin E (**5**) from inner bark of *Betula davurica* Pall [3], alnusdiol (**6**) from *Betula maximowicziana* Regel [2], and 3,5'-dihydroxy-4'-methoxy-3',4"-oxo-1,7-diphenyl-1-heptene (**7**) from *Betula platyphylla* var. japonica [1] (Figure 1) in Betulaceae.

Here, promastigotes of a forest type tropical leishmaniasis *Leishmania major*, which causes cutaneous leishmaniasis, was used for the screening.

As a result, regarding 50% inhibitory concentration (IC_{50}) (μg/mL) among seven diarylheptanoids, 1,7-*bis*[4-hydroxyphenyl]-3-hepten-5-one (**1**) was the highest 2 ± 0.2, followed by 3,5'-dihydroxy-4'-methoxy-3',4"-oxo-1,7-diphenyl-1-heptene (**7**) (3.9 ± 0.3), acerogenin E (**3**) (17 ± 0.9), 16-hydroxy-17-*O*-methylacerogenin E (**2**) (17 ± 1.2), 17-*O*-methyl-7-oxoacerogenin E (**5**) (28 ± 2.9), and 15-methoxy-17-*O*-methyl-7-oxoacerogenin E (**4**) (> 100) and alnusdiol (**6**) (> 100), respectively.

Then, comparing the results of 3 *vs*. 6, 4 *vs*. 5, and 2 *vs*. 3, it was found that the carbonyl group of C-9 is necessary for activity. Interestingly, regarding the biological activity of 2 and 3, the presence of substituents at C-4 was not related to activity at all. The bulkiness C-5 of 4 decreased the activity, but it is also necessary to take into account the steric differences between these compounds. Among 6 types of diphenyl type heptanoids (**2**, **3**, **4**, **5**, **6**, and **7**), cycle diphenyl ether type heptanoid (**7**) showed the highest insecticidal activity in Leishmania.

The above results showed that among the seven diarylheptanoids, linear and some cyclic diarylheptanoids showed remarkable activity. The C-9 carbonyl group was found to be essential for the activity of biphenyl-type diarylheptanoids [4].

2.2. Antitumor Activities

2.2.1. Antitumor Promoting Effects of Cyclic Diarylheptanoids (1)

In 2000, according to Ishisa *et al., roughly*, using Epstein Barr virus early antigen (EBA-EA) activation assay as a primary screening, the antitumor promoting effects on 11 kinds of cyclic diarylheptanoids (**8**, **9**, **10**, **11**, **12** - **18**) (Figure 2), with curcumin (**19**) (Figure 2) as a control, were examined on the activation inhibitory effect against Epstein Barr virus (EB virus) in Epstein Barr virus early antigen (EBA-EA) positive serum from a patient with nasopharyngeal carcinoma (NPC). Here, Epstein

Barr virus is the cause of infectious mononucleosis which is called "Kiss disease".

Subsequently, the two most powerful compounds 13-oxomyricanol (**11**) and myricanone (**8**) in the EBV-EA assay were also examined for the *in vivo* two-stage carcinogenesis-inhibiting effects on the promotion of mouse skin tumors.

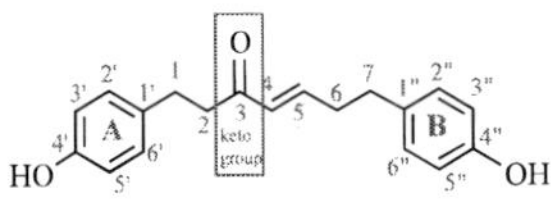

1,7-*bis*[4-hydroxyphenyl]-3-hepten-5-one (1)

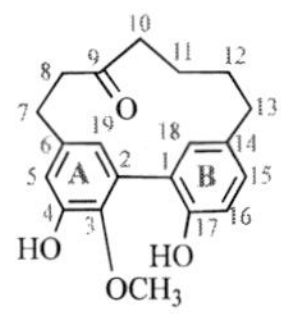

16-hydroxy-17-*O*-methylacerogenin E (2)

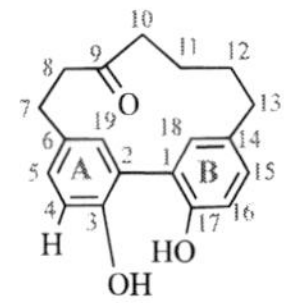

acerogenin E (3)

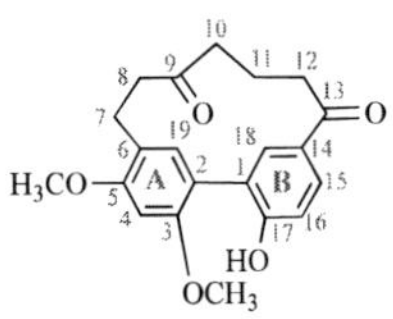

15-methoxy-17-*O*-methyl-7-oxoacerogenin E (4)

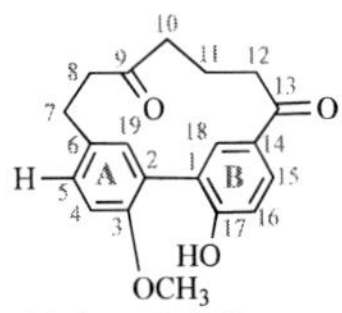

17-*O*-methyl-7-oxoacerogenin E (5)

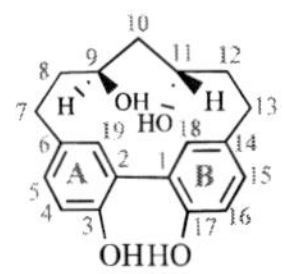

alnusdiol (6)

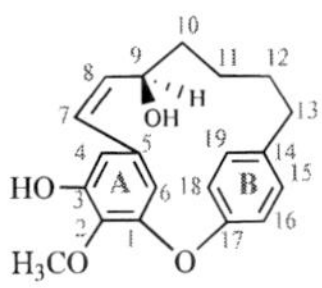

3,5'-dihydroxy-4'-methoxy-3',4"-oxo-1,7-diphenyl-1-heptene (7)

Figure 1. Seven diarylheptanoids - 1,7-*bis*[4-hydroxyphenyl]-3-hepten-5-one (1), 16-hydroxy-17-*O*-methylacerogenin E (2), acerogenin E (3), 15-methoxy-17-*O*-methyl-7-oxoacerogenin E (4), 17-*O*-methyl-7-oxoacerogenin E (5), alnusdiol (6), and 3,5'-dihydroxy-4'-methoxy-3',4"-oxo-1,7-diphenyl-1-heptene (7) - from *Betula spp.*

The eleven cyclic diarylheptanoids (**8, 9, 10, 11, 12 - 18**), including the seven synthetic cyclic diarylheptanoids (**12 - 18**) used in this study, were as follows:

Acerogenin A (**10**) (Figure 2) from *Acer nikoense*, myricanol (**9**) [5] (Figure 2), 13-oxomyricanol (**11**) [6], myricanone (**8**) (Figure 2) from *Myrica rubra* [5], synthetic Compound (**12**), synthetic Compound (**13**), synthetic Compound (**14**), synthetic Compound (**15**), synthetic Compound

(**16**), synthetic Compound (**17**) (Figure 2), synthetic myricalactam (**18**) [5], and curcumin (**19**).

First, regarding the inhibitory effects and the survival rate (values in parentheses) of Raji cells on total 11 different types of cyclic diarylheptanoids (**8**, **9**, **10**, **11**, **12** - **18**) against activation of EBV-EA induced by a protein kinase C (PKC) activator TPA (12-*O*-tetradecanoylphorbol-13-acetate. **20**) (Figure 3), 13-oxomyricanol (**11**) (71.8% inhibition)(Raji cell viability> 80%) and myricanone (**8**) (74.6% inhibition) (Raji cell viability> 80%) at 500 mol ratio/TPA(20 ng = 32 pmol/mL) showed a remarkable inhibition of over 70%. The inhibitory activity of these two plant-derived diarylheptanoids (13-oxomyricanol (**11**) and myricanone (**8**)) is almost the same as that(the inhibitory activity) of the control curcumin (**19**)(77.2% inhibition) (Raji cell viability > 80%). Here, curcumin (**19**) is known to be a strong anti-tumor promoter [7].

In addition, the inhibitory effect on EBV-EA activation is well known to correlate well with *in vivo* anti-tumor promoting activity [8]. For the above two reasons, two plant-derived diarylheptanoids (13-oxomyricanol (**11**) and myricanone (**8**)) suggest to be antitumor promoters.

Second, based on the results of the *in vitro* assay of all 11 types of cyclic diarylheptanoids (**8**, **9**, **10**, **11**, **12** - **18**) against EBV-EA and Raji cells above, furthermore, the *in vivo* inhibitory effects of two plant-derived diarylheptanoids (13-oxomyricanol (**11**) and myricanone (**8**)) were investigated by a two-stage carcinogenesis test in mouse skin, using a tumor-initiator 7,12-dimethylbenz[*a*]anthracene (DMBA. **21**) (Figure 3) and a tumor-promoter TPA (**20**) (Figure 3).

The results on inhibition of TPA(**20**)-induced tumor promotion by multiple doses of 13-oxomyricanol (**11**) and myricanone (**8**) were as follows: *First*, among all 11 types of cyclic diarylheptanoids (**8**, **9**, **10**, **11**, **12** - **18**), 13-oxomyricanol (**11**) and myricanone (**8**), which generally lack both a conjugated double bond and a β-diketone structure, are expected to be lower than the effect of curcumin (**19**).

Second, however, the effects of 13-oxomyricanol (**11**) and myricanone (**8**) were essentially as strong as the effect of acyclic diarylheptanoid curcumin (**19**). Therefore, cyclization of hydrogenated acyclic diarylheptanoids may restore antitumor promoting activity. This hypothesis may be useful for drug discovery studies of active cyclic diarylheptanoids, where cyclic diarylheptanoids may have higher activity than the corresponding acyclic diarylheptanoids.

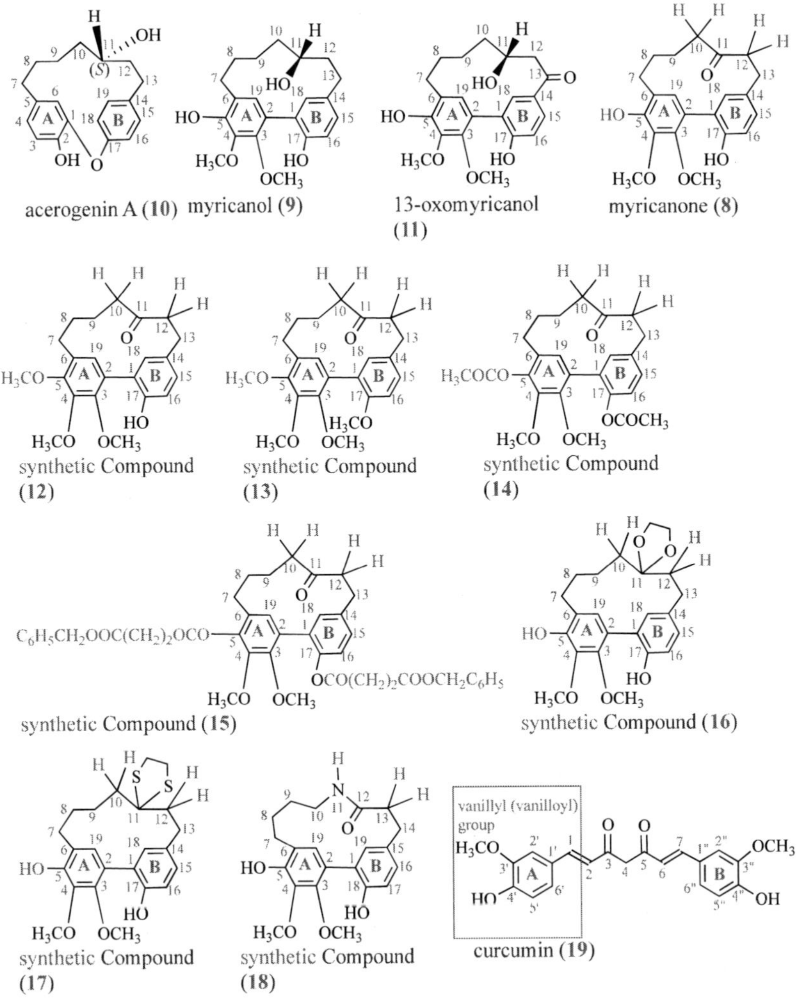

Figure 2. Eleven Curcuminoids (diarylheptanoid) and one curcumin (as control): acerogenin A (**10**), myricanol (**9**), 13-oxomyricanol (**11**), myricanone (**8**), synthetic Compound (**12**), synthetic Compound (**13**), synthetic Compound (**14**), synthetic Compound (**15**), synthetic Compound (**16**), synthetic Compound (**17**), synthetic Compound (**18**), and curcumin (**19**).

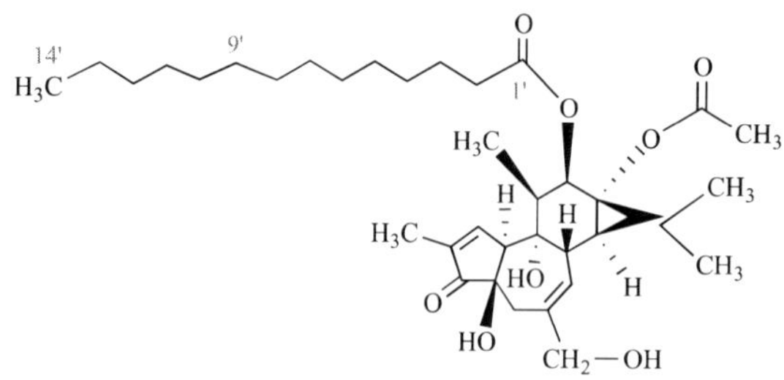

TPA (12-*O*-tetradecanoylphorbol-13-acetate. **20**)

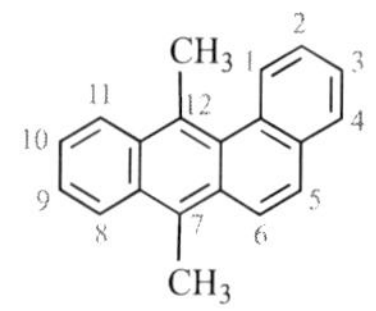

dimethylbenz[*a*]anthracene (DMBA. **21**)

Figure 3. TPA (12-*O*-tetradecanoylphorbol-13-acetate. **20**) and 7,12-dimethylbenz[*a*]anthracene (DMBA. **21**).

Third, comparing the antitumor-promoting activity of diarylheptanoids, the ketone at position 11 of the cyclic structure appears to be important for activity.

Fourth, esterification of 5 and 17-hydroxy groups with one bulky benzyl succinyl ester like synthetic Compound (**15**) caused further activity loss. Thus, the 5,17 hydroxy substitution pattern appears to be important for antitumor promoting activity.

From the above results, in conclusion, 13-oxomyricanol (**11**) and myricanone (**8**) showed similar inhibitory effects on tumor promotion. This fact suggests that cyclization of diarylheptanoids does not reduce antitumor promoting activity. In other words, cyclization of diarylheptanoids may increase the activity of hydrogenated acyclic diarylheptanoids. A comparison of cyclic diarylheptanoids is as follows: (1) The presence of a carbonyl moiety in cyclic diarylheptanoids is important for activity. (2) Activity was improved by introducing hydroxyl group into C-5 and C-17 [9]. These cyclic diarylheptanoids suggest the potential for new drug development into more powerful new anti-tumor promoters [10].

2.2.2. Antitumor Promoting Effects of Cyclic Diarylheptanoids (2)

In 2002, three linear diarylheptanoids and eleven cyclic diarylheptanoids were examined on potential antitumor promoters by using the *in vitro* short-term 12-*O*-tetradecanoylphorbol-13-acetate (TPA. **20**)-induced Epstein–Barr virus early antigen (EBV-EA) activation assay.

Each diarylheptanoid is follows (Figure 4) (Figure 4(continued 1):

Three linear diarylheptanoids are curcumin (**19**), (-)-centrolobol (**22**), and (-)-di-*O*-methylcentrolobol (**23**) (Figure 4).

Eleven cyclic diarylheptanoids are myricanone (**8**), 12-dehydroporson (**24**), porson (**25**), myricanone oxime (**26**), myricamine (**27**), acerogenin K (**28**), isomyricanone (**29**), acerogenin A (**10**), acerogenin C (**30**) (Figure 4), acerogenin C oxime (**31**), and galeon (**32**) (Figure 4(continued 1)).

Monomethylmyricanone (**33**) (Figure 4) related to myricanone (**8**).

First, on *in vitro* short-term 12-*O*-tetradecanoylphorbol-13-acetate (TPA. **20**) (Figure 4(continued 1))-induced Epstein–Barr virus early antigen (EBV-EA) activation, each diarylheptanoid concentration (mol ratio/TPA (**20**)) needed to inhibit 50% of positive control activated with TPA (**20**), *i.e.*, 50% inhibitory concentration (IC_{50}) was the highest in myricanone (**8**) 260, followed by 12-dehydroporson (**24**) (IC_{50}: 300), curcumin (**19**) (IC_{50}: 320) and (-)-centrolobol (**22**) (IC_{50}: 320), isomyricanone (**29**) (IC_{50}: 350), acerogenin K (**28**) (IC_{50}: 420) and (-)-centrolobol (**22**) (IC_{50}: 420), porson (**25**) (IC_{50}: 450) and acerogenin C oxime (**31**) (IC_{50}: 450), acerogenin A (**10**) (IC_{50}: 490) [10], myricanone oxime (**26**) (IC_{50}: 500), galeon (**32**) (IC_{50}: 580), acerogenin C (**30**) (IC_{50}: 620), and myricamine (**27**) (IC_{50}: 820), respectively.

The extended quinol structure of myricanone (**8**) is known to be essential for maintaining the antitumor promoting activity of cyclic diarylheptanoids [10]. Therefore, 12-dehydroporson (**24**) and porson (**25**) methylated at the 5-hydroxy group should have a lower anti-tumor promoting activity than curcumin (**19**). However, porson (**25**) showed a decrease in antitumor promoting activity as expected, 12-dehydroporson (**24**) showed essentially the same antitumor promoting activity as curcumin (**19**).

Three cyclic diarylheptanoids, 12-dehydroporson (**24**) (α-diketo group in position C-11, 12), porson (**25**) (α-ketole group in position C-12), and monomethylmyricanone (**33**) (ketone body in position C-11), were less active than the antitumor promoting activity of myricanone (**8**) from the structure comparison with myricanone (**8**) [10] reported previously. In other words, α-diketo moiety on cyclic diarylheptanoid showed to be important for antitumor promoting activity.

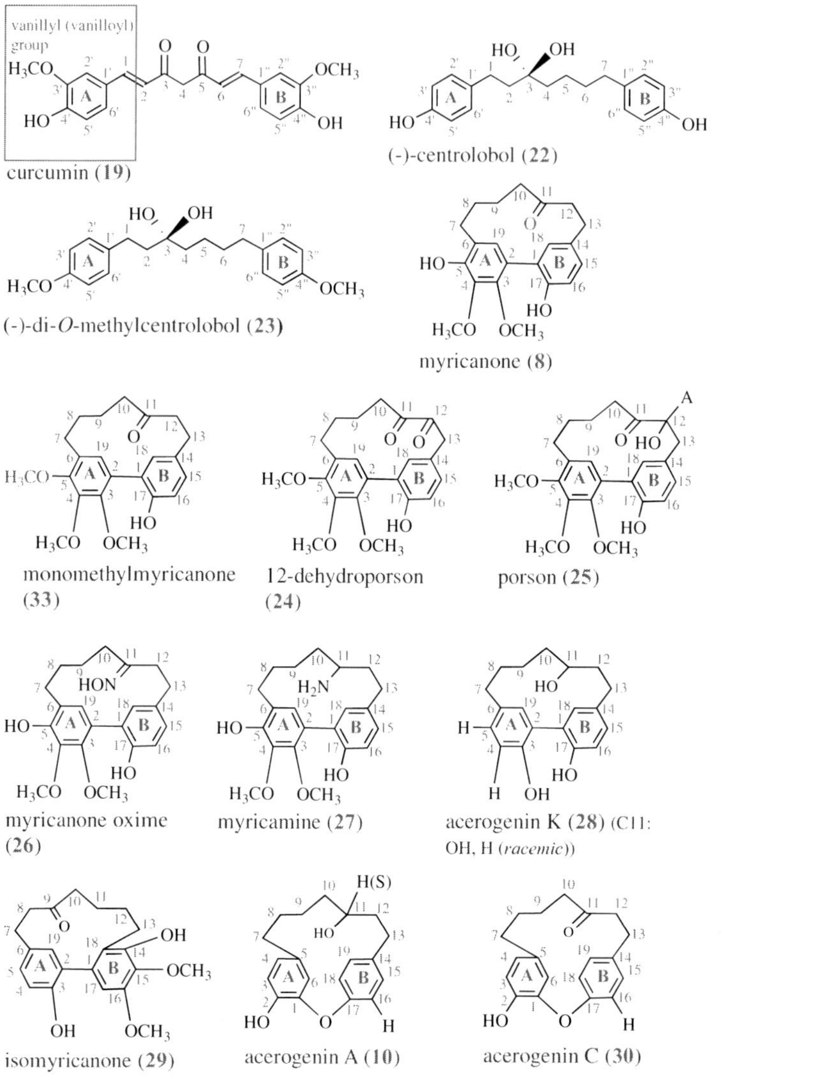

Figure 4. Three linear diarylheptanoids - curcumin (**19**), (-)-centrolobol (**22**), and (-)-di-*O*-methylcentrolobol (**23**), and nine cyclic diarylheptanoids - myricanone (**8**), 12-dehydroporson (**24**), porson (**25**), myricanone oxime (**26**), myricamine (**27**), acerogenin K (**28**), isomyricanone (**29**), acerogenin A (**10**), and acerogenin C (**30**). Monomethylmyricanone (**33**) related to myricanone (**8**).

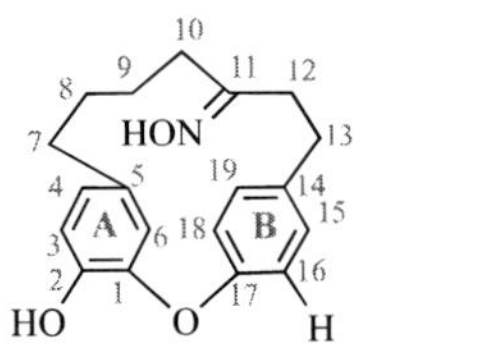

acerogenin C oxime (**31**)

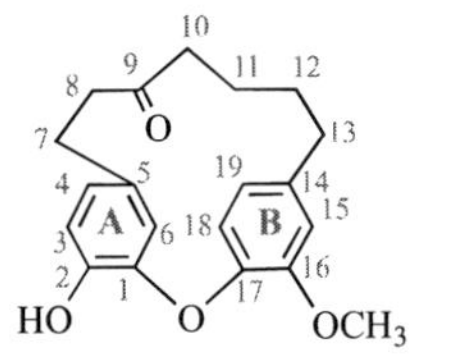

galeon (**32**)

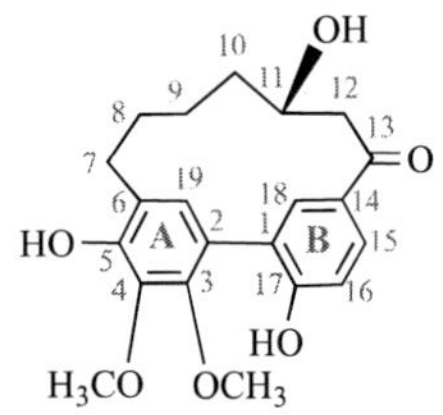

13-oxomyricanol (**11**)

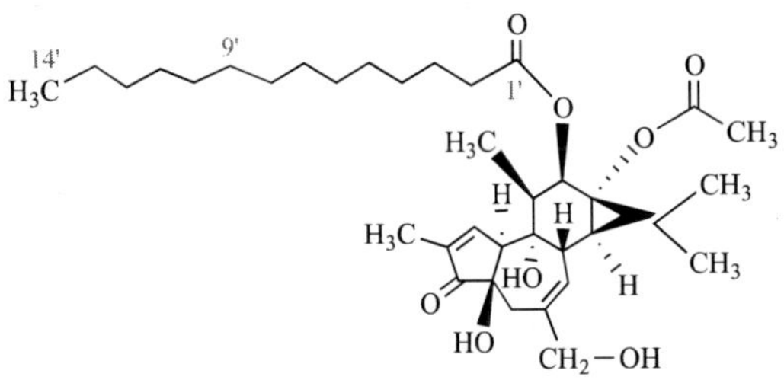

12-*O*-tetradecanoylphorbol-13-acetate (TPA. **20**)

(The four types of substructures of myricanone (**79**))

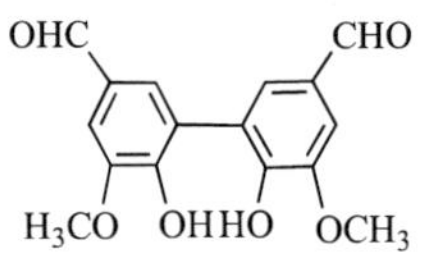

compound 15 (**34**)

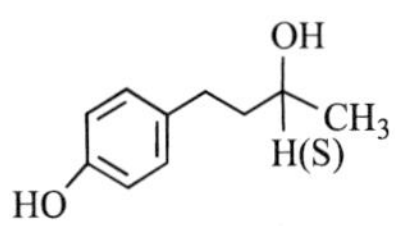

compound 16 (**35**)

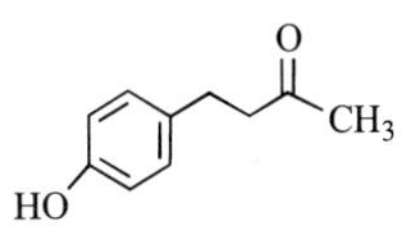

compound 17 (**36**)

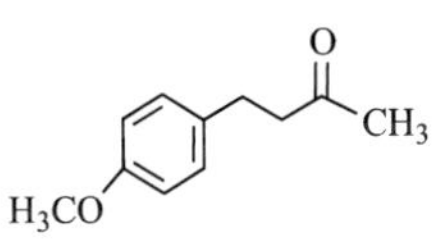

compound 18 (**37**)

Figure 4(continued 1). Two cyclic diarylheptanoids - acerogenin C oxime (**31**), and galeon (**32**). 12-*O*-Tetradecanoylphorbol-13-acetate (TPA. **20**) and 13-oxomyricanol (**11**). The four types of substructures (compound 15 (**34**), compound 16 (**35**), compound 17 (**36**), compound 18 (**37**)) of myricanone (**8**).

In contrast, the antitumor promoting activity of myricanone oxime (**26**) replaced the C-11 carbonyl group of myricanone (**8**) with an oxime, or myricamine (**27**) replaced the C-11 carbonyl group of myricanone (**8**) with an amine decreased. Furthermore, acerogenin K (**28**), which has a hydroxy group instead of a carbonyl group at C-11, reduced the antitumor promoting activity.

Also, the isomerization of myricanone (**8**), which gives the [7-*ortho*, *meta*-0] cyclophane structure isomyricanone (**29**), reduced the antitumor promoting activity.

The above results suggest that the 13-membered ring is important for antitumor promoting activity, probably due to steric factors.

The antitumor-promoting activity of four types of diphenyl ether-type cyclic diarylheptanoids (acerogenin A (**10**), acerogenin C (**30**), acerogenin C oxime (**31**), galeon (**32**)) was less active than the three types of biphenyl compounds (myricanone (**8**), 12-dehydroporson (**24**), 13-oxomyricanol (**11**) (Figure 4(continued 1)) [10].

In addition, (-)-centrolobol (**22**), a linear biosynthetic precursor of acerogenin A (**10**) and (-)-di-*O*-methylcentrolobol (**23**), showed moderate antitumor promotion activity.

Therefore, cyclization to diphenyl ether-type cyclic diarylheptanoids reduced antitumor promoting activity.

Also, the four types of substructures (compound 15 (34), compound 16 (**35**), compound 17 (**36**), compound 18 (**37**)) (Figure 4(continued 1)) of myricanone (**8**) were investigated for its antitumor promoting activity. As a result, these four types of partial structures - compound 15 (**34**) - compound 18 (**37**) - showed a decrease in antitumor promoting activity, and the importance of the 13-membered ring was emphasized.

Summarizing the above results, the following conclusions were drawn: (a) The presence of the α-diketo part of the side chain is important for antitumor promoting activity. (b) Replacing the side chain ketone with another substituent (amine, oxime, hydroxyl) reduced the antitumor promoting activity. (c) Cyclization as a *meta*- or *meta*-bridged biphenyl structure that generates a 13-membered ring rather than a diphenyl ether structure is important for antitumor promoting activity.

Second, regarding *in vivo* two-stage carcinogenicity study of mouse skin papilloma (melanoma spreading from the epidermis (outer layer of skin) to the dermal papillary layer (thin upper layer of dermis) induced by peroxynitrite ($ONOO^-$), an ion radical with strong oxidizing power, myricanone (**8**) showed the most active antitumor-promoting activity among 11 cyclic diarylheptanoids. Therefore, to elucidate the cancer prevention mechanism of myricanone (**8**), myricanone (**8**) was investigated for the antitumor effects on *in vivo* mouse skin carcinogenesis initiated by peroxynitrite ($ONOO^-$) and promoted by 12-*O*-tetradecanoylphorbol-13-acetate (TPA. **20**). Specifically, the incidence (%) of mice with papillomas and the average number of papillomas per mouse were measured.

First, regarding the time course of tumor formation in two Groups (I and II Groups), In Group I (control) (treated with peroxynitrite ($ONOO^-$) (390 nmol) + TPA (**20**) (1.7 nmol), the first papilloma mice (approximately 34%) appeared after 6 weeks. In Group II (treated with peroxynitrite ($ONOO^-$) (390 nmol) + myricanone (**8**) (0.0025%, 2 weeks) + TPA (**20**) (1.7 nmol)), the first papilloma mice (approx. 5%) appeared after 8 weeks.

The proportion of papilloma mice in Group I was 100% after 10 weeks. On the other hand, the proportion of papilloma mice in Group II was approximately 26% after 10 weeks and approximately 86% after 20 weeks.

Second, regarding the average number of tumors per mouse in the two Groups (I and II Groups), Group I produced about 8 papilloma per mouse after 20 weeks. Group II, on the other hand, had only about 5 papilloma per mouse. Therefore, treatment with myricanone (**8**) (0.0025%, 2 weeks) reduced the average number of tumors per mouse by approximately 38% after 20 weeks of promotion.

From the above results, myricanone (**8**) appears to be effective in inhibiting peroxynitrite-induced carcinogenesis in mouse skin. Here, peroxynitrite produced by the reaction of nitric oxide (NO) and superoxide is a powerful oxidant as well as nitrating agent and hydroxylating agent. Peroxynitrite causes tumor initiation. Combined with previous research results [10], these above results show that myricanone (**8**) plays a useful physiological role, including both antiinitiating activity and antipromoting activity against two-stage carcinogenesis.

Here, it suggests that curcumin I (**19**) is known to have strong antioxidant activity. Curcumin I (**19**) must be able to strongly block and neutralize reactive oxygen species (ROS), which are chemical carcinogens such as superoxide, peroxyl, hydroxy radicals and NO donors [11, 12].

Similar to this inhibitory action of curcumin I (**19**), the possible antioxidant effect of myricanone (**8**), a cyclic curcumin derivative, may be due to the inhibitory effect on peroxynitrite-induced carcinogenesis by myricanone (**8**).

In conclusion, among the diarylheptanoids, like the linear type curcumin I (**19**), the cyclic type myricanone (**8**) can also be expected to have substantial chemical carcinogenesis prevention properties. Myricanone (**8**) has the potential to become a valuable chemical prevention agent. Additional studies will be needed to elucidate the relationship between diarylheptanoid structure and the inhibitory effects on chemical carcinogenesis. However, diarylheptanoids are expected to develop new cancer preventives [13].

2.3. Anti-Inflammatory Effects of Cyclic Diarylheptanoids

In 2006, Akihisa *et al.*, aimed to search for potential antitumor promoters from natural resources, and confirmed one novel cyclic biphenyl ether type acerogenin M (**38**) along with nine known diarylheptanoids from stem bark of *Acer nikoense*. The 10 types of diarylheptanoids (Figure 5) are as follows:

- Cyclic biphenyl ether type (**38**, **10**, **38** - **44**): acerogenin M (**38**), acerogenin A (**10**) [14], aceroside I (**39**) [14], aceroside III (**40**) [15], (*R*)-acerogenin B (**41**) [16], aceroside B_1 (**42**) [16], acerogenin D (**43**) [17], aceroside IV (**44**) [18]
- Cyclic biphenyl type (**28**): acerogenin K (**28**) [19]
- Linear type (22): (-)-centrolobol (**22**) [20]

Regarding the anti-inflammatory effect between 7 diarylheptanoids (**10**, **39** - **42**, **44**, and **22**) from *Acer nikoense* and 2 controls (quercetin (**45**) and indomethacin (**46**)) (Figure 5(continued 1)) on TPA (**20**)-induced inflammation in mice, (*R*)-acerogenin B (**41**) (50% inhibitory dose (ID_{50}): 0.26 μg/ear) showed the highest inhibition of inflammation, followed by indomethacin (**46**) (ID_{50}: 0.30 μg/ear), acerogenin A (**10**) (ID_{50}: 0.32 μg/ear) and aceroside B_1 (**42**) (ID_{50}: 0.32 μg/ear), aceroside IV (**44**) (ID_{50}:

0.49 μg/ear), (-)-centrolobol (**22**) (ID_{50}: 0.66 μg/ear), aceroside III (**40**) (ID_{50}: 0.81 μg/ear), aceroside I (**39**) (ID_{50}: >1.0 μg/ear), and quercetin (**45**) (ID_{50}: 1.6 μg/ear), respectively.

From the results of these mice *in vivo* anti-inflammatory tests, diarylheptanoids from *Acer nikoense* stem bark are suggested to be useful as anti-inflammatory agents [21].

2.4. Inhibitory on Nitric Oxide Production of Cyclic Diarylheptanoids

In 2002, Tao *et al.*, isolated three novel biphenyl type diarylheptanoid glycosides together with ten known diarylheptanoid glycosides (Figure 6) (Figure 6(continued 1)) from the bark of Chinese *Myrica rubra.*

Each biphenyl type diarylheptanoid glycoside is as follows:

Three novel biphenyl diarylheptanoid glycosides: myricanol 11-*O*-β-D-glucopyranoside (**47**), myricanone 5-*O*-β-D-glucopyranoside (**48**), neomyricanone 5-*O*-β-D-glucopyranoside (**49**) (Figure 6)

Ten known diarylheptanoids: (+)-*S*-myricanol 5-*O*-β-D-glucopyranoside (**50**), (+)-*S*-myricanol (**51**), myricanol glucoside (**52**), myricanol (**9**), myricanone (**8**), myricanene A 5-*O*-α-L-arabinofuranosyl (1→6)-β-D-glucopyranoside (**53**) (Figure 6), myricanene A (**54**), myricanene B 5-*O*-α-L-arabinofuranosyl(1→6)-β-D-glucopyranoside (**55**), myricanene B (**56**), myricanane (**57**) (Figure 6(continued 1)).

Nitric oxide (NO) is produced by the oxidation of L-arginine (**58**) (Figure 6(continued 1)) by nitric oxide synthase (NOS). However, in the NOS family, inducible nitric oxide synthase (iNOS), in particular, is involved in pathological aspects associated with NO overproduction. And iNOS expressed in response to inflammatory cytokines involved as causative factors that cause various inflammatory symptoms *in vivo* such as interleukin-1β (IL-1β), tumor necrosis factor (TNF–α) and lipopolysaccharide (LPS) in various cell types of macrophages, endothelial cells and smooth muscle cells.

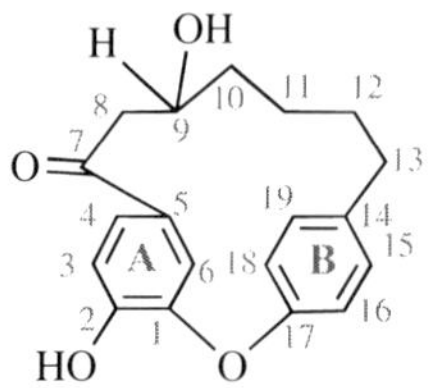

acerogenin M (**38**)

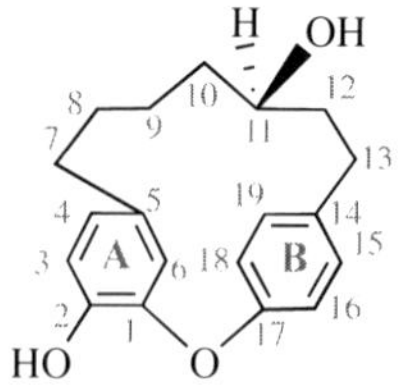

acerogenin A (**10**)

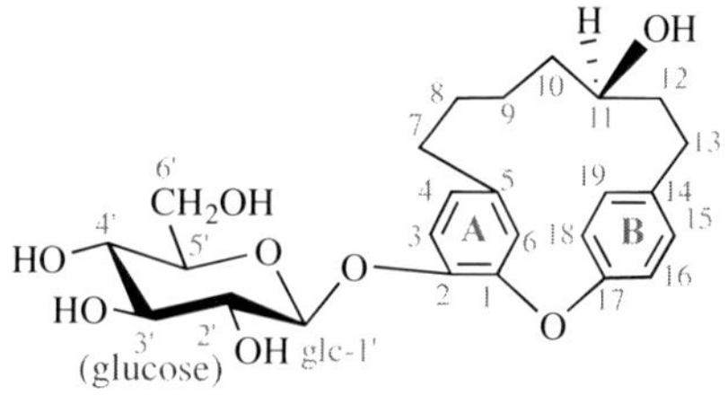

aceroside I (**39**)

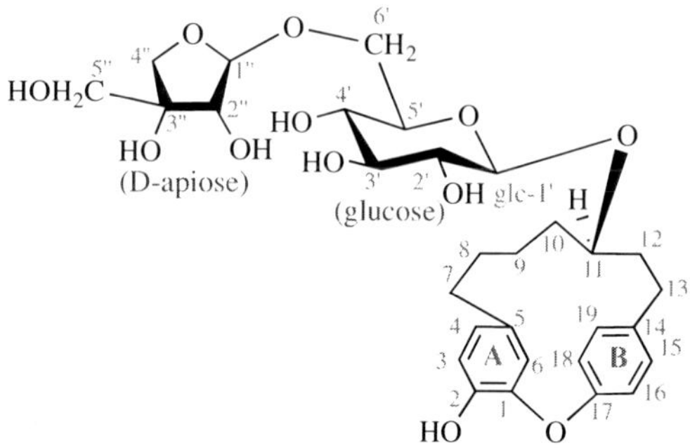

aceroside III (**40**)

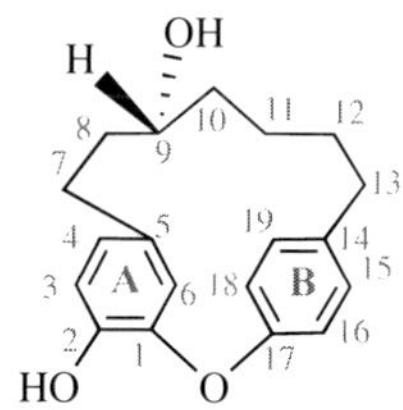

(*R*)-acerogenin B (**41**)

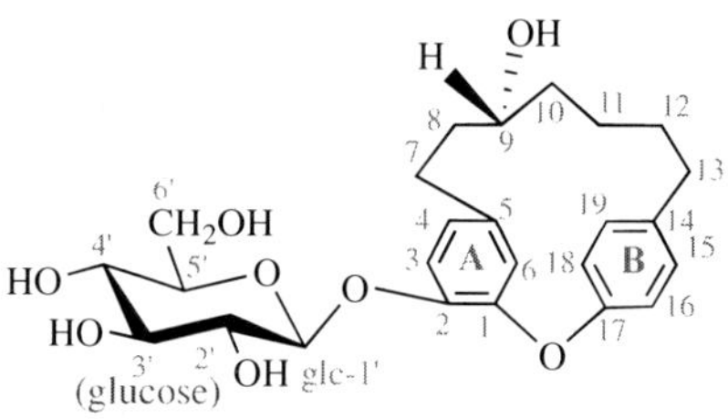

aceroside B_1 (**42**)

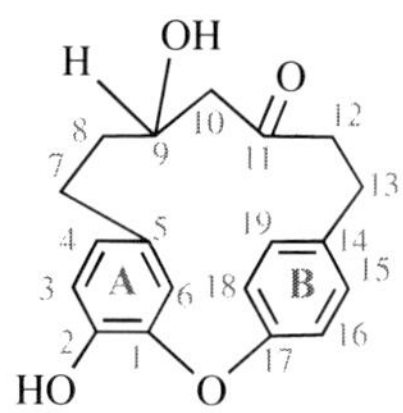

acerogenin D (**43**)

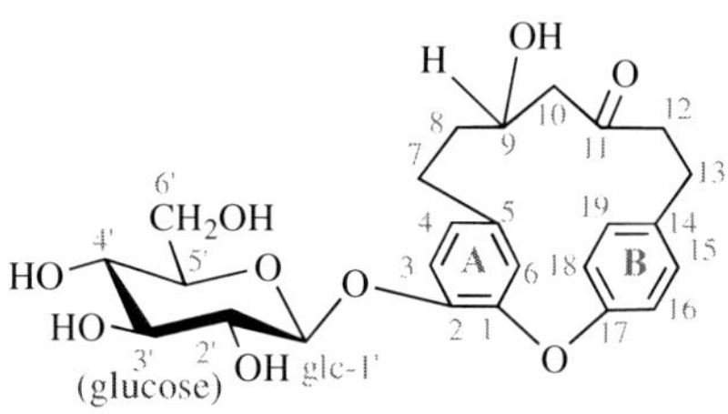

aceroside IV (**44**)

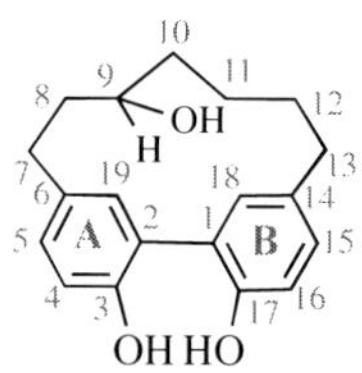

acerogenin K (**28**)

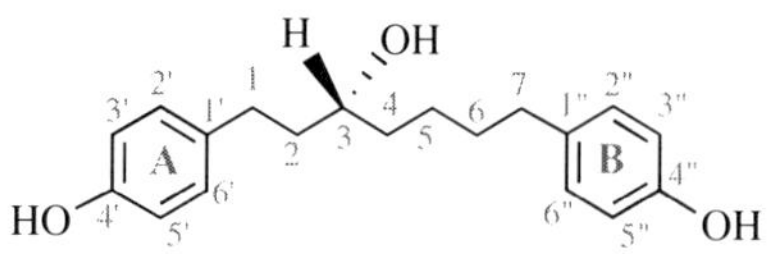

(-)-centrolobol (**22**)

Figure 5. One novel cyclic biphenyl ether type acerogenin M (**38**) along with nine known diarylheptanoids (**10**, **39**- **44**, **28**, **22**) from stem bark of *Acer nikoense*.

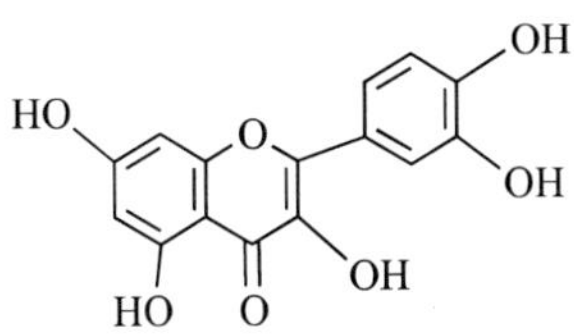

quercetin (**45**)

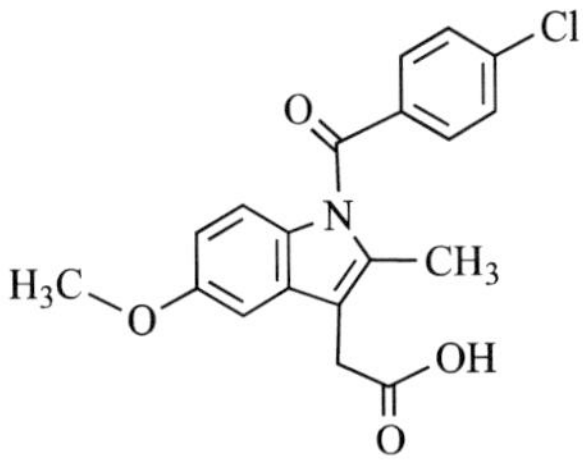

indomethacin (**46**)

Figure 5(continued 1). Two reference compounds (controls) (quercetin (**45**) and indomethacin (**46**)) for anti-inflammatory test on diarylheptanoids.

First, based on the above facts, two types of polyphenols ((-)-epigallocatechin (**59**) and (-)-epigallocatechin 3-*O*-gallate (EGCG. **60**)), and one nitric oxide synthase (NOS) inhibitor N^G-monomethyl-L-arginine (L-NMMA. **61**) (Figure 6(continued 1)) were used as control samples.

And regarding their inhibitory effect of diarylheptanoid glycosides from *Myrica rubra* against NO production in lipopolysaccharide (LPS)-activated mouse peritoneal macrophages, among 11 diarylheptanoid glycosides, (+)-*S*-myricanol (**51**) has shown the highest inhibitory effect (50% inhibitory concentration (IC_{50}) (μM): 19), followed by myricanol (**9**) (IC_{50} (μM): 23), myricanone (**8**) (IC_{50} (μM): 23) and myricanene A (**54**) (IC_{50} (μM): 23), myricanane (**57**) (IC_{50} (μM): around 26), (-)-epigallocatechin 3-*O*-gallate (**60**. control) (IC_{50} (μM): 27), a NOS inhibitor N^G-monomethyl-L-arginine (L-NMMA. **61**) (IC_{50} (μM): 28), myricanene B (**56**) (IC_{50} (μM): around 30), myricanene B 5-*O*-α-L-arabinofuranosyl (1→6)-β-D-glucopyranoside (**55**) (IC_{50} (μM): > 30), (-)-epigallocatechin (**59**. control) (IC_{50} (μM): 65), and (+)-*S*-myricanol 5-*O*-β-D-glucopyranoside (**50**) (IC_{50} (μM): > 100) and myricanene A 5-*O*-α-L-arabinofuranosyl(1→6)-β-D-glucopyranoside (**53**) (IC_{50} (μM): > 100), respectively.

From the above results, NO production inhibitory activity (IC_{50} (μM): 19-30) of six biphenyl diarylheptanoids ((+)-*S*-myricanol (**51**), myricanol (**9**), myricanone (**8**), myricanene A (**54**), myricanene B (**56**), and myricanane (**57**) was almost the same as the NO production inhibitory activity (IC_{50} (μM): 28) of N^G-monomethyl-L-arginine (L-NMMA. **61**), a non-selective NOS inhibitor.

However, four biphenyl-type diarylheptanoid glycosides (myricanone 5-*O*-β-D-glucopyranoside (**48**), (+)-*S*-myricanol 5-*O*-β-D-glucopyranoside (**50**), myricanol glucoside (**52**), myricanene A 5-*O*-α-L-arabinofuranosyl (1→6)-β-D-glucopyranoside (**53**)) were weak or no activities.

Here, the activity of glycosides is known to have a lower activity than their activity of the corresponding aglycons [**22**, **23**, **24**, **25**, **26**].

Then, for these reasons, since four biphenyl-type diarylheptanoid glycosides (myricanone 5-*O*-β-D-glucopyranoside (**48**), (+)-*S*-myricanol 5-*O*-β-D-glucopyranoside (**50**), myricanol glucoside (**52**), myricanene A 5-*O*-α-L-arabinofuranosyl(1→6)-β-D-glucopyranoside (**53**)) could hardly penetrate the cell membrane, it was presumed that their activity was low because these four biphenyl-type diarylheptanoid glycosides could not reach the active site.

Second, the inhibitory effects of two major diarylheptanoids (myricanol (**9**) and myricanone (**8**)) on inducible nitric oxide synthase (iNOS) induction were investigated. These two biphenyl diarylheptanoids (myricanol (**9**) and myricanone (**8**)) suppressed iNOS induction of LPS-activated macrophages. This suppression of iNOS induction was closely related to NO inhibition.

These results indicate that two diarylheptanoids (myricanol (**9**) and myricanone (**8**)) showed inhibitory activity against iNOS induction mainly in LPS-activated macrophages, and as a result, this suggests that NO production was also inhibited.

Considering the existence of a clear relationship between the inhibition of NO by the diarylheptanoid and the suppression of iNOS induction, the inhibitory activity of diarylheptanoids on NO production in LPS-activated macrophages provides one experimental fact to demonstrate the traditional effects of this natural remedy for the treatment of inflammation since ancient times [27].

In 2008, Wang J *et al.*, identified five novel cyclic diarylheptanoids (myricananin A (**62**), myricananin B (**63**), myricananin C (**64**), myricananin D (**65**), myricananin E (**66**)), two novel cyclic diarylheptanoids (acetonide of myricananin A (**67**) and acetonide of myricananin B (**68**)), and four known cyclic diarylheptanoids (12-hydroxymyricanone (**69**), alnusonol (**70**), myricatomentogenin ((+)-3',4"-epoxy-1-(4'-hydroxylphenyl)-7-(3"-hydroxyphenyl)heptane-3-one. **71**), and actinidione (**72**)) (Figure 7) from the root of *Myrica nana*, and several of these cyclic diarylheptanoids were tested for their inhibitory effect on nitric oxide (NO) release.

First, of eleven types of cyclic diarylheptanoids, except 3 types of cyclic diarylheptanoids (myricananin B (**63**), acetonide of myricananin A (**67**), myricatomentogenin (**71**)), the inhibitory effects (50% inhibitory concentration (IC_{50} (μM)) of 8 cyclic diarylheptanoids on nitric oxide (NO) production in lipopolysaccharide (LPS)-activated peritoneal macrophages, using a NOS inhibitor N^G-monomethyl-L-arginine (L-NMMA. **61**) (Figure 7) as a control, were as follows:

12-Hydroxymyricanone (**69**) was the highest IC_{50} (30.19 μM), followed by myricananin A (**62**) (IC_{50}: 45.32 μM), alnusonol (**70**) (IC_{50}: 46.18 μM), acetonide of myricananin B (**68**) (IC_{50}: 52.81 μM), myricananin C (**64**) (IC_{50}: 63.21 μM), N^G-monomethyl-L-arginine (L-NMMA. **61**) (IC_{50}: 64.24 μM), respectively. However, the other three types of cyclic diarylheptanoids (myricananin D (**65**), myricananin E (**66**), actinidione (**72**)) did not show an inhibitory effect.

Second, regarding the inhibitory effect of myricananin A (**62**) on inducible nitric oxide synthase (iNOS) induction of lipopolysaccharide (LPS)-activated peritoneal macrophages, myricananin A (**62**) (100 μM) suppressed iNOS expression in lipopolysaccharide (LPS)-activated peritoneal macrophages. Therefore, it was suggested that the mechanism of myricananin A (**62**) in suppressing nitric oxide (NO) production is mainly related to the inhibitory effect on iNOS induction. These results provided one clear pharmacological mechanism of action and also provided reasonable support for the use of traditional folklore remedies for burns [28].

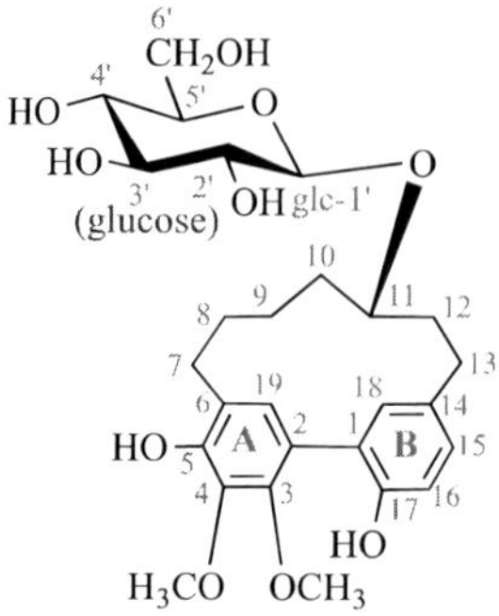

myricanol 11-*O*-β-D-glucopyranoside (**47**)

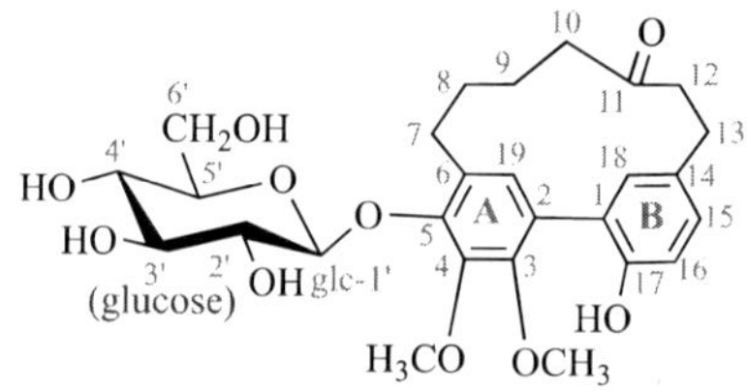

myricanone 5-*O*-β-D-glucopyranoside (**48**)

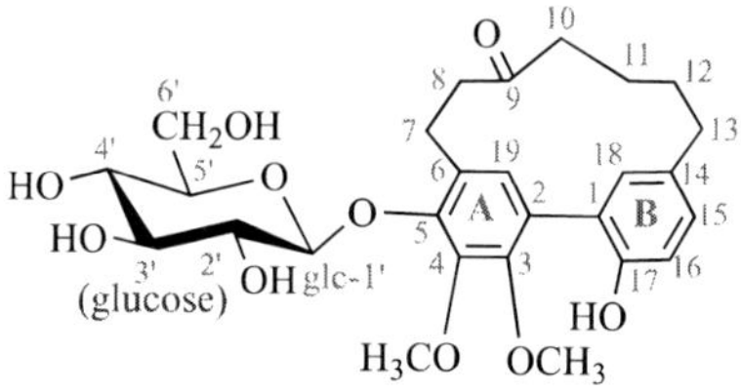

neomyricanone 5-*O*-β-D-glucopyranoside (**49**)

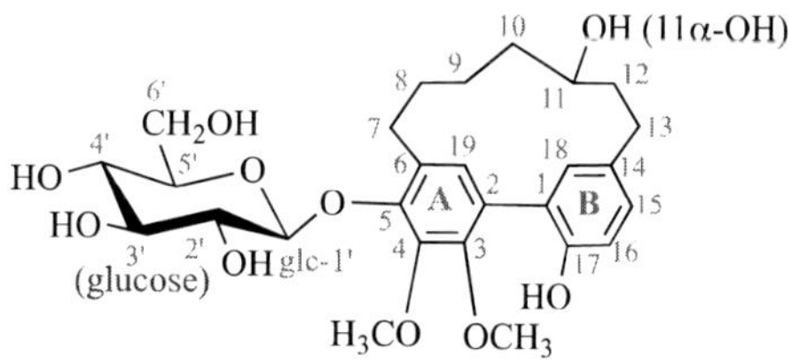

(+)-*S*-myricanol 5-*O*-β-D-glucopyranoside (**50**)

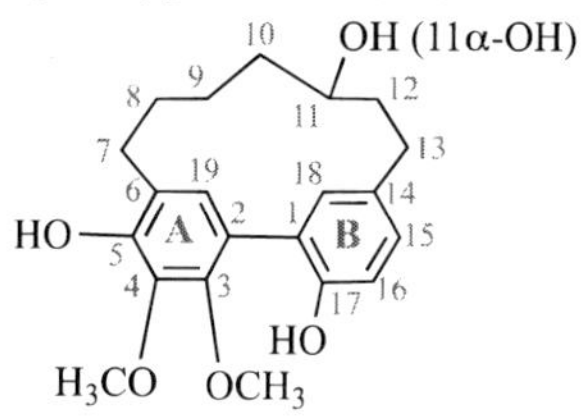

(+)-*S*-myricanol (**51**)

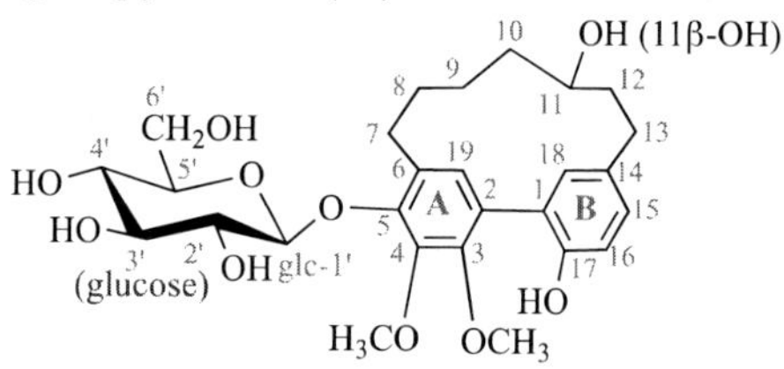

myricanol glucoside (**52**)

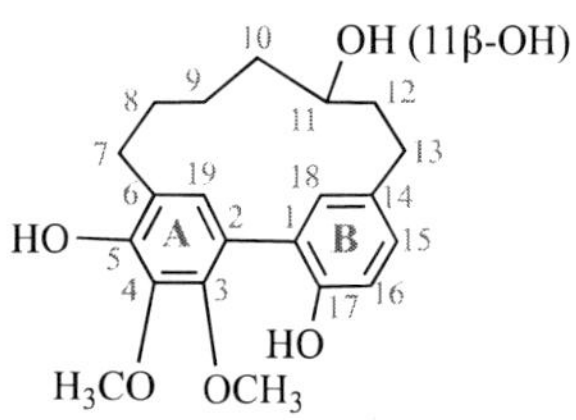

myricanol (**9**)

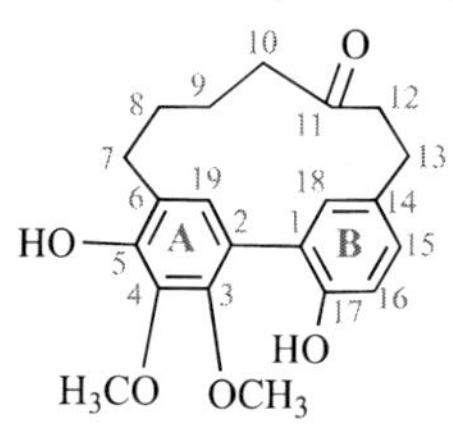

myricanone (**8**)

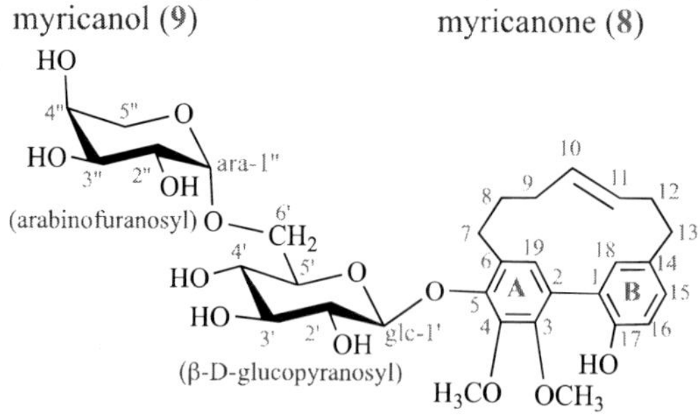

myricanene A 5-*O*-α-L-arabinofuranosyl(1→6)-β-D-glucopyranoside (**53**)

Figure 6. Diarylheptanoids (**51**, **9**, **8**) and their glycosides (**47**, **48**, **49**, **50**, **52**, **53**) from the bark of Chinese *Myrica rubra*.

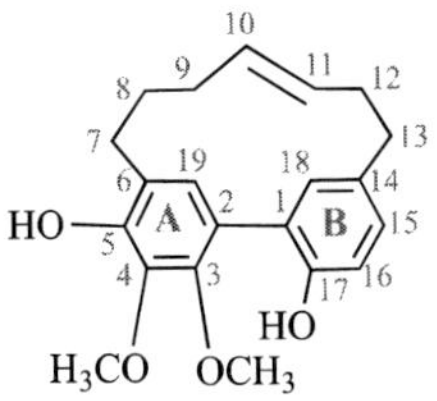

myricanene A (**54**)

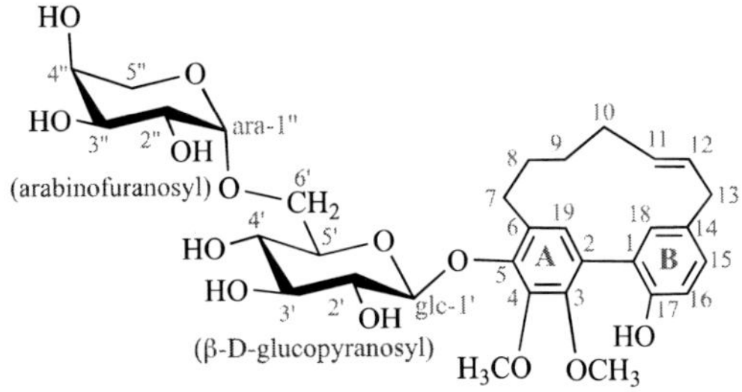

myricanene B 5-*O*-α-L-arabinofuranosyl(1→6)-β-D-glucopyranoside (**55**)

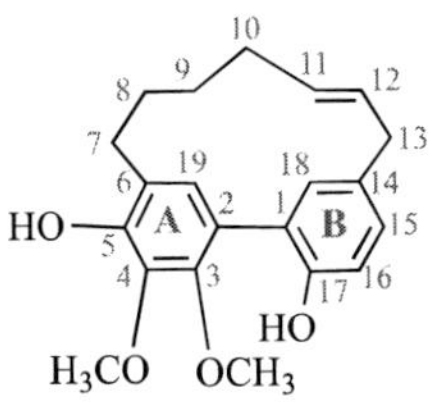

myricanene B (**56**)

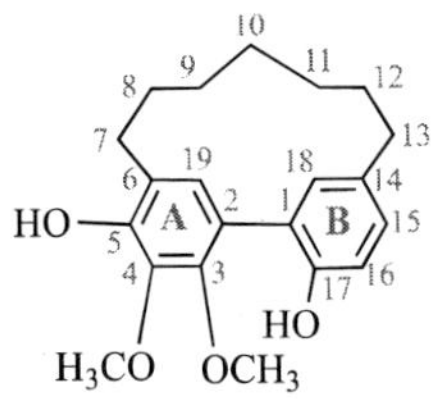

myricanane (**57**)

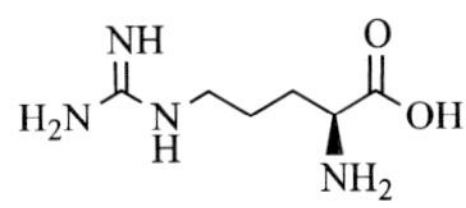

L-arginine (**58**)

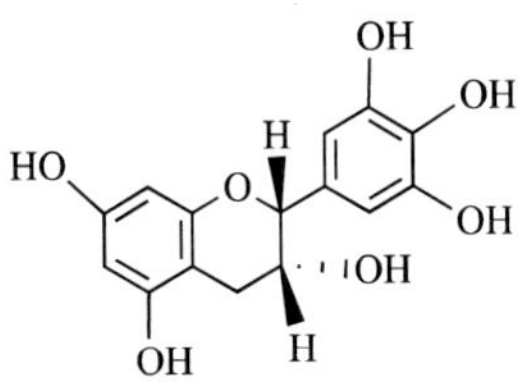

(-)-epigallocatechin (**59**)

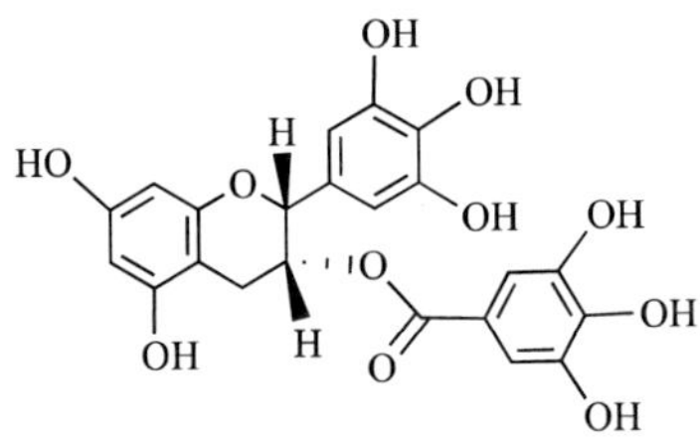

(-)-epigallocatechin 3-*O*-gallate (EGCG. **60**)

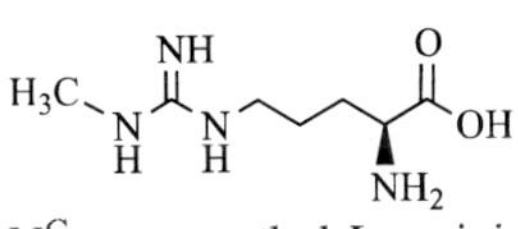

N^G-monomethyl-L-arginine (L-NMMA. **61**)

Figure 6(continued 1). Diarylheptanoids (**54**, **56**, **57**) and their glycosides (**55**) from the bark of Chinese *Myrica rubra*. L-Arginine (**58**). Three controls: (-)-epigallocatechin (EGCG. **59**), (-)-epigallocatechin 3-*O*-gallate (EGCG. **60**), and N^G-monomethyl-L-arginine (L-NMMA. **61**).

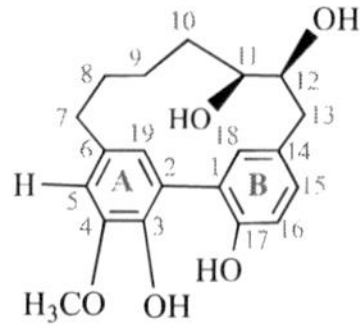
myricananin A (62)

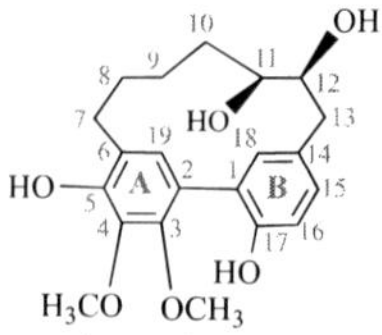
myricananin B (63)

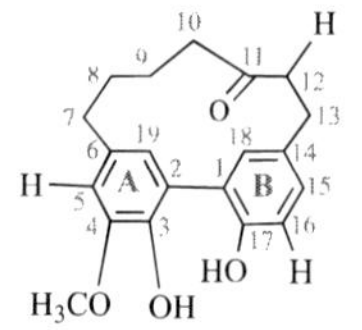
myricananin C (64)

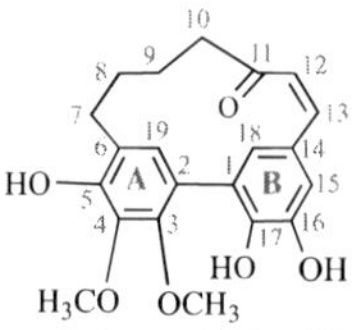
myricananin D (65)

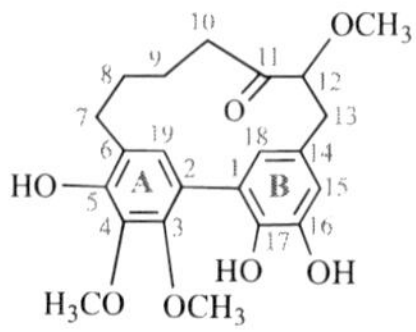
myricananin E (66)

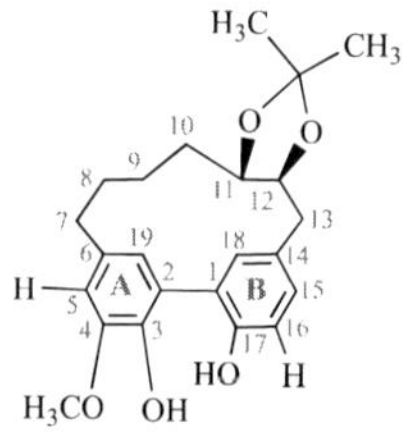
acetonide of myricananin A (67)

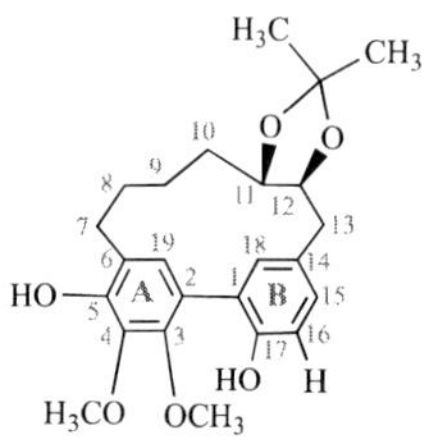
acetonide of myricananin B (68)

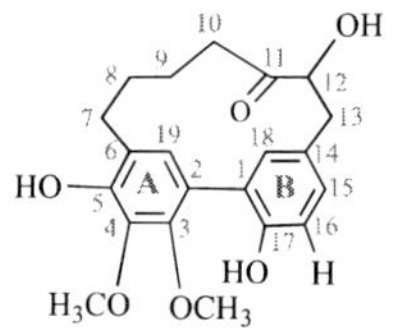
12-hydroxymyricanone (69)

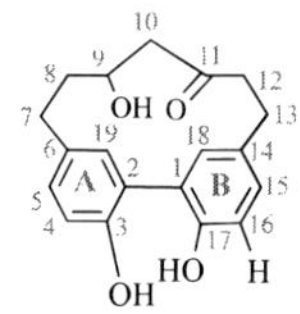
alnusonol (70)

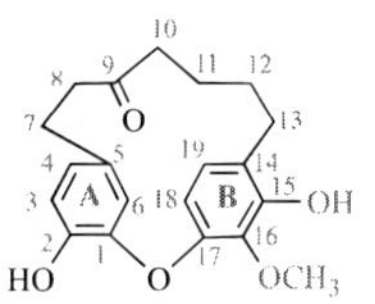
myricatomentogenin ((+)-3',4''-epoxy-1-(4'-hydroxylphenyl)-7-(3''-hydroxyphenyl)heptane -3-one. 71)

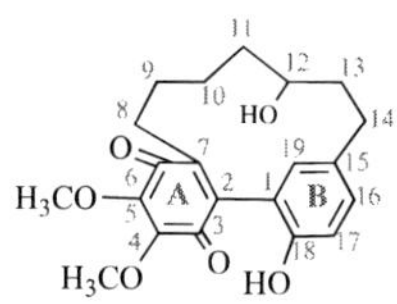
actinidione (72)

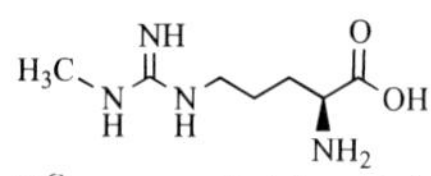
N^G^-monomethyl-L-arginine (L-NMMA. 61)

Figure 7. Eleven diarylheptanoids (62 - 72) from the root of *Myrica nana*. N^G-monomethyl-L-arginine (L-NMMA. 61).

Conclusion

Diarylheptanoids (curcuminoids) are found not only in plants but also in seaweed.

Chapter 3, biological activity of diarylheptanoids were typically described as follows: Leishmanicidal and antiprotozoal activities, antitumor activities, anti-inflammatory effects, and inhibitory on nitric oxide production.

References

[1] Fuchino H, Konishi S, Satoh T, Yagi A, Saitsu K, Matsumi T, Tanaka N. Chemical evaluation of *Betula species* in Japan .II. Constituents of *Betula platyphylla* var. japonica. *Chem. Pharm. Bull.* 44(5), 1033–1038, 1996.

[2] Fuchino H, Satoh T, Tanaka N. Chemical evaluation of *Betula species* in Japan. III. Constituents of *Betula maximowicziana* Regel. *Chem. Pharm. Bull.* 44(9), 1748-1753, 1996.

[3] Fuchino H, Satoh T, Shimizu M, Tanaka N. Chemical evaluation o*f Betula species* in Japan. IV. Constituents of *Betula davurica. Chem. Pharm. Bull.* 46(1), 166-168, 1998.

[4] Takahashi M, Fuchino H, Sekita S, Satake M. *In vitro* leishmanicidal activity of some scarce natural products. *Phytother. Res.* 18(7), 573-578, 2004.

[5] Inoue T. Constituents of *Acer nikoense* and *Myrica rubra*. On diarylheptanoids. *Yakugaku Zasshi* 113(3),181-97, 1993. In Japanese.

[6] Malterud KE, Anthonsen T. 13-Oxomyricanol, a new [7.0]-metacyclophane from *Myrica nagi. Phytochemistry* 19(4), 705-707, 1980.

[7] Huang MT, Ma W, Lu YP, Chang RL, Fisher C, Manchand PS, Newmark HL, Conney AH. Effects of curcumin, dimethoxy-curcumin, bisdemethoxycurcumin and tetrahydrocurcumin on 12-*O*-tetradecanoylphorbol-13-acetate-induced tumor promotion. *Carcinogenesis* 16(10), 2493-2497, 1995.

[8] Takasaki M, Konoshima T, Kozuka M, Tokuda H. Anti-tumor-promoting activities of euglobals from *Eucalyptus plants. Biol. Pharm. Bull.* 18(3), 435-438, 1995.

[9] Henle G, Henle W. Immunofluorescence in cells derived from Burkitt's lymphoma. *J. Bacteriol.* 91(3), 1248-1256, 1966.

[10] Ishida J, Kozuka M, Wang H, Konoshima T, Tokuda H, Okuda M, Yang Mou X, Nishino H, Sakurai N, Lee KH, Nagai M. Antitumor-promoting effects of cyclic diarylheptanoids on Epstein-Barr virus activation and two-stage mouse skin carcinogenesis. *Cancer Lett.* 159(2), 135-140, 2000.

[11] Masuda T, Hidaka K, Shinohara A, Maekawa T, Takeda Y, Yamaguchi H. Chemical studies on antioxidant mechanism of curcuminoid: analysis of radical reaction products from curcumin. *J. Agric. Food Chem.* 47(1), 71-77, 1999.

[12] Onoda M, Inano H. Effect of curcumin on the production of nitric oxide by cultured rat mammary gland. *Nitric Oxide* 4(5), 505-515, 2000.

[13] Ishida J, Kozuka M, Tokuda H, Nishino H, Nagumo S, Lee KH, Nagai M. Chemopreventive potential of cyclic diarylheptanoids. *Bioorg. Med. Chem.* 10(10), 3361-3365, 2002.

[14] Nagai M, Kubo M, Fujita M, Inoue T, Matsuo M. Studies on the constituents of Aceraceae plants. II. Structure of aceroside I, a glucoside of a novel cyclic diarylheptanoid from *Acer nikoense* Maxim. *Chem. Pharm. Bull.* 26(9), 2805-2810, 1978.

[15] Nagai M, Kubo M, Takahashi K, Fujita M, Inoue TN. Studies on the constituents of Aceraceae Plants. V. Two diarylheptanoid glycosides and anarylbutanol apiosylglucoside from *Acer nikoense*. *Chem. Pharm. Bull.* 31(6), 1923-1928, 1983.

[16] Morikawa T, Tao J, Toguchida I, Matsuda H, Yoshikawa M. Structures of new cyclic diarylheptanoids and inhibitors of nitric oxide production from Japanese folk medicine *Acer nikoense*. *J. Nat. Prod.* 66(1), 86-91, 2003.

[17] Nagumo S, Kaji N, Inoue T. Nagai, M. Studies on the constituents of Aceraceae plants. XI. Two types of cyclic diarylheptanoid from *Acer nikoense*. *Chem Pharm Bull* 41(7), 1255-1257, 1993.

[18] Kubo M, Nagai M, Inoue T. Studies on the constituents of Aceraceae plants. IV. Carbon-13 nuclear magnetic resonance spectra of acerogenin A, rhododendrol and related compounds, and structure of

aceroside IV from *Acer nikoense. Chem. Pharm. Bull.* 31(6), 1917-1922, 1983.

[19] Nagumo S, Ishizawa S, Nagai M, Inoue T. Studies on the constituents of aceraceae plants. XIII. Diarylheptanoids and other phenolics from *Acer nikoense. Chem. Pharm. Bull.* 44(5), 1086-1089, 1996.

[20] Nagai M, Kenmochi N, Fujita M, Furukawa N, Inoue T. Studies on the constituents of Aceraceae plants. VI. Revised stereochemistry of (-)-centrolobol, and new glycosides from *Acer nikoense. Chem. Pharm. Bull.* 34(3), 1056-1060, 1986.

[21] Akihisa T, Taguchi Y, Yasukawa K, Tokuda H, Akazawa H, Suzuki T, Kimura Y. Acerogenin M, a cyclic diarylheptanoid, and other phenolic compounds from *Acer nikoense* and their anti-inflammatory and anti-tumor-promoting effects. *Chem. Pharm. Bull.* 54(5), 735-739, 2006.

[22] Matsuda H, Murakami T, Kageura T, Ninomiya K, Toguchida I, Nishida N, Yoshikawa M. Hepatoprotective and nitric oxide production inhibitory activities of coumarin and polyacetylene constituents from the roots of *Angelica furcijuga. Bioorg. Med. Chem. Lett.* 8(16), 2191-2196, 1998.

[23] Yoshikawa M, Morikawa T, Toguchida I, Harima S, Matsuda H. Medicinal Flowers. II. Inhibitors of nitric oxide production and absolute stereostructurs of five new germacrane-type sesquiterpenes, kikkanols D, D monoacetate, E, F, and F monoacetate from the flowers of *Chrysanthemum indicum* L. *Chem. Pharm. Bull.* 48(5), 651-656, 2000.

[24] Matsuda H, Kageura T, Morikawa T, Toguchida I, Harima S, Yoshikawa M. Effects of stilbene constituents from rhubarb on nitric oxide production in lipopolysaccharide-activated macrophages. *Bioorg. Med. Chem. Lett.* 10(4), 323-327, 2000.

[25] Kageura T, Matsuda H, Morikawa T, Toguchida I, Harima S, Oda M, Yoshikawa M. Inhibitors from rhubarb on lipopolysaccharide-induced nitric oxide production in macrophages: Structural

requirements of stilbenes for the activity. *Bioorg. Med. Chem.* 9(7), 1887-1893, 2001.

[26] Matsuda H, Kageura T, Oda M, Morikawa T, Sakamoto Y, Yoshikawa M. Effects of constituents from the bark of *Magnolia obovata* on nitric oxide production in lipopolysaccharide-activated macrophages. *Chem. Pharm. Bull.* 49(6), 716-720, 2001.

[27] Tao J, Morikawa T, Toguchida I, Ando S, Matsuda H, Yoshikawa M. Inhibitors of nitric oxide production from the bark of *Myrica rubra*: Structures of new biphenyl type diarylheptanoid glycosides and taraxerane type triterpene. *Bioorg. Med. Chem.* 10(12), 4005-4012, 2002.

[28] Wang J, Dong S, Wang Y, Lu Q, Zhong H, Du G, Zhang L, Cheng Y. Cyclic diarylheptanoids from *Myrica nana* inhibiting nitric oxide release. *Bioorg. Med. Chem.* 16(18), 8510-8515, 2008.

In: *Curcuma longa* and Its Health Effects ISBN: 978-1-53618-083-1
Editor: Noboru Motohashi

Chapter 4

SELECTIVE EXTRACTION OF CURCUMIN

Noboru Motohashi[1,*], Anuradha Vanam[2,†], Jyothirmayi Vadapalli[3,‡] and Rao Gollapudi[4,≠]

[1]Meiji Pharmaceutical University, Tokyo, Japan
[2]Sri Venkateswara University, Tirupathi, AP, India
[3]Acharya Nagarjuna University, Nagarjunanagar, AP, India
[4]University of Kansas, Lawrence, Kansas, USA

ABSTRACT

Curcumin, one of diarylheptanoids, is one of the oldest and representative diarylheptanoids. However, curcumins are very similar in bulk (molecular weight), structural formula, and affinities such as adsorbents for high performance liquid chromatography (HPLC) columns, so it has been considered difficult to isolate them simply, easily and completely. Recently, in order to isolate curcumin and the analogs, various adsorbent bases and separation methods such as new adsorbent of a molecularly imprinted polymer (MIP), serum protein electrophoresis (SPE) and others have begun to be used. Then Polymer P1 (P1) and

* Corresponding Author's Email: noborumotohashi@jcom.home.ne.jp.
† Corresponding Author's Email: agollapdr@gmail.com.
‡ Corresponding Author's Email: jyothi.galactica@gmail.com.
≠ Corresponding Author's Email: gollapudirao@ku.edu.

analogs, and scanning electron microscopy (SEM), and so forth have been used for the higer specific selectivity of curcumin and absorbents.

Keywords: selective separation of curcumin, selective binding templates, *molecularly imprinted polymer (MIP)*, serum protein electrophoresis (SPE). Polymer P1 (P1), scanning electron microscopy (SEM), MMWNTs/MIPs, selective separation method, relative standard deviation (RSD), π-π-conjugation effect

CHEMICAL CONSTITUENTS IN SELECTIVE EXTRACTION OF CURCUMIN

curcumin	(**1**)
acrylamide	(**2**)
methacrylic acid	(**3**)
curcumin II	(demethoxycurcumin. (1*E*,6*E*)-1-(4-hydroxy-3-methoxyphenyl)-7-(4-hydroxyphenyl)hepta-1,6-diene-3,5-dione. **4**)
curcumin III	(bisdemethoxycurcumin. (1*E*,6*E*)-1,7-*bis*(4-hydroxy phenyl) hepta-1,6-diene-3,5-dione. **5**)

ABBREVIATIONS IN SELECTIVE EXTRACTION OF CURCUMIN

BET	Brauner-Emmet-Teller
dc	dielectric constant
HPLC	high performance liquid chromatography
IF	imprinting factor
MAA	methacrylic acid
MIP	*molecularly imprinted polymer*
MIPs	molecularly imprinted polymers
MMWNTs	magnetic phenyl modified multi-walled carbon nanotubes

NIP	non-molecularly imprinted polymer
P	functional polymer
P1	P1 polymer
P2	P2 polymer
P3	P3 polymer
P4	P4 polymer
P5	P5 polymer
P6	P6 polymer
RSD	relative standard deviation

1. INTRODUCTION

Curcumin, one of diarylheptanoids, is the oldest and representative of diarylheptanoids. However, curcuminns are very similar in bulk (molecular weight), structural formula, and affinities such as adsorbents for high performance liquid chromatography (HPLC) columns, so it has been considered difficult to isolate them simply, easily and completely. Recently, in order to isolate curcumin and analogs, various adsorbent bases and separation methods such as new adsorbent of a molecularly imprinted polymer (MIP), serum protein electrophoresis (SPE) and others have begun to be used. Then Polymer P1 (P1) and analogs, and scanning electron microscopy (SEM), and so forth have been used for the higer specific selectivity of curcumin and absorbents.

2. SELECTIVE EXTRACTION OF CURCUMIN

Due to the difficulty in extracting and purifying curcumin (**1**) (Figure 1) from ginger rhizomes, there are limited methods for analyzing curcumin (**1**). Currently, common extraction methods for curcumin (**1**) are high performance liquid chromatography (HPLC) combined with other auxiliary extraction techniques including microwave, ultrasound and supercritical carbon dioxide [1, 2].

These methods will certainly yield high-purity curcumin (**1**). However, the pretreatment of these methods is time consuming and complicated. Recently, many new advanced adsorbents for extraction have been developeda as follows.

Recently, as one new adsorbent, *a molecularly imprinted polymer (MIP)*, an artificial polymer with certain selectivity for the target analyte, has a certain recognition capability, mechanical and chemical stability, and simplicity. It has gained more and more attention due to its significant advantages, including its preparation.

MIPs are typically used to separate and concentrate target samples from complex proteins and are packed and used in serum protein electrophoresis (SPE) cartridges [3].

In general, conventional component extraction methods from natural compounds are not optimal analytical extraction methods because it takes a lot of time in the extraction procedure and contain interference components. On the other hand, *MIP analysis* excels in sample clean-up by selective extraction, and is suitable for removing and reducing unrelated components other than the target component in the final extract. In particular, *molecularly imprinted polymer (MIP)* is gaining importance as a simpler, more reliable and rapid separation method.

Based on the above facts, in 2011, Azizi *et al.*, selected six different types of porogens (P1-P6) to evaluate the impact on *MIP* interactions, and the quality of curcumin (**1**)-*molecularly imprinted polymer (MIP)* and investigated *porogen effect*, namely, *the effect of the aggregate of specific shapes and sizes* on the quality of curcumin (**1**)-*molecularly imprinted polymer (MIP)*. These *porogen effects* were examined in a comparison between curcumin (**1**) *molecularly imprinted polymer (MIP)* and curcumin (**1**) *non-molecularly imprinted polymer (NIP)*. Then, a *molecularly imprinted polymer (MIP)* was prepared for the purpose of efficient curcumin (**1**) separation as follows:

As a result, first, according to Brunauer-Emmet-Teller adsorption equation (BET adsorption isotherm. Brauner-Emmet-Teller (BET) equation. BET), regardless of the functional monomers of two types of acrylamide (AM. **2**) and methacrylic acid (MAA. **3**) (Figure 1), a less polar solvent chloroform ($CHCl_3$) (BET surface area (m^2/g): 10.14 (P3); 28.13 (P4)) gave the highest surface area among the three types of porogens such as tetrahydrofuran (THF), chloroform ($CHCl_3$), and acetonitrile (MeCN) solvents. Porous solvents such as chloroform ($CHCl_3$) are considered highly soluble solvents because they dissolve well in other components such as templates and polymers.

Furthermore, when a highly soluble solvent such as chloroform ($CHCl_3$) is used in polymer production, it tends to be easily separated later when compared to a low solubility solvent. Regarding the separation of functional polymer (P) from porous solvents, as the separation time increased, the polymer surface area increased. As the surface area of the functional polymer increases, the pore size decreases. On the other hand, as the surface area of functional polymer decreases, the pore size becomes larger with high porosity. Polymer P1 (P1) prepared using THF as the porogen had a maximum pore size (average pore diameter: 618.43 nm) and a minimum surface area (BET surface area: 0.03 m^2/g).

Second, P1 polymer (P1) (binding amount (172.15 μg/g) has the highest amount of curcumin (**1**) bound to polymer Q, P2 polymer (P2) (binding amount: 171.71 μg/g), P3 polymer (P3) (binding amount: 167.27 μg/g), P3 polymer (P3) (binding amount: 167.27 μg/g), P5 polymer (P5) (binding amount: 166.35 μg/g), P6 polymer (P6) (binding amount: 163.36 μg/g), and P4 polymer (P4) (binding amount: 162.46 μg/g), respectively.

According to scanning electron microscopy (SEM), curcumin (**1**)-*molecularly imprinted polymer (MIP)* had deeper holes than curcumin (**1**)-non-molecularly imprinted polymer (*NIP*). This deep hole is used as a selective site for curcumin (**1**). This deep hole allows a possibility to increase curcumin (**1**)-bound polymer binding for all prepared polymers because curcumin (**1**) can easily penetrate pore size holes during batch binding analysis. Nevertheless, the amount of curcumin (**1**) bound to polymer from batch binding analysis varied with the type of adsorbent.

Third, on Batch binding analysis for porogen selection, the selection of the appropriate porogen depends on the synthetic polymer template and its functional monomer that can provide sufficient cross-reactivity. Different porogens with different hydrogen bond capacities and dielectric constants of three types of tetrahydrofuran (THF), chloroform ($CHCl_3$), and acetonitrile (MeCN) markedly changed the amount of curcumin (**1**)-bound polymer binding. Three types of porogens of tetrahydrofuran (THF), chloroform ($CHCl_3$), and acetonitrile (MeCN) were used to synthesize six types of functional polymers such as Polymer 1 (P1) (functional monomer (fm): methacrylic acid (MAA)), P2 (fm: acrylamide (AM)), P3 (fm: MAA), P4 (fm: AM), P5 (fm: MAA), and P6 (fm: AM)). Of the three porogens, chloroform ($CHCl_3$) is a nonpolar solvent; tetrahydrofuran (THF) is a moderately polar solvent; acetonitrile (MeCN) is a polar solvent.

All curcumin (**1**)-molecularly imprinted polymer (*MIP*) binding levels (Q. μg/g) were higher than the corresponding curcumin (**1**)-non-molecularly imprinted polymer (*NIP*) binding levels (Q. μg/g). This fact means that curcumin (**1**)-molecularly imprinted polymer (*MIP*) has a binding site similar to curcumin (**1**), so *MIP* is more selective for curcumin (**1**) than *NIP*. *NIP* does not have a similar binding site as curcumin (**1**). However, *NIP* curcumin (**1**) binding levels (Q. μg/g) was derived from functional groups of functional monomers that could be recognized by curcumin (**1**) during Batch binding analysis. Still, the *NIP* curcumin (**1**) binding levels (Q. μg/g) was lower than the *MIP* curcumin (**1**) binding levels (Q. μg/g).

Among the three porogens, the highest curcumin (**1**) binding amount (Q. μg/g) is 172.15 μg/g of curcumin (**1**)-*molecularly imprinted polymer* (*MIP1*) prepared using THF as the porogen.

Compared to the dielectric constants of the three porogens, chloroform ($CHCl_3$) has the highest imprinting factor (IF) 1.29 (fm): MAA), followed by IF: 1.24 (fm: MAA) (THF)). These two functional monomers are each made from the same methacrylic acid (MAA). In general, for the synthesis of functional polymers, the non-polar solvents such as chloroform ($CHCl_3$) are selected as the porogen during polymerization. Nonpolar solvents usually have a low hydrogen-bonding capacity, which reduces the ability to interrupt the bonding interactions that occur between the polymer template and the functional monomer.

The medium polar solvent tetrahydrofuran (THF) is more efficient for recombination of curcumin (**1**) than the nonpolar solvent chloroform

($CHCl_3$). Hydrogen acceptor molecules such as curcumin (**1**) interact effectively with a hydrogen donor solvent THF having low dielectric constant. On the other hand, the structure of the functional polymer (P) also depends on the type of porogen used during the polymerization. A suitable porogen such as THF may moderately separate from the polymer during polymer polymerization. Such separation of THF from the polymer increases the selectivity and porosity of the polymer. Therefore, among polymer templates (P1-P6), the polymer template with porosity and sufficient binding sites gave a higher amount of binding (Q. μg/g) to curcumin (**1**).

This correlation also correlates well with gas adsorption experiments. Among the three types of porogens, the functional monomer methacrylic acid (MAA) had the highest imprint factor value (IF) 1.29 (chloroform ($CHCl_3$) with a dielectric constant 4.8), followed by IF 1.29 (dielectric constant 7.58), tetrahydrofuran (THF)), and IF 1.21 (acetonitrile (MeCN) with a dielectric constant 37.5). The functional monomer acrylamide (AM) possessed the highest imprint factor value (IF) 1.22 (acetonitrile (MeCN)), followed by IF 1.19 (tetrahydrofuran (THF)) and IF 1.17 (chloroform ($CHCl_3$)).

Amide groups have stronger hydrogen bonding ability in polar solvents such as acetonitrile (MeCN). Therefore, the hydrogen bonding ability of acetonitrile (MeCN) is higher than that of less polar solvents such as tetrahydrofuran (THF) and the nonpolar solvent chloroform ($CHCl_3$). As mentioned above, the imprinting factor value (IF) of functional monomer acrylamide (AM) increased with increasing dielectric constant such as 1F 1.17 (chloroform ($CHCl_3$): dielectric constant (dc) 4.8), 1F 1.19 (tetrahydrofuran (THF): dc 7.58), and 1F 1.22 (acetonitrile (MeCN): dc 37.5). This result suggests that curcumin (**1**) imprinting factor value (IF) to two kinds of functional monomers methacrylic acid (MAA) and acrylamide (AM) is greatly influenced by hydrogen bond strength.

From the many results above, among the 6 synthetic polymers (P1-P6), Polymer (P1) made from two components of tetrahydrofuran (THF) as the porogen and functional monomer methacrylic acid (MAA) showed the highest imprinting effect to curcumin (**1**). This high curcumin (1) imprinting effect was attributed to a high average pore size, as observed in a scanning electron microscope (SEM). Furthermore, to support this assessment, their imprinting factors (IFs) of six different types of polymers (P1 – P6) were examined by using four different types of adsorption solvents (chloroform ($CHCl_3$), tetrahydrofuran (THF), methanol (MeOH), and acetonitrile (MeCN)). As a result, P1 still gave the highest imprinting factor value (IF) of 1.29 [4].

In 2013, Kitabatake *et al.*, investigated the synthesis of monodispersed curcumin (**1**)-imprinted polymer by precipitation polymerization, and its application to the extraction of curcuminoids (diarylheptanoids) in turmeric.

First, monodisperse curcumin (**1**)-imprinted polymer (MIP) was synthesized by precipitation polymerization using a functional comonomer containing methacrylamide (MAM) and 4-vinylpyridine, divinylbenzene as a crosslinker, and a mixture of acetonitrile and toluene as the porogen.

Second, using methacrylamide (MAM) as a functional comonomer, two polymer molecules of monodisperse curcumin (**1**)-imprinted polymer (MIP) and monodisperse non-curcumin (**1**)-imprinted polymer (NIP) were formed. These two types of polymers, MIP and NIP were monodispersed and had a narrow particle size distribution (3.3 ± 0.09 and 3.5 ± 0.10 μm).

Third, in addition to shape recognition of narrow particle size, hydrophobic and hydrogen bonding interactions affected also the retention and molecular recognition of curcumin (**1**) on monodisperse curcumin (**1**)-imprinted polymer (MIP).

Fourth, when methacrylamide (MAM) is used as a functional comonomer, monodisperse curcumin (**1**)-imprinted polymer (MIP) could efficiently extract the three major turmeric curcuminoids (curcumin I (curcumin. diferuloylmethane. 1,7-*bis*-4-hydroxy-3-methoxyphenyl-1,6-heptadiene-3,5-dione. **1**), curcumin II (demethoxycurcumin. (1*E*,6*E*)-1-(4-hydroxy-3-methoxyphenyl)-7-(4-hydroxyphenyl)hepta-1,6-diene-3,5-dione. **4**), and curcumin III (bisdemethoxycurcumin. (1*E*,6*E*)-1,7-*bis*(4-hydroxyphenyl) hepta-1,6-diene-3,5-dione. **5**) (Figure 1) [5].

In 2015, Zhang *et al.*, confirmed three types of curcumin I (curcumin. diferuloylmethane. 1,7-*bis*-4-hydroxy-3-methoxyphenyl-1,6-heptadiene-

3,5-dione. **1**), curcumin II (demethoxycurcumin. (1*E*,6*E*)-1-(4-hydroxy-3-methoxyphenyl)-7-(4-hydroxyphenyl)hepta-1,6-diene-3,5-dione. **4**), and curcumin III (bisdemethoxycurcumin. (1*E*,6*E*)-1,7-*bis*(4-hydroxyphenyl) hepta-1,6-diene-3,5-dione. **5**) (Figure 1) from ginger poeder or kiwifruit root, by using a novel curcumin (**1**) molecularly imprinted polymers (MIPs) based on magnetic phenyl modified multi-walled carbon nanotubes (MMWNTs/MIPs) combining magnetic extraction and high-performance liquid chromatography (HPLC).

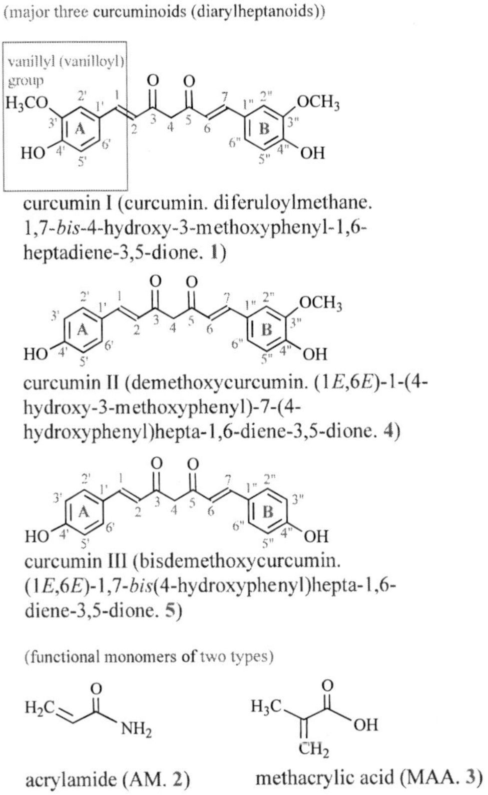

Figure 1. Major three curcuminoids (diarylheptanoids): curcumin I (curcumin. diferuloylmethane. 1,7-*bis*-4-hydroxy-3-methoxyphenyl-1,6-heptadiene-3,5-dione. **1**), curcumin II (demethoxycurcumin. (1*E*,6*E*)-1-(4-hydroxy-3-methoxyphenyl)-7-(4-hydroxyphenyl)hepta-1,6-diene-3,5-dione. **4**), and curcumin III (bisdemethoxycurcumin. (1*E*,6*E*)-1,7-*bis*(4-hydroxyphenyl)hepta-1,6-diene-3,5-dione. **5**).
Functional monomers of two types: acrylamide (AM. **2**) and methacrylic acid (MAA. **3**).

Here, phenyl groups grafted on MMWNTs/MIPs serve as auxiliary functional monomers for selective binding templates with the benzene ring in curcumin I (**1**), curcumin II (**4**), and curcumin III (**5**) *via* the π-π-conjugation effect.

Regarding selectivity of MMWNTs/MIPs, the adsorption capacity of the MMWNTs/MIPs towards curcumin (**1**) was higher when compared to that (adsorption capacity) of demethoxycurcumin (**4**) and bisdemethoxy-curcumin (**5**) (Figure 1). This means that phenyl groups grafted on MMWNTs / MIPs show higher selectivity for the template molecule curcumin.

After extraction by MMWNTs/MIPs, the ginger powder extract and kiwifruit root extract samples were directly detected by HPLC. As a result, recovery (%) of curcumin (**1**) was 99.3 – 100.5% (ginger powder extract), and 95.8 – 97.2% (kiwifruit root extract), respectively. The relative standard deviation (RSD) for recovery of these two extracts was less than 5.0%. Therefore, MMWNTs/MIPs for curcumin (**1**) is a highly selective separation method that gives accurate values that are fast and close to reality. The above results suggest that the use of MMWNTs/MIP is an effective method for quantitative analysis of curcumin (**1**) in extracts [6].

Conclusion

Many selective extraction methods for curcumin and its derivatives have been proposed. Until today, the separation of curcumin and its derivatives is very complex owing to their structural similarity an affinity.

In Chapter 4, high performance liquid chromatography (HPLC), *molecularly imprinted polymer (MIP)*, serum protein electrophoresis (SPE), and others have been tried in separation of curcumins. For example, MMWNTs/MIPs served greatly as auxiliary functional monomers for selective binding templates with the benzene ring in curcumin I (**1**), curcumin II (**4**), and curcumin III (**5**) *via* the π-π-conjugation effect.

Curcumin (**1**)-*molecularly imprinted polymer (MIP)* had deeper holes than curcumin (**1**)-non-molecularly imprinted polymer (*NIP*) in separation of curcumin and analogs. The usage of functional groups of functional monomers will play an important role. Then, this selectivity of curcumin can be expected to be very useful for a method to extract many curcuminoids similar to each other accurately and in a short time.

REFERENCES

[1] Mandal V, Mohan Y, Hemalatha S. Microwave assisted extraction of curcumin by sample-solvent dual heating mechanism using Taguchi L9 orthogonal design. *J. Pharm. Biomed. Anal.* 46(2), 322-327, 2008.

[2] Wakte PS, Sachin BS, Patil AA, Mohato DM, Band TH, Shinde DB. Optimization of microwave, ultra-sonic and supercritical carbon dioxide assisted extraction techniques for curcumin from *Curcuma longa*. *Sep. Purif. Technol.* 79(1), 50-55, 2011.

[3] Zhang ZH, Zhang ML, Luo LJ, Yang X, Hu YF, Zhang HB, Yao SZ. Synthesis and application of core-shell complex-imprinted polymer for the solid-phase extraction of melamine from dairy products. *J. Sep. Sci.* 33(17-18), 2854-2861, 2010.

[4] Azizi ES, Abmad MN, Islam AKMS, Arbain D, Tahir I. Porogen effect towards the quality of curcumin imprinted polymer. *Indonesian J. Chem.* 11(3), 207-211, 2011.

[5] Kitabatake T, Tabo H, Matsunaga H, Haginaka J. Preparation of monodisperse curcumin-imprinted polymer by precipitation polymerization and its application for the extraction of curcuminoids from *Curcuma longa* L. *Anal. Bioanal. Chem.* 405(20), 6555-6561, 2013.

[6] Zhang Z, Chen X, Rao W, Long F, Yan L, Yin Y. Preparation of novel curcumin-imprinted polymers based on magnetic multi-walled carbon nanotubes for the rapid extraction of curcumin from ginger powder and kiwi fruit root. *J. Sep. Sci.* 38(1), 108-114, 2015.

ABOUT THE EDITOR

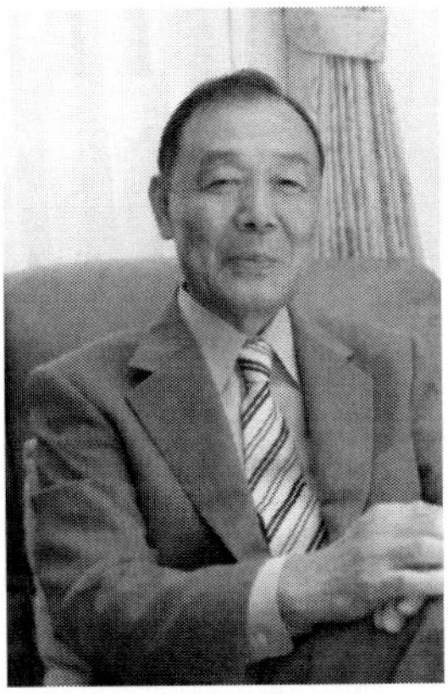

Noboru Motohashi

Foreign Examiner for Evaluation of the Ph.D.
Thesis in *Indian National University*, India;
Former Professor and Director (Elected Riji in Japanese)
of *Meiji Pharmaceutical University*, Tokyo Japan
E-mail: noborumotohashi@jcom.home.ne.jp.

Professional Appointments:

1966: Pharmaceutical Sciences, *Tohoku University*, Sendai, Japan (graduated school)

1985-1986: Visiting Professor of Department of Medicinal Chemistry, College of Pharmacy, *University of Kansas (KU)*, Lawrence, KS, USA

2006: Professor of *Meiji Pharmaceutical University*, Tokyo, Japan (retired)

2007: Advisor of *Meiji Pharmaceutical University*, Tokyo, Japan (retired)

2011: Elected Director (Riji in Japanese) of *Meiji Pharmaceutical University*, Tokyo, Japan (retired)

INDEX

B

C

D

E

F

G

H

I

J

K

L

M

N

O

P

Q

R

T

V

W

X

Z